Prevention of Kidney Disease and Long-Term Survival

Prevention of Kidney Disease and Long-Term Survival

Edited by
M. M. AVRAM

The Long Island College Hospital
Brooklyn, New York

Plenum Medical Book Company
New York and London

Library of Congress Cataloging in Publication Data

Main entry under title:

Prevention of kidney disease and long-term survival.

Includes bibliographies and indexes.
   1. Kidneys—Diseases—Prevention. I. Avram, Morrell M. [DNLM: 1. Nephrology—
Congresses. 2. Hemodialysis—Congresses. W3 300 P944 1981]
RC903.P73 1982   616.6′105   82-15036
ISBN-13: 978-1-4684-4201-4   e-ISBN-13: 978-1-4684-4199-4
DOI: 10.1007/978-1-4684-4199-4

© 1982 Plenum Publishing Corporation
Softcover reprint of the hardcover 1st edition 1982
233 Spring Street, New York, N.Y. 10013

Plenum Medical Book Company is an imprint of Plenum Publishing Corporation

For
Maria, Rella, Marc, Eric, Mathew, and David,
who are constantly in my loving thoughts and
whose ever-present example of hard work and
excellence inspires me toward achievement

Contributors

EDWARD M. ABRAMOWITZ, M.D., Division of Cardiology, The Long Island College Hospital, Brooklyn, New York

ROLAND J. ADAMSONS, M.D., Associate Professor, Department of Surgery, Downstate Medical Center, Brooklyn, New York

ALLEN C. ALFREY, M.D., Chief, Division of Nephrology, Veterans Administration Hospital; and Professor of Medicine, University of Colorado School of Medicine, Denver, Colorado

ABDUL G. ARSHAD, M.D., Department of Pathology, Downstate Medical Center, Brooklyn, New York

MORRELL M. AVRAM, M.D., Chief, The Avram Center for Kidney Diseases, Division of Nephrology, The Long Island College Hospital; Clinical Professor of Medicine, Department of Medicine, Downstate Medical Center; and Medical Director, Brooklyn Kidney Center and Nephrology Foundation of Brooklyn, Brooklyn, New York

DAVID S. BALDWIN, M.D., Professor of Medicine, Department of Medicine, New York University School of Medicine, New York, New York

HARRY BIENENSTOCK, M.D., Chief, Division of Rheumatology, The Long Island College Hospital; and Associate Clinical Professor of Medicine, Department of Medicine, Downstate Medical Center, Brooklyn, New York

BARRY M. BRENNER, M.D., Samuel A. Levine Professor of Medicine, Department of Medicine, Harvard Medical School; and Director, Renal Division, Brigham and Women's Hospital, Boston, Massachusetts

KHALID M. H. BUTT, M.D., Professor of Surgery, Department of Surgery, and Chief, Transplantation Service, Downstate Medical Center, Brooklyn, New York

VITO M. CAMPESE, M.D., Division of Nephrology, Department of Medicine, University of Southern California School of Medicine, Los Angeles, California

NANCY B. CUMMINGS, M.D., National Institute of Arthritis, Diabetes, and Digestive and Kidney Diseases, National Institutes of Health, Bethesda, Maryland

SEYMOUR S. CUTLER, M.D., Chief, Division of Pulmonary Medicine, The Long Island College Hospital; and Associate Professor of Medicine, Downstate Medical Center, Brooklyn, New York

WARREN D. DAVIDSON, M.D., Professor of Medicine, University of California Los Angeles School of Medicine, Los Angeles, California; and Harbor–UCLA Medical Center, Torrance, California

FRANK W. DIPILLO, M.D., Chief, Division of Hematology/Oncology, The Long Island College Hospital, Brooklyn, New York; and Clinical Associate Professor of Medicine, Downstate Medical Center, Brooklyn, New York

LEA EMMETT, R.N., Department of Surgery, Downstate Medical Center, Brooklyn, New York

PAUL A. FEIN, M.D., Division of Nephrology, The Long Island College Hospital; and Assistant Professor of Medicine, Department of Medicine, Downstate Medical Center, Brooklyn, New York

STANLEY S. FRANKLIN, M.D., Adjunct Professor of Medicine, University of California Los Angeles, School of Medicine, Los Angeles, California

ELI A. FRIEDMAN, M.D., Chief, Division of Nephrology, and Professor of Medicine, Department of Medicine, Downstate Medical Center, Brooklyn, New York

AMADO GAN, M.D., Division of Nephrology, The Long Island College Hospital; and Assistant Professor of Medicine, Department of Medicine, Downstate Medical Center, Brooklyn, New York

HARSH GANDHI, M.D., Division of Hematology/Oncology, The Long Island College Hospital, Brooklyn, New York

GILBERT F. GELFAND, M.D., Division of Rheumatology, The Long Island College Hospital, Brooklyn, New York

CARMELO GIORDANO, M.D., Professor of Medical Nephrology, Naples University, First School of Medicine, Naples, Italy

ALVIN I. GOODMAN, M.D., Professor of Medicine and Chief, Division of Nephrology, Department of Medicine, New York Medical College; and Director, Nephrology-Renal Unit, Westchester County Medical Center, Valhalla, New York

GERALD P. GRODSTEIN, M.D., Medical and Research Services, Veterans Administration Wadsworth Medical Center, Los Angeles, California

JOHN P. HAYSLETT, M.D., Chief, Section of Nephrology, and Professor of Medicine, Department of Internal Medicine, Yale University School of Medicine, New Haven, Connecticut

DAN A. HENRY, M.D., Medical and Research Services, Veterans Administration Wadsworth Medical Center, Los Angeles, California

SONDRA R. HIRSCH, R.N., Department of Medicine, Downstate Medical Center, Brooklyn, New York

GLADYS H. HIRSCHMAN, M.D., National Institute of Arthritis, Diabetes, and Digestive and Kidney Diseases, National Institutes of Health, Bethesda, Maryland

JOON H. HONG, M.D., Associate Department of Surgery, Downstate Medical Center, Brooklyn, New York

THOMAS H. HOSTETTER, M.D., Laboratory of Kidney and Electrolyte Physiology, Brigham and Women's Hospital, Boston, Massachusetts

MICHAEL IANCU, M.D., Division of Nephrology, The Long Island College Hospital; and Assistant Professor of Medicine, Downstate Medical Center, Brooklyn, New York

CARL M. KJELLSTRAND, M.D., Chief, Division of Nephrology, and Professor, Departments of Medicine and Surgery, University of Minnesota; and Nephrology Division, Regional Kidney Disease Program, Hennepin County Medical Center, Minneapolis, Minnesota

JOEL D. KOPPLE, M.D., Professor of Medicine and Public Health, University of California Los Angeles School of Medicine, Los Angeles, California

JOSEPH M. LETTERI, M.D., Chief, Division of Renal Diseases, Department of Medicine, Nassau County Medical Center; and Professor of Medicine, State University of New York at Stony Brook, Stony Brook, New York

CELIA S. LEVITZ, M.D., Assistant Professor of Medicine, Department of Medicine, Downstate Medical Center, Brooklyn, New York

NORMAN B. LEVY, M.D., Professor, Departments of Psychiatry, Medicine and Surgery, New York Medical Center; and Director, Division of Liaison Psychiatry, Westchester County Medical Center, Valhalla, New York

JOHN F. MAHER, M.D., Professor of Medicine, and Director, Division of Nephrology, Uniformed Services University of the Health Sciences School of Medicine, Bethesda, Maryland

GERI MANDEL, R.D.M.S., Division of Cardiology, The Long Island College Hospital, Brooklyn, New York

SHAUL G. MASSRY, M.D., Professor of Medicine, Division of Nephrology, Department of Medicine, University of Southern California School of Medicine, Los Angeles, California

RAO S. K. MUSUNURU, M.D., Division of Cardiology, The Long Island College Hospital, Brooklyn, New York

A. NOVOGRODSKY, M.D., Associate Professor of Biochemistry and Medicine, Rogosin Kidney Center, The New York Hospital–Cornell Medical Center, New York, New York

ABE N. PAHILAN, M.D., Division of Nephrology, The Long Island College Hospital, Brooklyn, New York

ISMAIL PARSA, M.D., Professor of Pathology, Department of Pathology, Downstate Medical Center, Brooklyn, New York

HELMUT G. RENNKE, M.D., Department of Pathology, Brigham and Women's Hospital, Boston, Massachusetts

GEORGE J. REZK, M.D., Division of Gastroenterology, The Long Island College Hospital, Brooklyn, New York

JOSEPH J. RICCA, M.D., Chief, Division of Gastroenterology, The Long Island College Hospital; and Associate Professor of Medicine, Downstate Medical Center, Brooklyn, New York

CHARLOTTE E. ROBERTS, R.D., Medical and Research Services, Veterans Administration Wadsworth Medical Center, Los Angeles, California

DAVID ROSENBLUM, M.D., Director, Diagnostic Radiology, Department of Radiology, The Long Island College Hospital; and Clinical Associate Professor of Radiology, Department of Radiology, Downstate Medical Center, Brooklyn, New York

A. L. RUBIN, M.D., Professor of Medicine, Biochemistry, and Surgery, Rogosin Kidney Center, The New York Hospital–Cornell Medical Center, New York, New York

WILLIAM J. SCARPA, M.D., Chief, Division of Cardiology, The Long Island College Hospital; and Associate Professor of Medicine, Department of Medicine, Downstate Medical Center, Brooklyn, New York

JOSEPH SCHLUGER, M.D., Director, Department of Medicine, The Long Island College Hospital; Associate Dean, Downstate Medical Center; and Professor of Clinical Medicine, Downstate Medical Center, Brooklyn, New York

BELDING H. SCRIBNER, M.D., Head, Division of Nephrology and Professor of Medicine, University of Washington School of Medicine, Seattle, Washington

GAURANG M. SHAH, M.D., Assistant Professor of Medicine, University of California Irvine, Irvine, California; and Veterans Administration Medical Center, Long Beach, California

MOHAMED H. SHAHJAHAN, R.C.P.T., Technical Director, Division of Respiratory Services, The Long Island College Hospital, Brooklyn, New York

RICHARD L. SIMMONS, M.D., Professor of Surgery, University of Minnesota Hospitals, Minneapolis, Minnesota

PAUL A. SLATER, M.D., Division of Nephrology, The Long Island College Hospital; and Assistant Professor of Medicine, Downstate Medical Center, Brooklyn, New York

KARIM B. SOLANGI, M.D., Division of Nephrology, Department of Medicine, New York Medical College, Valhalla, New York

KURT H. STENZEL, M.D., Professor of Biochemistry, Medicine, and Surgery, Rogosin Kidney Center, The New York Hospital–Cornell Medical Center, New York, New York

SANTOSH B. SUREKA, M.D., Division of Pulmonary Medicine, The Long Island College Hospital, Brooklyn, New York

ROBERT C. TOMFORD, M.D., Department of Medicine, Veterans Administration Medical Center, Denver, Colorado

MACKENZIE WALSER, M.D., Professor, Department of Pharmacology and Experimental Therapeutics and Department of Medicine, Johns Hopkins University School of Medicine, Baltimore, Maryland

STEPHEN A. WESELEY, M.D., Division of Nephrology, Department of Medicine, New York Medical College, Valhalla, New York

ROBERT L. WINER, M.D., Assistant Chief of Nephrology, Veterans Administration Medical Center, Long Beach, California; and Assistant Professor of Medicine, University of California Irvine, Irvine, California

ROBERT P. YATTO, M.D., Division of Gastroenterology, The Long Island College Hospital, Brooklyn, New York

Preface
Renal Failure Prevention and Treatment in the 1980s

It appears logical to juxtapose in this volume prevention—low cost and nonmorbid—with uremia therapy, which is very morbid and very high cost.

Treated uremic patients constitute an important, complex, and demanding group of survivors of a formerly universally fatal disease. Throughout the developed nations of the world, an increasing fraction of the health care budget is devoted to sustaining lives by dialytic therapy and renal transplantation. In the United States, for example, patients in renal failure comprise 0.2% of those eligible for support by Medicare, but consume 5.0% of the Medicare budget. Economic stresses in funding kidney patients have, in some countries such as Great Britain, forced a return to restrictive selection policies abhorrent to empathetic physicians. For third world residents, attention to nutrition, sanitation, and infections such as malaria must take a higher priority than costly uremia therapy. Thus the solution of one problem (retarding death from uremia) created several equally vexing other dilemmas (who should be treated and at what cost?). While sociologists, economists, and ethicists struggle with the new field of psychonephrology,[1] a group of investigators and clinicians convened to examine medical aspects of long-surviving treated uremic patients. These proceedings represent the first American analyis of those unique patients who have lived for ten or more years beyond what would have formerly been certain death in uremia.

Sponsored by the Long Island College Hospital's Department of Medicine and the newly established Avram Center for Kidney Diseases, conference participants met informally in Brooklyn Heights and then presented papers at New York's World Trade Center, a few miles distant. Specialists represented at the symposium included renal physiologists, nutritionists, psychiatrists, and kidney patients themselves. The search for the uremic toxin and its effects had been previously undertaken in an international symposium at the Long Island College Hospital.[2] The important derivative theme throughout the present volume is the exciting effort to prevent renal failure, thereby avoiding the cost and suffering of uremia therapy.

I am deeply appreciative of the enthusiasm and hard work displayed by the contributors—all my friends—who traveled from the major universities in the United States to the Long Island College Hospital, and for preparing the splendid material contained in this volume.

I hope the format used will make this a far more meaningful reading experience.

M. M. Avram, M.D.

REFERENCES

1. Levy N: *Psychonephrology*, Plenum Medical, New York, 1981.
2. Avram MM: *Parathyroid Hormones in Kidney Failure*, Parathyroid Hormones in Uremia: Toxin or Bystander, International Symposium, Brooklyn, May 3, 1979, S Karger, New York, Basel, 1980.

Acknowledgments

We wish to acknowledge the support of the Long Island College Hospital, the Department of Medicine, the Avram Center for Kidney Diseases, and the National Kidney Foundation of New York. The symposium was cosponsored by the New York Society of Nephrology, the New York State Kidney Disease Institute, and Kings County Medical Society.

Cheers for Hilary Evans of Plenum Press for most helpful suggestions.

My thanks are also due to Mrs. David J. LeBeau for her technical assistance in making this book possible.

Contents

Section I

Nutrition and Divalent Ion in Retarding Progression

Nephrologists have always been fascinated by the possibility of retarding progression of renal disease with simple alimentary maneuvers. This now appears possible by manipulation of diet or reduction of phosphate level in rat and humans.

Dietary manipulation as a means of treating renal insufficiency has been a major component of uremia therapy whenever alternative approaches such as hemodialysis were unavailable. The earliest regimens for management of acute renal failure, introduced during World War II, depended on a low protein, high fat and carbohydrate diet to retard development of uremic signs and symptoms. Early and repetitive hemodialysis proved superior to the tenuous state allowed by dietary therapy in acute renal failure. In chronic uremia, again before dialysis was generally available, a very low protein diet, containing 20 g or less, was found by some workers to protract life as endogenous renal function fell to as low as 3 ml/min. But, as regular hemodialysis was initiated at a creatinine clearance of 5 ml/min, or higher, dependence on dietary therapy became less attractive. There is today additional reason to consider a low protein diet in progressive renal insufficiency. Based on animal experiments and limited early clinical trials reviewed in this section, it appears that a protein-restricted diet may actually retard the onset of renal failure in some circumstances. Whether phosphorus or protein or the end products of protein catabolism are responsible for loss of nephrons is still speculative. What is both evident and stimulating is the realization that intervention during the course of renal disease may prove fruitful in maintaining a longer useful life before uremia supervenes.

In opening the section on prevention of renal failure, Kopple provides a masterful survey of the value of dietary nitrogen restriction as a means of both delaying the onset of dialytic therapy and retarding renal deterioration. His own inpatient and outpatient trials of high biological value protein diet, providing 0.55 to 0.60 g of protein/kg body weight per day to

1

one group, and 20 to 21 g/day of protein and of a mixture of nine essential amino acids to another group, had been ongoing for 15 weeks. His results indicate that chronically uremic patients from diverse socioeconomic backgrounds would adhere to a rigid outpatient dietary prescription. Kopple urges that nephrologists who believe low protein diets are "not clinically beneficial, acceptable, or adhered to . . . " reconsider their position as "further studies in this area are strongly indicated." Walser, in fact, assembled studies substantiating Kopple's position. Walser concluded that: "These studies provide convincing (though uncontrolled) evidence that phosphate restriction and calcium supplementation can slow the progress of renal failure." A relentless progression of uremic bone disease plagues the long-term dialysis patient.

Alfrey and Tomford provide telling data showing that phosphate may be a renal toxin, at least in experimental renal disease in the rat. These workers found that "phosphate depletion prevents progressive renal failure," which may, in part, explain the beneficial effects of a reduced protein diet low in phosphate.

Giordano's study shows a " . . . marked amelioration of acidosis during the low protein diet" and that "improvement of blood pH and plasma bicarbonate lasts for many years" with adherence to a low-protein diet. It is his conclusion that " . . . long term low protein diet is accompanied by a net improvement of acid–base balance in chronic uremia."

These are exciting new data that may substitute phosphate control for pharmacologic agents or invasive uremia therapy such as dialysis and transplantation.

M.M.A.

1

Low-Protein Diets and the Nondialyzed Uremic Patient

JOEL D. KOPPLE, CHARLOTTE E. ROBERTS,
GERALD P. GRODSTEIN, GAURANG M. SHAH,
ROBERT L. WINER, WARREN D. DAVIDSON, DAN A. HENRY,
AND STANLEY S. FRANKLIN

It is accepted that in patients with chronic renal failure, dietary control of salt and water balance and diuretics should be used to prevent depletion or excessive retention of salt and water.[1] Similarly, there is little argument concerning the need to control dietary potassium, phosphorus, and magnesium intake, to provide calcium and vitamin supplements, and to use phosphate binders in such patients.[1,2] Thus the controversy concerning the value of dietary therapy in chronic uremia relates to the management of protein intake to postpone dialysis therapy and optimize nutritional status.

It seems clear that accumulation of nitrogenous metabolites plays a major role in the pathogenesis of the uremic syndrome. This observation is based on findings that patients with symptomatic uremia usually undergo a reduction in symptoms when they are fed a protein-restricted diet. Conversely, an increase in protein intake may engender or intensify many uremic symptoms. Also, hemodialysis, which primarily removes small molecules (e.g., less than 400 daltons), including many metabolites of protein and amino acids, causes marked improvement in uremic symptoms even in patients who are in good water and mineral balance and are not acidotic. Hence it is probable that some of the toxic molecules that are removed by dialysis are metabolic products of protein or amino acids.

JOEL D. KOPPLE, CHARLOTTE E. ROBERTS, GERALD P. GRODSTEIN, WARREN D. DAVIDSON, DAN A. HENRY, AND STANLEY S. FRANKLIN ● Medical and Research Services, Veterans Administration Wadsworth Medical Center, Los Angeles, California, Department of Medicine and Public Health, University of California Los Angeles, California. GAURANG M. SHAH AND ROBERT L. WINER ● Veterans Administration Medical Center, Long Beach, California; and University of California Irvine, Irvine, California.

Despite these considerations, most nephrologists in the United States are reluctant to prescribe carefully controlled low-nitrogen diets for patients with advanced chronic renal failure who are not undergoing dialysis therapy. In general, their reticence is based on the following reasons: (1) Adherence to these diets is difficult, time-consuming, and unpleasant for the patient and the patient's family. (2) Patient compliance is so poor that such treatment may be ineffective. (3) Low-nitrogen diets may promote malnutrition. (4) These diets may not maintain patients as free of uremic symptoms as does treatment with dialysis and higher protein intakes.

On the other hand, if uremic patients could comfortably accept treatment with low-nitrogen diets, and adhere closely to these diets, it is possible that they would be maintained in better clinical condition prior to beginning dialysis treatment. In addition, if such low-nitrogen diets could safely delay the need for dialysis treatment, there could be improvement in the patients' quality of life and a reduction in the enormous costs of dialysis therapy. Moreover, there is the possibility that appropriate dietary therapy during the predialysis period could prevent wasting and malnutrition, which are frequent complications of renal failure.[3-5]

To demonstrate that such dietary therapy is safe and effective, however, the following theses would need to be demonstrated: (1) Patients will adhere adequately to the dietary prescription. (2) The diet will not be excessively burdensome to the patient or family. (3) The dietary therapy will maintain or improve nutritional status. (4) The diet will maintain the patient at least as well as dialysis treatment with higher protein intakes and better than with a combination of no dialysis treatment and less well-controlled dietary therapy; the patient should be better maintained with regard to uremic symptoms, superimposed illnesses, degree of rehabilitation, and mortality.

It is surprising that despite the great interest in the therapy of patients with end-stage renal disease, there has never been a prospective controlled comparison of the response to management with low-nitrogen diets as compared with either maintenance dialysis treatment with higher protein intakes or a more *laissez-faire* approach to dietary therapy. Indeed, there are still relatively few controlled prospective comparisons of two or more low-nitrogen diets.[6-11]

A study that compares the effects of dietary therapy with maintenance dialysis treatment should also determine under what conditions dietary therapy is not sufficient for the uremic patient. Hence such a study, by necessity, would evaluate the clinical indications for dialysis therapy, an important clinical question that has never been investigated in a prospective fashion.

MODERN EXPERIENCE WITH DIETARY THERAPY

Early Experience

The modern era of dietary protein management in chronic renal failure began with the observations by Giordano, who fed diets containing small quantities of essential amino acids to chronically uremic patients. His studies were based on observations known for many years that humans and other animals can utilize ingested urea or ammonium salts for synthesis of amino acids and protein.[12,13] However, only nonessential amino acids may be synthesized, at least in the quantities sufficient for bodily needs, and hence dietary intake of the essential amino acids is still necessary. Giordano reasoned that if uremic patients ingest diets providing low quantities of essential amino acids and virtually no nonessential amino acids, they can utilize their endogenous urea pool as a source of nonessential nitrogen. He therefore fed chronically uremic patients 16–18 g/day of primarily essential amino acids, sometimes with added urea.[13] There was a marked fall in serum urea nitrogen (SUN). Nitrogen balance became neutral or positive in some patients, although often only after an extended period of negative nitrogen balance.

In expanding on this concept of feeding uremic patients low quantities of nitrogen with abundant essential amino acids, Giovannetti and co-workers[14,15] fed uremic patients high-energy diets containing almost no nitrogen to deplete the labile pool of tissue amino acids and proteins and thereby enhance the propensity to conserve nitrogen. After the plasma urea decreased, the diet was supplemented with small amounts of primarily high biological value protein, which provided the recommended daily allowance for all essential amino acids. Nitrogen balance became positive in two patients after addition of the protein. However, the authors' data suggest that substantial protein depletion may have occurred while the patients were ingesting the protein-deficient diet.

Therapeutic results with the Giordano–Giovannetti diet were initially very encouraging.[13–20] The SUN often fell markedly. Uric acid and inorganic phosphate levels often diminished. Red cell production appeared to improve; hemoglobin and hematocrit fell more slowly in some patients and stabilized or even rose in others. Anorexia, nausea or vomiting, singultus, pruritus, and drowsiness decreased daramatically. Many patients became almost euphoric. Serum creatinine, serum albumin, and renal function did not change except as a result of the underlying disease.

Giovannetti and Maggiore[14]; Berlyne, Shaw, and Nilwarangkur[16]; and Kluthe et al.[20], reported that patients live longer, although no prospective controlled studies were carried out. However, it was their impression that the quality of life rather than its duration was most benefited. Terminally, Berlyne and Shaw's patients became acidotic, hyperkalemic, anxious, and agitated, and died suddenly without any return of uremic symptoms.[21]

On the other hand, several groups of investigators found that nitrogen balance was often negative with these diets. Herndon et al.[22] reported that minimum protein needs in chronically uremic patients were 0.5 and 0.7 g/day (*vide supra*); the quality of dietary protein varied and an allowance of 0.56 $g/m^2/day$ was made for unmeasured losses. Ford et al.[23] gave meat as the major source of dietary protein and reported a protein requirement of 0.5g/kg/day; Bostrom et al.[24], reported neutral nitrogen balance in three uremic patients ingesting 40 g of protein/day. Wright et al.[25] found that nitrogen balance was initially negative in all six patients receiving a 20 g protein diet and became neutral in only a single case.

Kopple and co-workers[6,7,26] conducted a series of experiments comparing diets providing 20 and 40 g/day of primarily high biological value protein. In two outpatient studies, chronically uremic patients felt as well when they ingested the higher protein diets as with the 20 g protein diet.[6,26] Moreover, nitrogen balance studies with isocaloric diets indicated that nitrogen balance was significantly more positive with the 40 g protein diet, potassium balance correlated with nitrogen balance, and body weight increased only with this diet as compared with the 20 g protein diet.[7] SUN was only slightly greater with the former diet. In these metabolic studies, when the GFR was above 4.0 ml/min, symptoms were well controlled with the 40 g protein diet.

Several investigators report neutral or positive nitrogen balances in some but not most patients fed 18–25 g protein/day.[19,27] Most of these researchers did not indicate that they corrected for unmeasured nitrogen losses. It is now the consensus of most investigators that diets for chronically uremic patients that provide 25 g/day or less of protein primarily of high quality may lead to malnutrition.

Experience with Amino Acid and Ketoacid Diets

Since the original work of Giordano[13] with amino acid diets, a number of investigators have examined the use of amino acid or ketoacid diets for patients with advanced renal failure.[8–11,28–40]

The interest in these semisynthetic diets was stimulated by several considerations: (1) chronically uremic patients fed very-low-protein diets— e.g., 18–25 g/day—appear to develop wasting; (2) there is evidence that diets providing low quantities of amino acids may be utilized more efficiently as compared with low-protein diets[28,30]; (3) amino acid diets may be more effective at normalizing extracellular and intracellular amino acid concentrations than low-protein diets.[38,39]

Bergström et al.[29] found that uremic patients fed 2.6 g/day of essential amino acid nitrogen frequently were in negative nitrogen balance. Kopple and Swendseid[30] compared the effects of a diet providing 22 g of primarily high-quality protein with 21 g of the eight classical essential amino acids in three chronically uremic patients. With each diet, balance was neutral in one patient and negative in two. However, with the amino acid diet, both nitrogen intake and urea nitrogen appearance (a term defined by Walser et al.[40] as the sum of urinary urea nitrogen excretion and change in body urea nitrogen) were lower, indicating more efficient utilization as compared with protein diets. Moreover, with the amino acid diet plasma levels of nonessential amino acids were, in general, well maintained, suggesting that adequate amounts of these amino acids were being formed.

Schloerb[28] and Bergström and co-workers[31] fed low-protein diets supplemented with essential amino acids to uremic patients and found greater nitrogen retention as compared with the low-protein diets.[28,31] Schloerb[28] found nitrogen balance to be slightly more positive with the former diets as compared with isonitrogenous diets containing protein as the sole source of nitrogen. Norée and Bergström[32] evaluated 26 uremic adults for at least three months while they received 16–20 g of unselected protein supplemented with about 14–21 g of essential L-amino acids. Despite the low creatinine clearances (mean, 3.9 ml/min; range, 2.0–8.5), all improved, and some were partly or fully rehabilitated. In another study of 12 such patients, there was no progression of neuropathy. Although nitrogen balance was well maintained in most patients, particularly in women,[31] a number of their patients were in negative balance. The unselected protein in these diets also enhanced their appeal to the patient. These investigators believe that many uremic patients with residual renal function who would normally require dialysis therapy may be treated equally effectively with these carefully defined diets.[31,32]

Other investigators have now reported clinical experience with the "Swedish diet."[8,11,34] Some workers observed increased levels of plasma essential amino acids and certain proteins as compared with low nitrogen diets alone. Bergström and co-workers also[38] reported a more normal pattern of intracellular muscle amino acid concentrations with these diets, but the effect was short lived. More recently, the last investigators have administered a new essential amino acid preparation in which, using tryptophan as the reference amino acid, the proportion of threonine and valine was increased, tyrosine was added, and the relative amounts of the other essential amino acids were reduced.[39] The authors report that during long-term treatment with this new formulation, muscle intracellular amino acid abnormalities associated with malnutrition were normalized and the patients attained neutral or positive nitrogen balance. More work is necessary on this important observation. Giordano, De Santo, and Pluvio[36] also report more positive nitrogen balance with modifications of the formulation of amino acids or of ketoacids and amino acids.

We investigated the metabolic response to four diets in nine nondialyzed chronically uremic patients with a glomerular filtration rate [mean of creatinine and urea clearances, 7.3 ± 4.3 (SD) ml/min].[8] The patients were assigned in random sequence to one or more of four diets. The diets provided each day 0.55–0.60 g/kg of protein (38.6 ± 2.7 g protein) primarily of high biological value (HBV-protein, eight studies), 43.6 ± 6.2 g of essential and nonessential amino acids in the egg pattern, and 3.0 g of miscellaneous protein (egg pattern AA, six studies), 20.7 g of the nine essential amino acids (including histidine) with 21.8 g of mixed-quality protein (EAA-protein, five studies), and 30.2 ± 1.9 g of the nine essential amino acids and 3.0 g of miscellaneous protein (EAA, five studies). The HBV-protein diet is our standard low-protein diet. The egg pattern AA diet was evaluated because egg contains the highest quality protein of any naturally occurring food, and it was therefore thought that the amino acid pattern in egg might be particularly nutritious. The EAA-protein diet is the Swedish diet. The EAA diet provided an amount of nine essential amino acids and protein (0.47 g/kg), which is similar to the recommended daily allowance of high biological value protein for normal adults.[41] The essential amino acids in the EAA-protein and EAA diets were proportioned according to the Rose formulation with histidine added.

The results indicate that among the four diet groups, mean nitrogen balances, measured after patients had equilibrated with the diets, were neutral and not different from each other (Figure 1). In a few individual patients, however, nitrogen balance was negative, particularly in those fed the EAA-protein or EAA diets. Urea nitrogen appearances tended to be lower with the EAA-protein diet and were lowest with the EAA diet (Figure 2). There were several differences among the patients with regard to their plasma essential and nonessential amino acids with each of the four diets.[8] Serum proteins did not differ among the four groups. However, in comparison with normal subjects, the uremic patients fed the HBV-protein and EAA-protein diets had decreased plasma total essential amino acids, and the essential/nonessential ratios were low with each diet group, except for the EAA diet. With each diet, there was decreased serum total protein, albumin, and, except for the egg pattern AA diet, transferrin. Body weight increased only with the HBV-protein diet. Uremic symptoms were not very different with the four diets, particularly when the GFR was

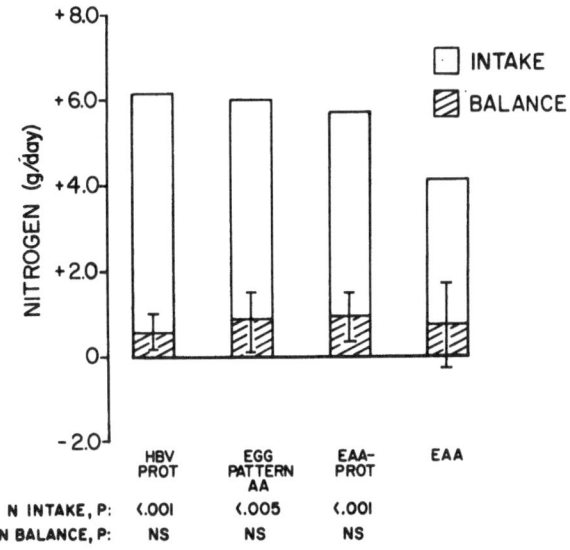

Figure 1. Mean nitrogen intakes and balances in chronically uremic patients fed HBV-protein, egg pattern AA, EAA-protein, and EAA diets. The nitrogen balances (± standard deviation) are calculated from data obtained after equilibration or near equilibration on the diets and are adjusted for changes in body urea content but not for unmeasured nitrogen losses, which are estimated to be about 0.5 g/day. The p values refer to the statistical significance of the differences between nitrogen intake or balance with a given diet as compared with the EAA diet. (From Kopple[8]; reproduced with permission of the editors of the *Proceedings* of the VIIth International Congress of Nephrology.)

4–5 ml/min or higher. Patients selected the HBV-protein diet as their dietary treatment of choice, and the EAA-protein diet was the second choice. These results suggest that, of the four diets, the HBV-protein diet may be preferable when the GFR is above 4-5 ml/min. With a GFR of about 2–5 ml/min in patients who are not receiving dialysis therapy, the EAA-protein or EAA diet seems preferable; the former diet is much better tolerated for extended periods of time.

Alpha-ketoacid and α-hydroxyacid analogues of essential amino acids have also been utilized for treatment of uremic patients.[9–11,34–36,40,42–44] Since these compounds lack the α-amino nitrogen and are rapidly converted to amino acids *in vivo*,[45–47] administering them may be almost tantamount to giving amino acids without increasing the nitrogen load. Several investigators have shown that in normal and uremic subjects nitrogen balance is improved by adding ketoacid analogues of phenylalanine, valine, or tryptophan to diets deficient in these essential amino

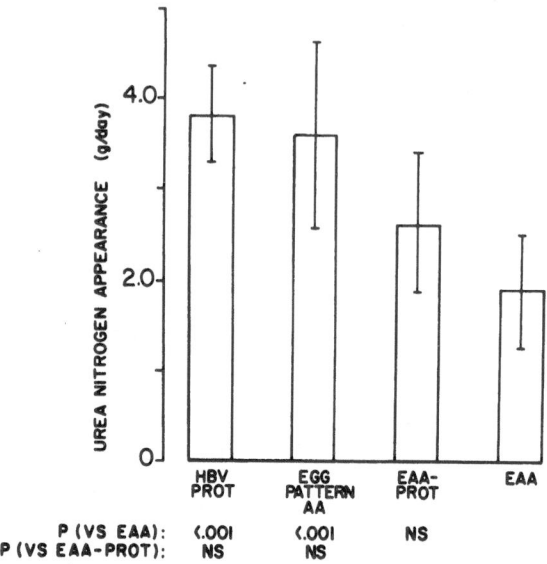

Figure 2. Mean urea nitrogen appearances (± standard deviation) in chronically uremic patients fed the HBV- protein, egg pattern AA, EAA-protein, and EAA diets. Data were obtained after equilibration or near equilibration on the diets. The *p* values refer to the statistical significance of the differences between a given diet and either the EAA diet or the EAA-protein diet. (From Kopple[8]; reproduced with permission of the editors of the *Proceedings* of the VIIth International Congress of Nephrology.)

acids.[42,43,47] Giordano et al.[43] also demonstrated incorporation of exogenously administered ammonium-N^{15} into phenylalanine and valine in protein under these conditions.

Walser and co-workers[40,44] administered low-protein diets supplemented with the ketoacid salts of five essential amino acids and the other four essential L-amino acids—threonine, lysine, histidine, and tryptophan—to patients with far-advanced renal failure. Occasionally, seven ketoacids were used. Urea appearance was remarkably low in many patients, and nitrogen balance was often neutral or positive even with nitrogen intakes of less than 4.0 g/day. Patients were frequently studied with a low protein diet that was supplemented with 14 g/day of the salts of five ketoacids and 2.3 g of four essential amino acids.[40,44] This diet appears to maintain more positive nitrogen balances with lower urea nitrogen appearances as compared with low-protein diets providing the essential amino acids. Subjects have been evaluated clinically with these diets for many months, and Walser reports that uremic symptoms improve even with preterminal levels of renal function.

Renal function stabilized or increased in several uremic patients fed ketoacid diets, and Walser et al.[40,44] suggested that the ketoacids may be responsible. Other investigators have not confirmed this finding, and it is possible that low serum phosphorus levels or a low calcium/phosphorus product with the ketoacid diets may be responsible for the improvement in renal function.[48-50]

Walser and co-workers[40,44] and Sapii et al.[46] also reported that ketoacid diets, and particularly the branched chain ketoacid analogues, can improve nitrogen balance. Similar observations have also been made for the branched chain amino acids and the effect is probably due to anabolic actions of leucine and α-ketoisocaproic acid (keto-leucine).

Recently, Abras and Walser described the results of treating four uremic patients who received, for one to two months, low-nitrogen preparations by continuous infusion through a nasogastric tube.[54] These formulations provided 28 g of six amino acids and 17 g of four nitrogen-free amino acid analogues. Patients also ingested three small meals per day and received a total (food plus infusion) of 33 kcal/kg/day and 3.4 g N/day. Mean nitrogen balance was positive, and the urea nitrogen appearance was very low, averaging 1.2 g/day.

Several other investigators have recently reported results in renal failure with low protein diets that are supplemented usually with five ketoacids or hydroxyacids and four essential amino acids.[9-11,34-36,40,42-44,51-54] Their observations can be summarized as follows:

1. Nitrogen balance is improved, and serum proteins and plasma amino acids are more normal as compared with the Swedish diet.[34,40,44]
2. Nitrogen balance is rather similar with the ketoacid diet as compared with the Swedish diet,[52] but adaptation to the low-nitrogen intake may occur more readily with the ketoacid diet.[51]
3. In outpatient studies there are reports of both little or no advantage[11] and substantial benefits[34] to treatment with diets providing low quantities of protein, essential amino acids, and ketoacids as compared with low protein and essential amino acids (the Swedish diet).
4. When protein and amino acid intake is about 40 g/day, addition of ketoacids provides no clear-cut improvement in nitrogen balance, urea nitrogen appearance, or clinical status.[10,53] Hence, for the ketoacids or hydroxyacids to be well utilized, they probably must be administered with diets providing less than 40 g of protein per day.

Many of these comparative studies suffer from lack of proper controls, from variations in amino acid or ketoacid formulations, or from poor documentation of actual intake.

CURRENT RESEARCH NEEDS
CONCERNING LOW-NITROGEN DIETS

It is unfortunate that despite the extensive literature concerning low-nitrogen diets in chronic renal failure, there is not a single report that carefully documents the extent to which outpatients have adhered to their prescribed diet. Thus, when investigators report that patients placed on very-low-nitrogen diets are well nourished, it is possible that their good nutrition reflects the fact that the patients ingested a somewhat higher protein intake than they were prescribed. Since diets that are slightly higher in protein content may also maintain patients relatively free of uremic symptoms (e.g., the 0.55–0.60 g/kg protein diet),[6-8] it is even possible, although not demonstrated that the good clinical and nutritional status of such patients might even be related to deviation from the diets. Indeed, the serum urea nitrogen/serum creatinine ratios (*vide infra*) of patients in many of the foregoing studies suggest that their dietary nitrogen intake was greater than prescribed. It is important to recognize that a diet providing 0.50–0.60 g of protein/kg/day provides only 1 to 2 g of nitrogen per day more than most of the essential amino acid or ketoacid and protein diet. Thus it is possible that the beneficial effects that some uremic outpatients have experienced with specialized diets could be related to the intake of a relatively low-nitrogen diet (e.g., 0.55–0.60 g of protein/kg/day) rather than to a specific amino acid or ketoacid formulation. It would seem that the only way to resolve this question would be careful documentation of nitrogen intake.

Assessment of Nitrogen Intake

In the past the standard method for assessing dietary compliance in outpatient studies has been dietary interviews supplemented by the dietary diaries. The inaccuracy of this technique is well documented, particularly with patients who are highly trained in therapeutic diets. Such patients can misrepresent their dietary intake in a sophisticated manner if they choose to do so. Fortunately, for assessment of the dietary protein intake there are two other methods, the SUN/serum creatinine ratio and the urea nitrogen appearance (UNA).

Serum Urea Nitrogen/Serum Creatinine Ratio

The SUN/serum creatinine ratio can also be used to assess the dietary protein intake of the uremic patient. This ratio correlates directly with the dietary protein intake in chronically uremic patients who are not undergoing dialysis therapy.[55] Thus, from knowledge of a patient's SUN and serum creatinine, one can estimate the dietary protein intake of a chronically uremic patient during the previous several days. However, several factors can increase the SUN/serum creatinine ratio independently of protein intake. These include catabolic stress and a urine output of 1,500 ml/day, which leads to decreased urea clearance. In women, children, and very wasted men, their reduced muscle mass is associated with less creatinine production, and hence the SUN/creatinine ratio will be higher for any given protein intake. Also, when dietary protein intake is changed to a substantial degree, a period of two to three weeks may be necessary before the SUN stabilizes and the SUN/serum creatinine ratio will reflect the new protein intake.

Urea Nitrogen Appearance

The urea nitrogen appearance (UNA) appears to be the most accurate method for estimating total nitrogen output or nitrogen intake under clinical conditions. UNA is the amount of urea, during a given period of time, that is lost from the body (i.e., in urine, dialysate, or other outputs) or that accumulates in the body. UNA is calculated from the following equation[56]:

UNA (grams/day) = urinary urea N (grams/day)

+ dialysate urea N (grams/day)

+ change in body urea N (grams/day)

Change in body urea nitrogen is calculated as follows:

Change in body urea N (grams) = $(SUN_f - SUN_i$, grams/liter$) \times BW_i$ (kg)

$\times$ 0.60 + $(BW_f - BW_i$, kg$)$

$\times SUN_f$(grams/liter)$\times$ 1.0

where i and f are the initial and final values of the period of measurement, SUN is serum urea nitrogen, and BW is body weight. The fraction of body weight that is water is represented by 0.60. A greater number may be used if the patient is lean or edematous, and a lesser number may be employed if the patient is obese or very young. The assumption is made that, in a uremic patient, any change in BW occurring during a one- to three-day interval is due to gain or loss of water. Therefore, the fraction of weight change that represents gain or loss of water is taken as 1.0. Collection periods for measurement of UNA usually vary from one to five days.

Sargent and co-workers[57] have devised a useful method for estimating UNA, incorrectly referred to as urea generation, in patients undergoing maintenance hemodialysis. This technique is based on the known dialysance of a given dialyzer at a given dialysate flow and blood flow, the renal clearance of urea, and the SUN and body weight at the beginning and end of one hemodialysis and the beginning of the next one. The term UNA is considered preferable to urea generation because some urea is degraded each day in the gastointestinal tract and the released ammonia is largely reconverted to urea in the liver. Hence, unless kinetic studies of urea metabolism are performed, it is not possible to calculate the urea generation exactly. Since UNA indicates the total amount of urea nitrogen that is lost from the body or that accumulates, it is the measure of urea production that is most useful clinically.

Urea is quantitatively the major nitrogenous product of protein and amino acid metabolism. Production of most of the other major products of nitrogen metabolism (i.e., creatinine, uric acid, guanidines) is relatively constant, and the synthesis of these compounds does not vary markedly with the rate of protein breakdown or of nitrogen intake. Therefore, the UNA should reflect the rate of net protein breakdown, and an adjustment

Figure 3. Relationship between total nitrogen output and urea nitrogen appearance in 12 studies in normal subjects ($\square$),[60] $y = 0.97$ X $- 1.28$, $r = 0.99$; 11 studies in patients with chronic renal failure ($\triangle$) from Cottini, et al.[61]; three studies from our laboratory (*), $y = 0.95$ X -1.56, $r = 0.99$; and 26 studies in patients undergoing maintenance hemodialysis ($\bullet$),[62] $y = 0.96$ X $- 1.74$, $r = 0.97$. The solid line depicts the regression analysis for these combined data for normal subjects, patients with chronic renal failure, and those undergoing hemodialysis, $r = 0.98$. Data from 12 studies in patients undergoing continuous ambulatory peritoneal dialysis, who lose protein into dialysate,[59] are indicated by X, $r = 0.96$. The values from patient 3 ($\bigcirc$), who had low-grade peritonitis and abnormally increased protein losses, are omitted from the regression analysis. (From Blumenkrantz et al.[59]; reproduced with permission from the editor of Kidney International.)

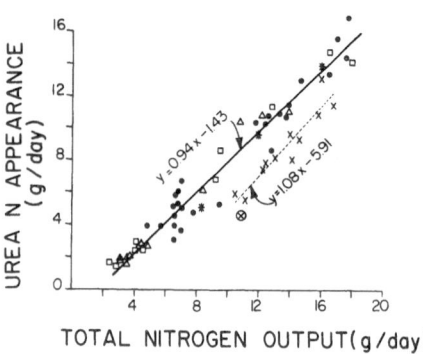

can be made in the values to account for the nonurea nitrogen losses. Indeed, we recently evaluated this question in 13 normal subjects and 28 nondialyzed chronically uremic patients who were studied for a combined total of over 2,000 days in our clinical research unit. The data indicated that there was a close correlation between UNA and total nitrogen output, calculated as the sum of urinary nitrogen, fecal nitrogen, and change in body urea nitrogen.[58]

In patients who are clinically stable and in protein balance, nitrogen output should equal nitrogen intake. Under these circumstances, UNA should also indicate nitrogen or protein intake. Indeed, observations from our metabolic balance studies indicate that there is a fairly high correlation between UNA and nitrogen intake,[58] although the correlation is not as close as between UNA and nitrogen output. Thus, in uremic patients who are clinically stable, it should be possible to monitor nitrogen intake from the UNA.

There are several factors that can alter the relationship between UNA and nitrogen intake or output. These include protein losses into urine or from peritoneal dialysis or increased urinary ammonia excretion due to an acid load.[59] In these individuals the UNA may underestimate total nitrogen output or nitrogen intake. Figure 3 gives an example of the relation between UNA and total nitrogen output and how this relationship may be altered in patients undergoing continuous ambulatory peritoneal dialysis who lose protein, amino acids, and peptides into dialysate.

COMPLIANCE OF CHRONICALLY UREMIC PATIENTS WITH LOW NITROGEN DIETS

We have used the close relationship between UNA and dietary nitrogen intake to evaluate the degree of compliance of chronically uremic patients with low-nitrogen diets. This study is part of a larger project to investigate the response of chronically uremic patients fed one of two nitrogen diets with regard to their acceptance of the diet, compliance with the diet, control of uremic toxicity, nutritional status, and overall clinical condition.

All patients accepted into the study were at least 18 years old and had chronic renal failure with a GFR between 4 and 12 ml/min. Patients were excluded from the study if they had vasculitis, collagen diseases (except for rheumatoid arthritis), active malignancy (other than basal cell carcinoma), liver failure, or marked abnormal psychosocial disorders or organic or functional mental disease that would prevent compliance with the dietary regimen.

Table I. Essential Amino Acid Content of 30 Tablets[a]

Amino acid	Grams per 30 tablets
L-Histidine	1.65
L-Isoleucine	2.1
L-Leucine	3.3
L-Lysine acetate	3.4[b]
Equivalent to L-lysine	2.4[c]
L-Methionine	3.3
L-Phenylalanine	3.3
L-Threonine	1.5
L-Tryptophan	0.75
L-Valine	2.4
Total Essential Amino Acids	20.7
Total Nitrogen	2.6

[a] Quantity of amino acids present in 30 tablets (Aminess®, Cutter Laboratories).
[b] Quantity of lysine acetate.
[c] Quantity of free lysine.

Patients were assigned by a table of random numbers to treatment with one of two diets: a diet providing 0.55–0.60 g of protein/kg body weight/day, which contained protein primarily of high biological value (HBV-protein diet), or a diet providing 20–21 g/day of protein and, with one exception, 20.7 g/day of a mixture of nine essential amino acids (Aminess®, courtesy of Cutter Laboratories) (EAA-protein diet). This essential amino acid mixture was provided in 30 tablets per day. One woman who weighed only 48.3 kg was prescribed 10.35 g/day of the essential amino acids. The amino acid composition of Aminess tablets is shown in Table I. The prescribed daily protein intake was increased by 1.0 g of primarily high-quality protein for each gram of urinary protein loss greater than 2.0 g/day. Prescribed nitrogen intake with the HBV-protein and EAA-protein diets averaged 6.3 and 5.8 g/day respectively. All patients were prescribed at least 35 kcal/kg/day unless their dry body weight was greater than 115% of normal, in which case energy intake was reduced. The food was provided in three meals with or without an evening snack. Prescribed phosphorus intake was 900 mg/day or less, and patients received aluminum hydroxide gel. All patients received multivitamin and calcium supplements, and medicines were given as clinically indicated.

The study protocol contained four steps or phases through which the patient passed in the following sequence: (1) During the "Identification Phase" contact with the patient was established and informed consent was obtained. (2) During the "Initiation Phase" baseline data were obtained and the patient was assigned in random fashion to one of the two low nitrogen diets. (3) During the "Control Phase" the patient underwent intensive training in dietary therapy and began to prepare and follow the diet. This phase lasted for at least two weeks, and the patient was not allowed to leave the Control Phase until his or her UNA was within two standard deviations of predicted values on two consecutive visits. The predicted values were determined from UNA measurements made in patients fed the HBV-protein or EAA-protein diets in our clinical research center.[8] (4) During the "Experimental Phase" the patient's nutritional, biochemical, clinical, and psychosocial responses to dietary treatment were monitored for up to 12–13 weeks. Patients were usually evaluated by the nephrologist and dietitian at weekly intervals during the Control Phase and every other week during the Experimental Phase.

For the UNA measurement, urine was collected for a 24-hour period, which ended the morning of the clinic visit. The determination of the change in body urea nitrogen was modified as follows: The SUN and body weight were measured at the time of each clinic visit and were used as the final values. Patients did not have blood drawn or body weight measured at the beginning of the urine collection. Instead, the SUN and the body weight from the previous visit, one or two weeks earlier, were used for the estimation of the initial SUN and body weight. The differences between the initial and final measurements of SUN and body weight were each divided by the number of days between the initial and final measurements. The sum of the dividend and the final measurement of SUN or body weight was then used as the initial value for calculation of the change in body urea nitrogen. It is assumed that over the period of study any inaccuracies in this method for measuring UNA will tend to cancel out. Urea was measured with a Technicon AutoAnalyzer or a Beckman BUN Analyzer.

The patients who entered this study came from a wide spectrum of socioeconomic and educational backgrounds. All patients were instructed and followed by the same dietitian and by one of five nephrologists who had undergone special training in the implementation of the study protocol.

For comparison, the expected UNAs with the HBV-protein and EAA-protein diets were derived from a study of eight patients fed the HBV-protein diet and five patients fed the EAA-protein diet in a metabolic unit for an average of 19.1 ± 3.9 days and 23.0 ± 6.2 days, respectively,[8] as shown in Figure 2. Characteristics of patients and these diets have been previously described.[8]

Preliminary data from the outpatient study are currently available from 13 patients fed the HBV–protein diet for 15 ± 4 weeks and ten patients fed the EAA-protein diet for 16 ± 4 weeks. These periods of time include both the Control and the Experimental Phases of the study. The patients came from a variety of socioeconomic and cultural backgrounds. The preliminary data indicate that the grand mean for the UNA (average from the Experimental Phase) was 4.3 ± 1.2 g N/day with the HBV-protein diet and 4.1 ± 1.1 g N/day with the EAA-protein diet. These UNA values are not different from each other and are similar to the UNA of patients fed the HBV-protein diet and EAA-protein diet under metabolic conditions (Figure 2). Indeed, the mean values for the UNA in the outpatient studies are well within two standard deviations of the UNA of the patients living in the metabolic unit. Anthropometric measurements and serum total protein and albumin concentrations were normal and did not change during the study with the two diets.

These results indicate that chronically uremic patients from different socioeconomic backgrounds adhere well to low-nitrogen diets that provide each day 0.55 or 0.60 g/kg of primarily high biological value protein or 20 g of protein and 20.7 g of essential amino acids. With each diet, the grand mean of the UNA, and hence the actual quantity of nitrogen ingested, was low and similar to the other diet. The data also indicate that the actual quantity of nitrogen ingested was close to the prescribed nitrogen intake. In general, patients who entered the Experimental Phase were willing to accept the restrictions of these diets in return for careful management of their metabolic and nutritional status, and possibly a greater period of time without dialysis treatment.

The preponderance of time spent on the dietary management was by the dietitian, and this form of treatment was therefore cost-effective. A comparison of the number of patients contacted by the investigators concerning this study and the patients who finished the study suggests that probably at least 25% to 45% of clinically stable chronically uremic patients may be treated with these diets for a period of weeks to months. These figures exclude patients with catabolic stress or with a rapidly falling GFR who are not candidates for long-term dietary therapy.

Since these preliminary data indicate that many chronically uremic patients will adhere closely to low nitrogen diets, will not object to the dietary control, do not become malnourished, and feel well with these diets, we believe that further studies in this area are strongly indicated. It is proposed that controlled prospective studies be carried out that will compare the response of chronically uremic patients fed such low-nitrogen diets with those who are allowed the more *ad libitum* diets commonly recommended by nephrologists and with those who are started earlier on maintenance dialysis therapy and who eat the protein intake typically prescribed for dialysis patients.

SUMMARY

Many reports suggest that carefully designed low-nitrogen diets can maintain nondialyzed chronically uremic patients relatively free of uremic symptoms and well nourished. However, many nephrologists believe that such diets are not clinically beneficial, acceptable, or adhered to by the patient. In order to demonstrate that a low-nitrogen diet is effective for management of patients with chronic renal failure, the diet should satisfy the following criteria: (1) it must be well tolerated; (2) patients must be able to adhere relatively closely to the diet; and (3) the diet must maintain patients in a better clinical or nutritional state than less well-controlled diets and in at least as good a clinical and nutritional state as dialysis therapy and intake of larger protein intakes. A major problem with the study of low-nitrogen diets in nonhospitalized patients is the difficulty in ascertaining compliance with the prescribed diets. The urea nitrogen appearance (UNA) may be used to assess the patient's actual nitrogen intake. Under most circumstances, if a patient is not very catabolic or anabolic the UNA will accurately indicate the average nitrogen intake. Using measurements of UNA, we conducted a preliminary study to assess the degree of dietary adherence in nondialyzed clinically stable chronically uremic patients assigned in random fashion to one of two low nitrogen diets—a diet providing 0.55–0.60 g of primarily high-quality protein/kg/day or a diet providing 20 g/day of protein of miscellaneous quality and 20.7 g/day of the nine essential amino acids. Patients initially underwent training in dietary therapy and after compliance with the diet was demonstrated, they were followed for up to 13 weeks with the diet. At present, 13 patients have been treated with the former diet and ten patients with the latter diet. The results indicate that most patients who entered the study accepted the diets well. The UNA data indicate that, in general, patients adhered closely to the prescribed nitrogen intake. Anthropometric measurements and serum proteins were usually normal and did not change during the study. Patients, in general, felt well during the study. Thus clinically stable chronically uremic patients appear capable of adhering to low nitrogen diets for extended periods of time and fare well with this therapy.

REFERENCES

1. Walser M: Conservative management of the uremic patient, in Brenner BM, Rector FC Jr (eds): The Kidney, Philadelphia, WB Saunders Co, 1981, pp 2383–2424.
2. Kopple JD, Swendseid ME: Vitamin nutrition in patients undergoing maintenance hemodialysis. Kidney Int 7:S79–84, 1975.

3. Kopple JD: Abnormal amino acid and protein metabolism in uremia. *Kidney Int* 14:340–348, 1978.

4. Blumenkrantz MJ, Kopple JD, Gutman RA, et al: Methods for assessing nutritional status of patients with renal failure. *Am J Clin Nutr* 33:1567–1585, 1980.

5. Guarnieri G, Faccini L, Lipartiti T, et al: Simple methods for nutritional assessment in hemodialyzed patients. *Am J Clin Nutr* 33:1598–1607, 1980.

6. Kopple JD, Sorenson MK, Coburn JW, et al: Controlled comparison of 20-g and 40-g protein diets in the treatment of chronic uremia. *Am J Clin Nutr* 21:553–564, 1968.

7. Kopple JD, Coburn JW: Metabolic studies of low protein diets in uremia. I. Nitrogen and potassium. *Medicine* 52:583–595, 1973.

8. Kopple JD: Treatment with low protein and amino acid diets in chronic renal failure, in *Proceedings VIIth International Congress of Nephrology, Canada, June 18–23.* S Karger, 1978, pp 497–507.

9. Kampf D, Fischer H-CH, Kessel M: Efficacy of an unselected protein diet (25 g) with minor oral supply of essential amino acids and keto analogues compared with a selective protein diet (40 g) in chronic renal failure. *Am J Clin Nutr* 33:1673–1677, 1980.

10. Hecking E, Andrzejewski L, Prellwitz W: Double-blind crossover study with oral α-ketoacids in patients with chronic renal failure. *Am J Clin Nutr* 33:1678–1681, 1980.

11. Frohling PT, Schmicker R, Vetter K, et al: Conservative treatment with ketoacid and amino acid supplemented low-protein diets in chronic renal failure. *Am J Clin Nutr* 33:1667–1672, 1980.

12. Kies C: Nonspecific nitrogen in the nutrition of human beings. *Fed Proc* 31:1172–1177, 1972.

13. Giordano C: Use of exogenous and endogenous urea for protein synthesis in normal and uremic subjects. *J Lab Clin Med* 62:231–246, 1963.

14. Giovannetti S, Maggiore Q: A low-nitrogen diet with proteins of high biological value for severe chronic uraemia. *Lancet* 1:1000–1003, 1964.

15. Monasterio G, Giovannetti S, Maggiore Q: The place of the low protein diet in the treatment of chronic uremia. *Panminerva Med* 7:479–484, 1965.

16. Berlyne GM, Shaw AB, Nilwarangkur S: Dietary treatment of chronic renal failure. Experiences with a modified Giovannetti diet. *Nephron* 2:129–147, 1965.

17. Shaw AB, Bazzard FJ, Booth EM, et al: The treatment of chronic renal failure by a modified Giovannetti diet. *Q J Med* 34:237–253, 1965.

18. Franklin SS, Gordon A, Kleeman CR, et al: Use of balanced low-protein diet in chronic renal failure. *JAMA* 202:477–484, 1967.

19. Snyder D, Merrill JP: "Conservative" management of chronic renal failure with a selected protein diet. *Trans Assoc Am Phys* 74:409–418, 1966.

20. Kluthe R, Oechslen D, Quirin H, et al: Six years' experience with a special low-protein diet, in Kluthe R, Berlyne G, Burton B (eds): *Uremia, An Internationl Conference on Pathogenesis, Diagnosis and Therapy.* Stuttgart, Georg Thieme Verlag, 1972, p 250.

21. Berlyne GM, Shaw AB: Giordano-Giovannetti diet in terminal renal failure. *Lancet* 2:7–9, 1965.

22. Herndon RF, Freeman S, Cleveland AS: Protein requirements in chronic renal insufficient patients. *J Lab Clin Med* 52:235–246, 1958.

23. Ford J, Phillips ME, Toye FE, et al: Nitrogen balance in patients with chronic renal failure on diets containing varying quantities of protein. *Br Med J* 1:735–740, 1969.

24. Boström H, Edgren B, Engelke B: Experience with the Giovannetti diet in chronic uraemia. *Scand J Urol Nephrol* 1:171–180, 1967.

25. Wright PL, Brereton PJ, Snell DEM: Effectiveness of modified Giovannetti diet compared with mixed low-protein diet. *Metabolism* 19:201–213, 1970.

26. Kopple JD, Shinaberger JH, Coburn JW, et al: Evaluating modified protein diets for uremia. *J Am Diet Assoc* 54:481–481, 1969.

27. Hood CEA, Beale DJ, Housley J, et al: Dialysed egg as nitrogen source in dietary control of chronic renal failure. *Lancet* 1:479–482, 1969.

28. Schloerb PR: Essential L-amino acid administration in uremia. *Am J Med Sci* 252:650–659, 1966.

29. Bergström J, Fürst P, Josephson B, et al: Factors affecting the nitrogen balance in chronic uremic patients receiving essential amino acids intravenously or by mouth. *Nutr Metab* (suppl)14:162–170, 1972.

30. Kopple JD, Swenseid ME: Nitrogen balance and plasma amino acid levels in uremic patients fed an essential amino acid diet. *Am J Clin Nutr* 27:806–812, 1974.

31. Bergström J, Fürst P, Norée L-O: Treatment of chronic uremic patients with protein-poor diet and oral supply of essential amino acids. *Clin Nephrol* 3:187–194, 1975.

32. Norée L-O, Bergström J: Treatment of chronic uremic patients with protein-poor diet and oral study of essential amino acids. II. Clinical results of long-term treatment. *Clin Nephrol* 3:195–203, 1975.

33. Kopple JD: Treatment of renal failure with defined-formula diets, in Shils ME (ed): *Defined-Formula Diets for Medical Purposes.* Chicago, American Medical Association, 1977, pp 113–123.

34. Heidland A, Kult J, Rökel A, et al: Evaluation of essential amino acids and keto acids in uremic patients on low-protein diet. *Am J Clin Nutr* 31:1784–1792, 1978.

35. Bauerdick H, Spellerberg P, Lamberts B: Therapy with essential amino acids and their nitrogen-free analogues in severe renal failure. *Am J Clin Nutr* 31:1793–1796, 1978.

36. Giordano C, DeSanto NG, Pluvio M: Nitrogen balance in uremic patients on different amino acid and keto acid formulations—A proposed reference pattern. *Am J Clin Nutr* 31:1797–1801, 1978.

37. Young GA, Chem C, Oli HI, et al: The effects of calorie and essential amino acid supplementation on plasma proteins in patients with chronic renal failure. *Am J Clin Nutr* 31:1801–1807, 1978.

38. Alvestrand A, Bergstrom J, Furst P: Effect of essential amino acid supplementation on muscle and plasma free amino acids in chronic uremia. *Kidney Int* 14:323–329, 1978.

39. Furst P, Alvestrand A, Bergstrom J: Effects of nutrition and catabolic stress on intracellular amino acid pools in uremia. *Am J Clin Nutr* 33:1387–1395, 1980.

40. Walser M, Coulter AW, Dighe S, et al: The effect of ketoanalogues of essential amino acids in severe chronic uremia. *J Clin Invest* 52:678–690, 1973.

41. Food and Nutrition Board, National Research Council: Protein and amino acids, in *Recommended Dietary Allowances*, ed 9. Washington D.C., National Academy of Sciences, 1980, pp 39–54.

42. Richards P, Houghton BJ, Brown CL, et al: Synthesis of phenylalanine and valine by healthy and uraemic men. *Lancet* 2:128–134, 1971.

43. Giordano C, Phillips ME, DeSanto NG, et al: Utilisation of ketoacid analogues of valine and phenylalanine in health and uraemia. *Lancet* 1:178–182, 1972.

44. Walser M: Ketoacids in the treatment of uremia. *Clin Nephrol* 3:180–186, 1975.

45. Walser M, Lund P, Ruderman NB, et al: Synthesis of essential amino acids from their α-keto analogues by perfused rat liver and muscle. *J Clin Invest* 52:2865–2877, 1973.

46. Sapir DG, Owen OE, Pozefsky T, et al: Nitrogen sparing induced by a mixture of essential amino acids given chiefly as their keto-analogues during prolonged starvation in obese subjects. *J Clin Invest* 54:974–980, 1974.

47. Rudman D: Capacity of human subjects to utilize keto analogues of valine and phenylalanine. *J Clin Invest* 50:90–96, 1971.

48. Collier VU, Mitch W, Walser M: The effect of spontaneous or induced lowering of plasma CA × P product on progression of chronic renal failure (CRF). *Clin Res* 26:564A, 1978.

49. Ibels LS, Alfrey AC, Haut L, et al: Preservation of function in experimental renal disease by dietary restriction of phosphate. *N Engl J Med* 298: 122–126, 1978.

50. Walser M: Does dietary therapy have a role in the predialysis patient? *Am J Clin Nutr* 33:1629–1637, 1980.

51. Abras E, Walser M: Continuous enteral alimentation with a formula high in branched-chain compounds in severe chronic renal failure. *Clin Res* 29:262, 1981 (abst).

52. Bergström J, Ahlberg M, Alverstrand A, et al: Metabolic studies with keto acids in uremia. *Am J Clin Nutr* 31:1761–1766, 1978.

53. Burns J, Cresswell E, Ell S, et al: Comparison of the effects of keto acid analogues and essential amino acids on nitrogen homeostasis in uremic patients on moderately protein-restricted diets. *Am J Clin Nutr* 31:1767–1775, 1978.

54. Ell S, Fynn M, Richards P. et al: Metabolic studies with keto acid diets. *Am J Clin Nutr* 31:1776–1783, 1978.

55. Kopple JD, Coburn JW: Evaluation of chronic uremia. Importance of serum urea nitrogen, serum creatinine, and their ratio. *JAMA* 227:41–44, 1974.

56. Grodstein GP, Blumenkrantz MJ, Kopple JD: Nutritional and metabolic response to catabolic stress in uremia. *Am J Clin Nutr* 33:1411–1416, 1980.

57. Sargent J, Gotch F, Borah M, et al: Urea kinetics: A guide to nutritional management of renal failure. *Am J Clin Nutr* 31:1696–1702, 1978.

58. Grodstein G, Kopple JD: Urea nitrogen appearance, a simple and practical indicator of total nitrogen output. *Kidney Int* 16:953, 1979 (abst).

59. Blumenkrantz MJ, Kopple JD, Moran JK, et al: Nitrogen and urea metabolism during continuous ambulatory peritoneal dialysis. *Kidney Int* (in press).

60. Staffee WP, Goldsmith RS, Pencharz PB, et al: Dietary protein intake and dynamic aspects of whole body nitrogen metabolism in adult humans. *Metabolism* 25:281–297, 1976.

61. Cottini EP, Gallina DL, Dominguez JM: Urea excretion in adult humans with varying degrees of kidney malfunction fed milk, egg or amino acid mixture: Assessment of nitrogen balance. *Nutrition* 103:11–19, 1973.

62. Borah MF, Schoenfeld PY, Gotch FA, et al: Nitrogen balance during intermittent dialysis therapy of uremia. *Kidney Int* 14:491–500, 1978.

2

Delay of Progression of Renal Failure

MACKENZIE WALSER

It has become traditional to view chronic renal failure as a process that progresses inexorably toward the point at which no significant amount of renal function remains. Occasional patients seem not to progress or even to improve, but these are infrequent exceptions to the general rule. Because of the generality of this observation, it also has become traditional to accept this inexorable progression as an inevitable phenomenon. Generally it is assumed that unless the etiologic agent can be removed, for example, by discontinuing analgesic intake in analgesic nephropathy or by controlling blood pressure in hypertensive nephropathy, continuing damage to the remaining nephrons by the disease process will occur.

In certain types of renal disease, this seems likely to be true. For example, the renal damage caused by diabetes would seem to be a continuing process, although Dr. Friedman, in Chapter 7, offers some clues as to how to reduce the extent of this process. But in the more common forms of chronic renal disease, including glomerulonephritis and interstitial nephritis, our knowledge of the underlying disease process is not great enough to be able to state with any assurance that the process is continuing to damage nephrons. The alternative possibility, that uremia is itself nephrotoxic, is equally consistent with the available data. Furthermore, if some aspect of the uremic state damages the kidney and can be brought under control by appropriate measures, these same measures might well slow progression even in diseases such as diabetes where the fundamental etiologic process cannot be removed.

In Chapter 3, Drs. Alfrey and Tomford summarize data supporting a role of phosphate in contributing to the progression of experimental renal failure in rats. I would like to summarize data that point to a role of both calcium and phosphate in contributing to the progession of chronic renal failure in humans.

MACKENZIE WALSER ● Department of Pharmacology and Experimental Therapeutics and Department of Medicine, Johns Hopkins University School of Medicine, Baltimore, Maryland.

Our interest in the possibility of delaying or reversing progression in renal failure was aroused by the observation that occasional patients, when placed on a low-protein diet supplemented by ketoanalogues of essential amino acids, showed an unmistakable change in the rate of progression of their renal failure, coincident with normalization of serum calcium and phosphorus concentrations.[1,2]

My former colleague, Dr. Mitch, was stimulated to develop a quantitative technique whereby the rate of progression would be assessed. He found that the reciprocal of plasma creatinine concentration, plotted against time in individual patients, declined linearly in about 90% of cases.[3] This observation has now been repeatedly confirmed.[4-10] The simplest explanation would be that nephrons are destroyed at a constant rate. If creatinine output remained constant, a linear fall in creatinine clearance with time would thus translate into a linear fall in reciprocal plasma creatinine with time. Recent evidence shows that creatinine clearance does indeed fall linearly with time in chronic renal failure.[11]

However, creatinine output decreases progressively as renal failure becomes more severe, and may fall to as little as one third of normal.[12-15] How then can the decline in reciprocal plasma creatinine remain linear?

The fall in creatinine output is not caused by a decline in creatinine production or lean body mass. Creatinine production per kilogram of body weight remains normal.[16] Degradation of creatinine, presumably by intestinal bacteria, causes the fall in creatinine output. The rate of degradation rises as plasma creatinine increases. Mathematically it can be shown[17] that a linear fall with time in creatinine clearance coupled with degradation increasing in proportion to the plasma creatinine concentrations still leads to a linear fall with time in reciprocal plasma creatinine concentration.

Thus we have a rational technique for following the progression of renal failure applicable to most patients. There still remain a few in whom the fall in plasma creatinine with time is not linear. In some of these there is an obvious clinical explanation for a change in the rate of progression, but in others no explanation can be found. Thus a large group of patients should be studied over many months before any firm conclusions can be drawn as to the effects of any specific form of therapy on progression. No such study has been conducted, but it is appropriate now to examine less complete data bearing on this question in order to examine how best to design a study to determine whether nutritional therapy can delay progression.

First, what are the prospects of halting progression in the near-end-stage patient? Slowing progession at this point may delay the onset of dialysis a few months, or possibly years, but for such an approach to have

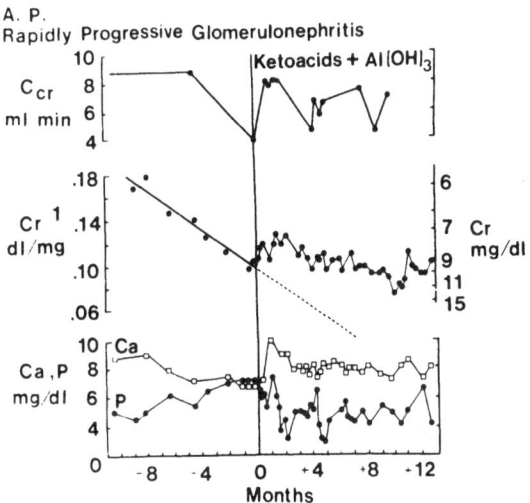

Figure 1. Effect of controlling serum phosphate concentration on the progression of renal failure in a patient with biopsy-proved "rapidly progressive glomerulonephritis." Prior to nutritional therapy (initiated at the vertical line), progression was occurring at a constant rapid rate, as indicated by reciprocal serum creatinine. Control of serum phosphate by a protein- and phosphate-restricted diet supplemented with ketoacids and Al(OH)$_3$ arrested progression for over one year; serum phosphate was normal or slighly low. (Reprinted with permission from Walser et al.[20])

wide utility it would be necessary to show that some patients would be kept off dialysis more or less indefinitely. Retrospective analysis of changing serum creatinine in patients we have managed conservatively showed that progression was faster when the serum Ca × P product was above 33 mg^2/dl^2 than when it was 33 mg^2/dl^2 or less.[18] In these patients low products occurred spontaneously, since no specific attempt was made to induce hypophosphatemia.

We then attempted to slow or stop progression in end-stage patients by techniques aimed at reducing the progressive accumulation of calcium and phosphate deposits in the kidney that we believe contribute to functional deterioration. These were pilot studies in seven patients using each patient's historical plasma creatinine results to assess whether a change in progression was achieved. Phosphate intake was restricted to 400–600 mg/day and an aluminum hydroxide preparation* designed to maximize phosphate-binding capacity[19] plus calcium supplement was administered. When this outpatient regimen was unsuccessful in maintain-

*Controphos, Doyle Pharmaceutical Company.

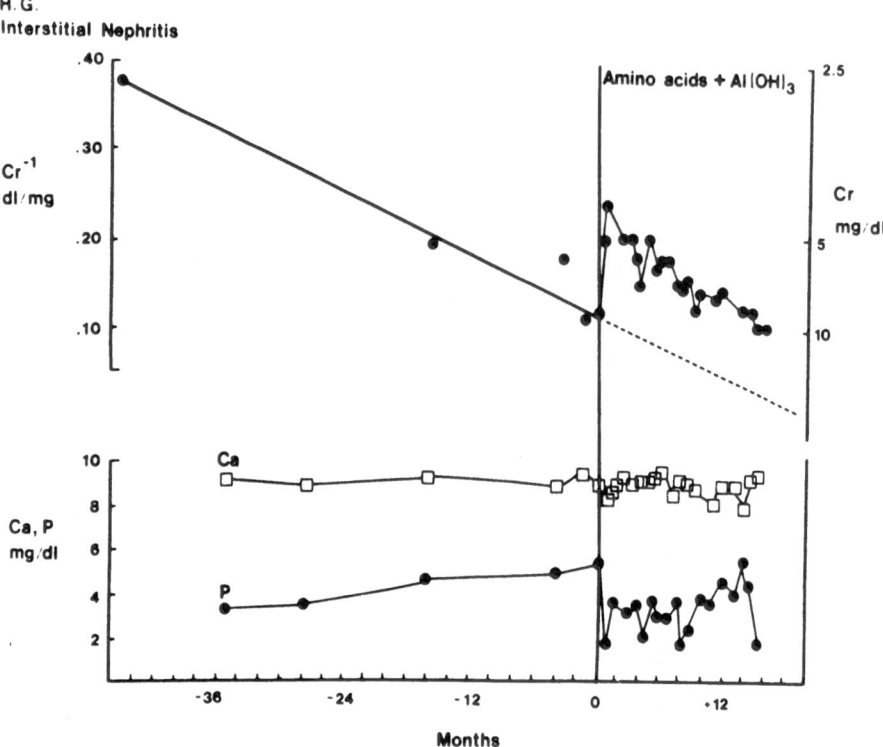

Figure 2. A second example of arrested progression with a protein- and phosphate-restricted diet supplemented with essental amino acids and Al(OH)$_3$. Serum phosphate was maintained at about 3 mg/dl, on the average. (Reprinted with permission from Walser et al.[20])

ing a low normal serum phosphate, the patients were hospitalized and placed on a very low phosphate intake (about 200 mg/day) for a few days to bring serum phosphate down.

In seven patients studied in this manner, promising results were obtained in only two (Figures 1 and 2).[20] The others, who included a diabetic and a case of pyelonephritis, continued to progress at more or less the same rate.[21] Compliance with this restrictive regimen was also a problem.

Despite the difficulties attendant on the use of this regimen, the evidence suggests that control of plasma calcium and phosphate may retard progression in some cases of end-stage renal failure. The converse also seems to be the case. Retrospective analysis[22] of two reports[23,24] in which calcium carbonate was administered to severe chronic uremic patients in an attempt to conrol acidosis showed that those patients whose plasma calcium/phosphate product rose during $CaCO_3$ therapy also exhibited an increase in serum creatinine.

In moderate renal failure, more promising results have been obtained. Barsotti et al.[11] have recently reported the effects on progression of administering a very low phosphorus (300 mg/day) and protein (0.2 g/kg per day of vegetable origin) intake, supplemented with calcium (1,700 mg/day) and a mixture of ketoanalogues and essential amino acids. Twelve chronic uremics with an initial creatinine clearance of about 12 ml/min were studied. After some nine months on 0.5 g/kg/day of high biological value, these patients were shifted to the above regimen. Creatinine clearances were measured monthly before and after the change. The average rate of decrease of creatinine clearance fell from 0.5 ± 0.2 ml/min/mo to 0.03 ± 0.5 ml/min/mo for 4–12 months (Figure 3). Thus progression was nearly stopped, on the average. The authors suggest that

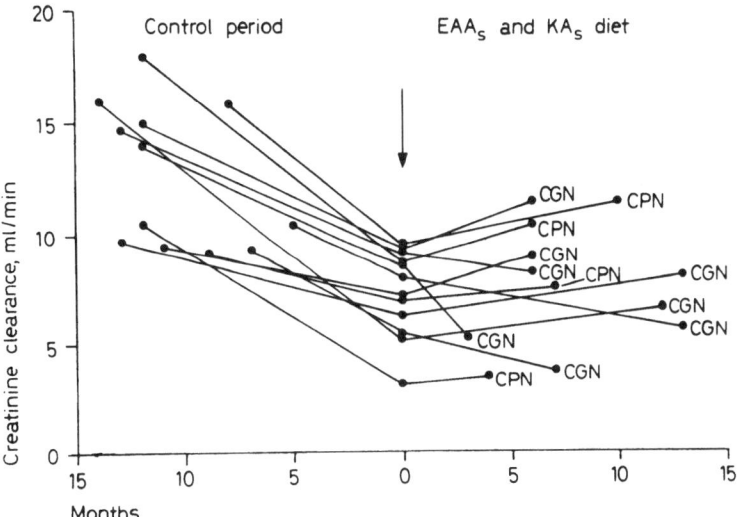

Figure 3. The decline in creatinine clearance during a control period on protein restriction alone and during a period of more severe protein and phosphate restriction plus supplementation with essential amino acids, ketoanalogues, and calcium in 12 patients with chronic renal failure. Each of the straight lines was obtained from monthly measurements of 24-hour creatinine clearance. The correlation coefficients between clearance and time were all high (−0.881 to −0.995). The diagnoses in each patient are shown at the right of the figure (CGN: chronic glomerulonephritis; CPN: chronic pyelonephritis). (Reprinted with permission from Barsotti et al.[11])

this effect was probably due to an accompanying fall in plasma phosphate (from 5.3 ± 0.8 mg/dl to 4.0 ± 0.9 mg/dl).

In early renal failure the results of phosphate restriction and calcium supplementation are even more impressive. Johnson et al. [25] applied these measures to 27 patients with an average serum creatinine of 4.5 mg/dl. In the ensuing 27 months serum creatinine rose to an average of 4.9 mg/dl, indicating almost no progression. Maschio et al. [26] administered 0.4–0.6 g/kg of protein, 500–700 mg of phosphate, and 900–1,500 mg of calcium daily to 18 patients with an average initial plasma creatinine of 4.3 ± 0.8 mg/dl. A few patients also received vitamin D or its analogues. After 5–13 years, plasma creatinine had risen to an average of only 8.2 ± 1.9 mg/dl. Isolated osteomalacia was detectable on bone biopsy in half. In a group of 200 patients with very early renal failure (plasma creatinine 1.6–2.8 mg/dl) given the same regimen (without vitamin D), plasma creatinine scarcely changed in two years. Plasma phosphate remained low normal in both groups (about 3 mg/dl).

These studies provide convincing (though uncontrolled) evidence that phosphate restriction and calcium supplementation can slow the progress of renal failure. Clearly these measures become more difficult to apply as the disease becomes more severe.

What remains is to perform a prospective randomized trail of a regimen designed along these lines. Such a study must include a large number of patients with different types of renal disease and must continue long enough to permit firm conclusions as to the effect, if any, of such regimens on progression rate in each type of renal disease.

ACKNOWLEDGMENT. Supported by USPHS Research Grant, AM-18020.

REFERENCES

1. Walser M: Keto-analogues of essential amino acids, in *Clinical Nutrition Update: Amino Acids*. Chicago, American Medical Association, 1977, p 183.
2. Walser M, Sapir DG, Mitch WE, et al: Evidence for an anabolic action of essential amino acid analogues in uremia and starvation. *Zeit Ernahrung Suppl* 119:S5, 1977.
3. Mitch WE, Buffington GA, Lemann J, et al: A simple method of estimating progression of chronic renal failure. *Lancet* 2:1326, 1976.
4. Rutherford WE, Blondin J, Miller JP, et al: Chronic progressive renal disease: Rate of change of serum creatinine concentration. *Kidney Int* 11:62, 1977.
5. Leumann EP: Progression of renal insufficiency in pediatric patients: Estimation from serum creatinine. *Helv Paediatr Acta* 33:25, 1978.
6. Arbus GS, Bacheyie GS: Method for predicting when children with progressive renal disease may reach high serum creatinine levels. *Pediatrics* 67:871, 1981.

7. Reimold EW: Use of serum creatinine to predict terminal renal failure in chronic progressive renal disease in children. *Kidney Int* 16:936, 1979.

8. Gretz N. Huber W, Gretz T, et al: Zur Anwendung mathematischer Modelle für die Verlaufsbeschreibung der chronischen Niereninsuffizienz. *Nieren- und Hochdruckkrankheitin* 9:117, 1980.

9. Jones RH, Hayakawa H, Mackay JD, et al: Progression of diabetic nephropathy. *Lancet* 1:1105, 1979.

10. Talwalkar YB, Mandel S: Monitoring the progression of chronic renal failure. *Lancet* 1:366, 1977.

11. Barsotti G, Guiducci A, Ciardella F, et al: Effects on renal function of a low-nitrogen diet supplemented with essential amino acids and ketoanalogues and of hemodialysis and free protein supply in patients with chronic renal failure. *Nephron* 27:113, 1981.

12. Mitch WE, Walser M: A proposed mechanism for reduced creatinine excretion in severe chronic renal failure. *Nephron* 21:248, 1978.

13. Doolan PD, Alpen EL, Theil GB: A clinical appraisal of the plasma concentration and endogenous clearance of creatinine. *Am J Med* 32:65, 1962.

14. Enger E, Blegen EM: The relationship between endogenous creatinine clearance and serum creatinine in renal failure. *Scand J Clin Lab Invest* 16:273, 1964.

15. Goldman R: Creatinine excretion in renal failure. *Proc Soc Exp Biol Med* 85:446, 1954.

16. Mitch WE, Collier, VU, Walser M: Creatinine metabolism in chronic renal failure. *Clin Sci* 58:327, 1980.

17. Walser M: Conservative management of the uremic patient, in Brenner BM, Rector, FC (eds): *The Kidney*, volume II. Philadelphia, WB Saunders, 1981, p 2383.

18. Collier VU, Mitch WE, Walser M: Effects of spontaneous or induced lowering of plasma CA × P product on progression of chronic renal failure (CRF). *Clin Res* 26:564A, 1978.

19. Rutherford E, King S, Perry B, et al: Use of a new phosphate binder in chronic renal insufficiency. *Kidney Int* 17:528, 1980.

20. Walser M, Mitch WE, Collier VU: Essential amino acids and their nitrogen-free analogues in the treatment of chronic renal failure, in Schreiner G (ed): *Controversies in Nephrology*. Washington, DC, Georgetown University Division of Nephrology, 1979.

21. Walser M, Mitch WE, Collier VU: The effect of nutritional therapy on the course of chronic renal failure. *Clin Nephrol* 11:66, 1979.

22. Walser M: Calcium carbonate-induced effects on serum Ca × P product and serum creatinine in renal failure: A retrospective study, in SG Massry, Ritz E, John H (eds): *Phosphate and Minerals in Health and Disease*. New York, Plenum Press, 1980, p 281.

23. Makoff D, Gordon A, Franklin SS, et al: Chronic calcium carbonate therapy in uremia. *Arch Intern Med* 123:15, 1969.

24. Berlyne GM: Calcium carbonate and uremic acidosis. *Isr J Med Sci* 7:1235, 1971.

25. Johnson WJ, Goldsmith RS, Jowsey J, et al: The influence of maintaining normal serum phosphate and calcium on renal osteodystrophy, in Norman AW (ed): *Vitamin D and Problems Related to Uremic Bone Disease*. Bern, Walter de Gruyter, 1975, p. 561.

26. Maschio G, Oldrizzi L, Tessitore N, et al: Effects of dietary protein and phosphorus restriction on the progression of early renal failure. *Kidney Int* (in press).

3

Phosphate and Prevention of Renal Failure

ALLEN C. ALFREY AND ROBERT C. TOMFORD

When a critical level of renal functional deterioration has occurred from a variety of different renal diseases, there is almost invariable progression to total loss of renal function. Ahlmen[1] found that the median time for renal impairment to progress to end-stage disease after the plasma creatinine had increased to 5 mg/dl was six months in patients with diabetic nephropathy, ten months in patients with glomerulonephritis, and 14 months in patients with nonobstructive pyelonephritis.

It has largely been assumed that this progressive functional deterioration is inevitable and that little can actually be done to prevent this phenomenon. However, there is increasing evidence that this may not necessarily be the case and that there may be ways of retarding or preventing functional loss.[2,3] In view of the frequency with which calcification is found in end-stage kidneys,[4,5] it seems possible that renal parenchymal calcification could be a late common pathogenetic mechanism that accelerates the rate of functional deterioration. To test this possibility a number of studies have been performed in our laboratory over the past three years.

METHODS AND RESULTS

Prevention of Functional Deterioration

Remnant Kidney Model. Studies were initially carried out using the remnant kidney model of chronic renal failure in rats.[2] If a critical amount of renal tissue is removed, there is subsequent deterioration of the

ALLEN C. ALFREY ● Division of Nephrology, Veterans Administration Hospital; and Department of Medicine, University of Colorado School of Medicine, Denver, Colorado. ROBERT C. TOMFORD ● Department of Medicine, Veterans Administration Medical Center, Denver, Colorado.

remaining renal parenchyma and the animal ultimately dies of uremia.[6,7] To determine if this is a consequence of renal parenchymal calcification, animals were placed on a low phosphorus diet (ICN 0.05% P) six weeks prior to establishing the remnant kidney. A second group of animals with remnant kidneys was placed on an identical diet with a proportion of sodium phosphate to sodium biphosphate (4:1 by weight) added to give it a normal phosphorus content (0.5% P).

The effect on renal function is shown in Figure 1. It can be appreciated that animals on a regular phosphorus diet had a progressive rise in plasma creatinine after six weeks. In contrast, the animals maintained on a phosphorus-restricted diet actually had a slight improvement in plasma creatinine over the 24-week study period. Survival was also markedly different in the two groups of animals. All of those on the normal phosphorus diet had died by the 168th day of study whereas only three of the phosphorus-restricted group died during the study period.

Kidney calcium content was 13 ± 1 mmol/kg in the P-restricted animals as compared with 251 ± 53 mmol/kg in the non-P-restricted animals. Similarly, kidney histology was essentially normal in the P-

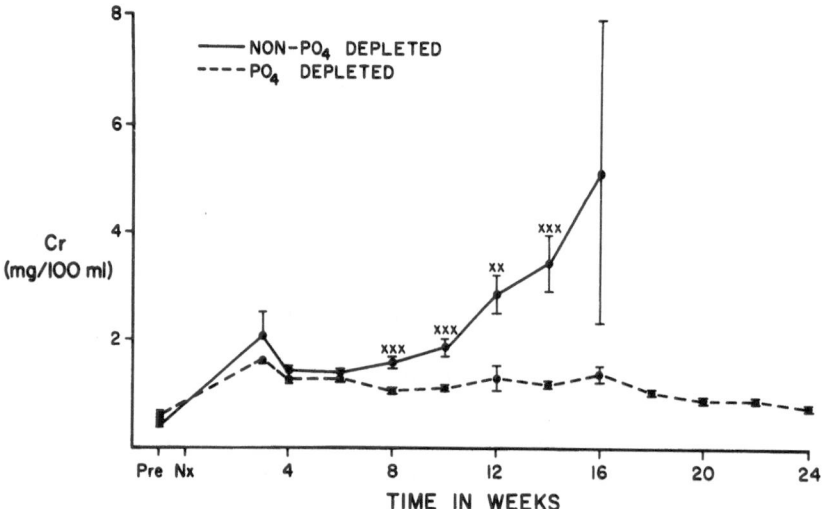

Figure 1. Effect of phosphate restriction on renal function as determined by plasma creatinine levels in the remnant kidney model. Animals placed on a phosphate-deficient diet had a rise in plasma creatinine early during the course of the disease similar to that seen in nonrestricted animals. However, after eight weeks plasma creatinine tended to fall in the restricted animals in contrast with the nonrestricted animals, who had a progressive rise in plasma creatinine levels. XXX denote $p < 0.05$. (From Alfrey AC et al.[8])

restricted animals in contrast with extensive tubulo-interstitial disease present in the kidney remnant in the nonrestricted animals.

A second study was carried out to determine the effect of P restriction at a time when disease was well established.[8] Thirty days after the remnant kidney was initiated animals were divided into two groups. One group was placed on a P-restricted diet and the second group was placed on an identical diet with P added to give it a phosphorus content of 0.5%. During the study period ten of the 15 animals in the phosphate-supplemented group died and all had progressive renal functional deterioration (Figure 2). In contrast animals placed on the P-restricted diet at 30 days had no mortality during the remaining 45 days of study and actually had improvement of renal function. Not only did function improve but phosphate restriction had major effects on proteinuria, suggesting reversal of glomerular damage. In all of the phosphorus-restricted animals, after 45 days on the low P diet, urine protein fell, at times to the normal range ($<$ 20 mg/day). In contrast, four surviving animals maintained on normal P intake had either no change or a slight increase in proteinuria when studied at the same time period (Figure 3).

Nephrotoxic Serum Nephritis. Phosphorus restriction has also been shown to have a beneficial effect on an experimental model of chronic glomerulonephritis.[3] The model employed was nephrotoxic serum

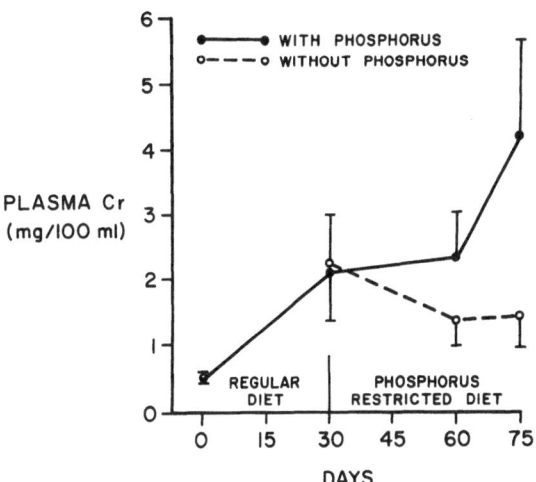

Figure 2. Effect of phosphate restriction begun 30 days after establishing the renal remnant. Plasma creatinine progressively rose in nonrestricted animals whereas it fell in the phosphate restricted group. (From Alfrey AC et al.[8])

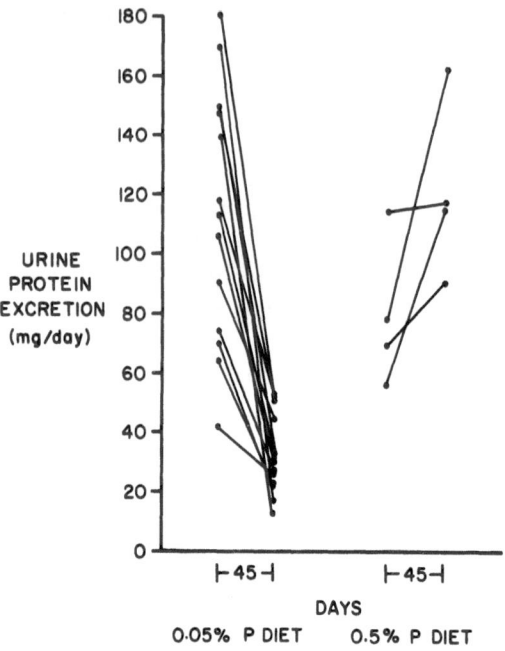

Figure 3. Effect of phosphate restriction on proteinuria. Urine protein was measured 30 days after the renal remnant was established and 45 days after the animals had been on the experimental diets. Protein excretion fell in all animals on the phosphate-restricted diet. In contrast, animals on a phosphate-supplemented diet had a slight increase in proteinuria over a similar time period. (From Alfrey AC et al.[8])

nephritis. Antirat glomerular basement membrane antibodies were produced in rabbits by immunizing them repeatedly with purified rat glomerular basement membrane in complete Freund's adjuvant. The uninephrectomized rats were preimmunized with rabbit gamma globulin five days prior to being injected with nephrotoxic serum. At 30 days postinjection the rats were randomized into two groups. Group A, 13 animals, was continued on a regular phosphorus diet. Group B, 11 animals, was changed to the identical diet without added phosphorus (0.05% P). The subsequent course was markedly different in the two groups of animals, as shown in Figure 4. Group A animals had progressive loss of renal function whereas Group B animals maintained near-normal renal function throughout the study period. The difference in plasma creatinine had reached statistical significance by the 11th week and remained so over the duration of the study. At the conclusion of the study 12 of the 13 animals in Group A had died whereas only three of the 11 animals in Group B were dead ($p < 0.001$). On histologic examination all animals in Groups A and B showed intense linear staining of the glomerular capillary loops by antirat IgG. However, light microscopy was strikingly different in the two groups. Group A animals had crescentic glomerulonephritis and severe interstitial disease with tubular dilatation and atrophy and marked inflammatory cell infiltration. In contrast, Group B animals had a mild

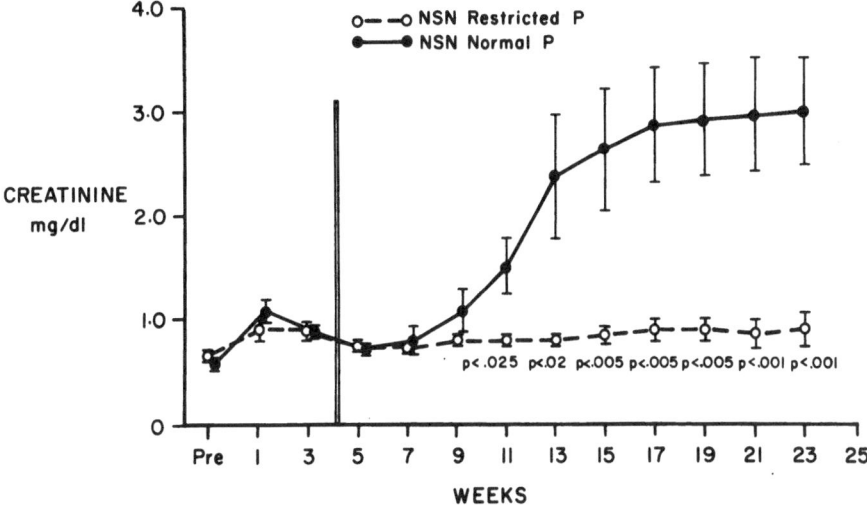

Figure 4. Effect of phosphate restriction on plasma creatinine levels in nephrotoxic serum nephritis. Progressive rise in plasma creatinine only occurred in the animals receiving phosphate-supplemented diet. (From Karlinsky MK et al.[3])

proliferative glomerulonephritis without crescents and intact tubules and interstitium.

Kidney calcium content was also significantly higher in Group A animals as compared with Group B (30 $\pm$ 6 versus 18 $\pm$ 1 mmol/kg, $p <$ 0.001).

Effect of Parathyroidectomy (PTX) and Thyroparathyroidectomy (TPTX). To determine whether the protective effect of phosphorus restriction was mediated through the suppression of parathyroid hormone secretion, ten PTX animals and 11 TPTX animals were compared with nine control animals with nephrotoxic serum nephritis. At the conclusion of the study, when five of nine control animals and six of ten PTX animals had died of uremia, all TPTX animals were alive and their plasma creatinine levels were significantly lower than either of the other groups [0.9 $\pm$ 0.3 mg/100 ml as compared with 4.8 $\pm$ 0.6 mg/100 ml in the controls and 4.3 $\pm$ 0.5 mg/100 ml in the PTX animals ($p < 0.01$)].

DISCUSSION

These studies clearly show that phosphorus restriction is protective of renal function and histologic damage in two distinct types of experimental renal disease. It has been known for years that if a critical amount of renal tissue is removed in a variety of species, the remaining renal tissue will ultimately be destroyed.[6,7] The reason for this phenomenon has not been ascertained. However, it has been established that renal function is maintained better if animals are placed on a low-protein diet.[9] It seems possible that in association with the reduction in protein that phosphorus is also restricted, which explains the protective effect of these diets. Animals in this study were maintained on a normal protein diet (24% beef fibrin) and the only variable was phosphorus. This would suggest that phosphorus is necessary for mediating structural damage, functional deterioration, and proteinuria in this experimental model of renal failure. Phosphorus restriction not only prevented damage to the renal remnant, but it also was able to reverse damage after the disease was well established.

Of even more relevance to human disease is the finding that phosphorus restriction is of equal benefit in preventing functional deterioration and histologic damage in experimental glomerulonephritis, nephrotoxic serum nephritis.[3] There are two distinct pathogenetic phases of this disease. The immediate heterologous phase is though to result from the deposition of rabbit immunoglobulins on rat glomerular basement membrane, which produces glomerular damage. The second, or autologous, phase results from the rat forming antibodies against the rabbit protein attached to the glomerular basement membrane. It would appear that phosphorus restriction primarily affects the autologous phase of this disease.

The mechanism by which phosphorus deprivation exerts its protective effect in these two types of experimental diseases remains to be elucidated. Initially it was felt that phosphorus restriction by producing hypercalcemia would suppress parathyroid hormone secretion, thus preventing renal parenchymal calcification and interstitial injury. Although recent studies have shown that thyroparathyroidectomy[10] is as effective as phosphorus restriction in preventing functional deterioration in nephrotoxic serum nephritis, selective parathyroidectomy has no beneficial effects on the course of this disease.[11] Furthermore, interstitial disease and early functional deterioration precede renal parenchymal calcification.[11] Thus it would appear that neither parathyroid hormone nor renal parenchymal calcification is important in initiating renal functional deterioration and histologic damage in this disease. However, it is possible that late in the course of renal failure these factors may play a role in accelerating functional deterioration.

Additional studies are required to determine how thyroidectomy and phosphorus depletion are similar and whether their protective effects on the prevention of renal functional deterioration are mediated through common mechanisms. Furthermore, at this time it is unknown whether phosphate depletion or merely phosphate restriction is required for this protective effect to be manifested.

In spite of these limitations, it is apparent that phosphate depletion and thyroid ablation are extremely effective in preventing progressive renal failure in nephrotoxic serum nephritis. When the mechanism(s) of this protective effect is elucidated it is hoped that we will have more insight with regard to the factors that promote functional deterioration in the diseased kidney and that we will be able to modify the course of human renal failure.

SUMMARY

We have carried out studies to determine methods of reducing the rate of renal functional deterioration in experimental renal disease. It was initially found that phosphorus restriction prevented functional deterioration and histologic damage in the remnant kidney model of chronic renal failure. It was subsequently shown that phosphorus restriction, besides preventing functional damage, could reverse structural changes and proteinuria, when it was instituted 30 days after the remnant kidney was established and progressive disease had commenced. Furthermore, it was shown that phosphorus restriction was equally protective in nephrotoxic serum nephritis.

To determine if this protective effect was mediated through suppression of parathyroid hormone secretion, studies were carried out in thyroparathyroidectomized and parathyroidectomized rats with nephrotoxic serum nephritis. Under these conditions it was found that whereas the thyroparathyroidectomized animals were protected from renal functional deterioration, parathyroidectomy had no beneficial effect.

It is concluded that thyroid ablation and phosphate depletion prevent progressive renal failure in experimental renal disease. This protective effect appears not to be mediated through either PTH suppression or the prevention of renal parenchymal calcification.

REFERENCES

1. Ahlmén J: Incidence of chronic renal insufficiency. *Acta Med Scand* (suppl)582:1, 1975.
2. Ibels LS, Alfrey AC, Haut L, et al: Preservation of function in experimental renal disease by dietary restriction of phosphate. *N Engl J Med* 298:122–126, 1978.
3. Karlinsky ML, Haut L, Buddington B, et al: Preservation of renal function in experimental glomerulonephritis. *Kidney Int* 17:293–302, 1980.

4. Ibels LS, Alfrey AC, Huffer WE, et al: Calcification in end-stage kidneys. *Am J Med* 71:33–37, 1981.

5. Kuzela DC, Huffer WE, Conger JD, et al: Soft tissue calcification in chronic dialysis patients. *Am J Pathol* 86:403–424, 1977.

6. Morrison AB: Experimentally induced chronic renal insufficiency in the rat. *Lab Invest* 11:321 –331, 1962.

7. Chanutin A, Ferris EB, Jr: Experimental renal insufficiency produced by partial nephrectomy. *Arch Intern Med* 49:767–787, 1932.

8. Alfrey Ac, Karlinsky M, Haut L: Protective effect of phosphate restriction on renal function, in Massry SG, Ritz E, Jahn H (eds): *Phosphate and Minerals in Health and Disease,* New York, Plenum Press, 1980, p 209.

9. Lalich JJ, Burkholder PM, Paik WCW: Protein overload nephropathy in rats with unilateral nephrectomy. *Arch Pathol* 99:72, 1975.

10. Tomford RC, Karlinsky ML, Buddington B, et al: The effect of parathyroidectomy on nephrotoxic serum nephritis. *Am Soc Nephrol* 12:19A, 1979.

11. Tomford RC, Karlinsky ML, Buddington B, et al: The effect of thyroparathyroidectomy and parathyroidectomy on renal function and the nephrotic syndrome in rat nephrotoxic serum nephritis. *J Clin Invest* 68:655–664, 1981.

4

Improvement of Acidosis in Long-Term Dietary Treatment of Chronic Renal Failure

CARMELO GIORDANO

In chronic renal failure there is reduced capability to excrete titrable acid, particularly in the form of ammonia. Consequently, a slow but progressive depletion of cations initiates from the body with consumption of buffer reserves and generation of acidosis.

With a fixed amount of residual nephron population the degree of acidosis will be related to the balance of proton generation that ultimately will be a direct consequence of the degree of protein intake.

Last year, at the first Symposium on the Pathobiology of Uremic Patients treated for ten years or more, we presented data suggesting that dietary managment of chronic renal failure could have lasted as long as ten years.[1] This exceptional human material, unique in its gender, has been reconsidered in the light of finding data on acid-base balance.

The purpose of this chapter is to present data related to acidosis collected from a group of patients given a protein-restricted diet for a very long time.

METHODS

A group of 18 patients suffering from chronic renal failure with a mean serum creatinine of 2.9 mg/dl $\pm$ 0.51 had been studied before commencing the dietary treatment. After four to six years, 16 of these patients who had been on continous dietary treatment could be studied again. At that time the serum creatinine was 4.5 mg/dl $\pm$ 0.70. After ten

CARMELO GIORDANO • Department of Medical Nephrology, Naples University, First School of Medicine, Naples, Italy.

years, four patients were still on dietary treatment and their mean serum creatinine was 8.9 mg/dl ± 1.6.

Dietary treatment was a low protein diet relatively rich in energy supply as detailed elsewhere.[1] Determination of plasma amino acid concentration was performed on a Beckman amino acid analyzer Mod. 120 A and 120C following the procedure of Stein and Moore.[2] The total amount of nitrogen in the urine was assayed by the Kjeldahl procedure and urinary ammonia with the usual recommendations.[3] Blood pH was measured in the morning in a blood sample taken in fasting and resting conditions after warming of the forearm with a warmed wool pad. Bicarbonate concentration was calculated in the usual manner.

RESULTS

Table I reports the concentration of the amino acids that are of major interest to ammonia production. It is evident that in the years after initiating the protein-restricted diet, while the glutamine concentration increases, glutamic acid decreases and aspartic acid increases.

Table II is related to the urinary content of nitrogen and ammonia in the patients before and during the long standing dietary treatment. It is shown that although the urinary pH remains unchanged there is a marked diminution of urinary ammonia as well as total urinary nitrogen.

Table III indicates that blood pH that was clearly acidotic at the beginning of dietary treatment ameliorates and strengthens within the normal range over the years. Similarly, plasma bicarbonate improves with diet, getting close to normal values with time.

Table I. Plasma Amino Acids[a]

	At start	After 5 years	After 10 years	Normal values
Glutamine	2.48 ± 0.40	5.73 ± 0.65[b]	6.48 ± 0.60	7.80 ± 0.50
Glutamic acid	2.90 ± 0.35	1.33 ± 0.11[b]	1.22 ± 0.23	0.80 ± 0.15
Aspartic acid	0.21 ± 0.10	0.29 ± 0.12	0.48 ± 0.12[b]	0.60 ± 0.10
Alanine	2.03 ± 0.31	1.80 ± 0.18[b]	2.70 ± 0.20	3.40 ± 0.75
Glycine	2.30 ± 0.70	2.0 ± 0.27	2.15 ± 0.21	1.90 ± 0.48
Patient's serum creatinine	2.9 ± 0.5	4.5 ± 0.7	8.9 ± 1.6	1.0 ± 0.2
n	18	18	4	10

[a] Measured in milligrams per deciliter.

[b] Significantly different from normal values ($p \leq 0.05$).

Table II. Urinary Total Nitrogen (UTN), Urinary Ammonia (UA)
and Urinary pH (UpH)

	At start	After 5 years	After 10 years
UTN mg	4730 ± 2.1	3200 ± 0.65	2600 ± 0.48
UA mEq	21 ± 5.8	7 ± 1.42	5.2 ± 0.51
UpH	5.5 ± 0.4	5.3 ± 0.25	5.5 ± 0.12
n (out of 18)	6	8	4

DISCUSSION

It is a well-established fact that 43% of urinary ammonia derives from the amidic group of glutamine and some 18% from the aminic group of the same amino acid,[4] whereas glutamic acid, alanine, and glycine account for an additional 10% or so.[3]

The increase in glutamine concentration during a protein-restricted diet is to be considered a positive dietary effect since this amino acid is the major contributor to urinary ammonia. However, the fact that there is a reduced amount of ammonia in the urine of our subjects during the dietary period may signify that there was no need for excreting any larger amount, which is linked with the fact that at the same time blood pH rises to normal and plasma bicarbonate gets close to normal.

The mitigation of acidosis is an interesting feature of dietary therapy that was long obscured, because a low-protein diet at first was recommended with methionine supplementation,[5] and thus, if anything, low protein was associated with acidosis.

The present study demonstrates that, on the contrary, a low protein diet is accompanied by a net improvement of acid-base balance in patients with chronic renal failure at an earlier or at an advanced stage.

The remarkable effect of the diet reduces the depletion of cations and restores the potassium pool[6] and adds a valuable therapeutic force to dietary management with low protein intake of long duration.

Table III. Blood pH and Plasma Bicarbonate Concentration

	At start	After 4–6 years	After 10 years
Blood pH	7.21 ± 0.06	7.40 ± 0.05	7.38 ± 0.07
Plasma bicarbonate mEq	15 ± 1.4	20 ± 1.1	21 ± 1.0
n	18	18	4

REFERENCES

1. Giordano C: Prolongation of survival for a decade or more by low protein diet, in Giordano C, Friedman EA (eds): *Uremia—Pathobiology of Patients Treated for 10 Years or More*. Milan, Wichtig, 1981, pp 4–7.
2. Stein WH, Moore S: The free amino acid of human blood plasma. *J Biol Chem* 211:915–926, 1954.
3. Stone WJ, Balagura S, Pitts RF: Diffusion equilibrium for ammonia in the kidney of the acidotic dog. *J Clin Invest* 46:1603–1613, 1967.
4. Pitts RF, Pilkington LA, De Haas JCM: N^{15} tracer studies on the origin of urinary ammonia in the acidotic dog, with notes on the enzymatic synthesis of labeled glutamic acid and glutamines. *J Clin Invest* 44:731–743, 1965.
5. Berlyne GM, Hocken AG: The dietary treatment of chronic renal failure, in Berlyne GM (ed): *Nutrition and Renal Diseases*. Edinburgh/London, Livingston, 1968, pp 38–54.
6. Giordano C, Esposito R, De Pascale C, et al: Dietary treatment in renal failure. *Proceedings Third International Congress in Nephrology, Washington, 1966*. Basel/New York, Karger, 1967, vol. 3, pp 214–229.

Section II

Glomerular Damage and Its Prevention

Most patients we treat for chronic uremia have "idiopathic" or glomerulonephrotic disease. By understanding causal mechanisms of these morbid states we can now prevent, retard, and treat more logically.

In the previous section the promise of dietary alteration as a tool in retarding renal deterioration was explored. This section provides further evidence that progressive renal damage need not be inevitable. Appreciation of the injurious effects of glomerular hyperfiltration, and hypertension, suggests that future clinical regimens will be structured to minimize these threats to renal integrity and function. Should further data confirm that hyperfiltration is important to human renal disease, then an old mystery will be partly solved. It has been unclear why, consequent to any renal damage, as in obstruction that is relieved or cortical necrosis, further nephron loss occurs. These conditions, as is true for all damaged kidneys, are associated with a decreased nephron mass, and thus relative glomerular hyperfiltration. The deleterious effects of hyperfiltration have thus far been experimentally shown only in the rat but they now become eminently applicable to humans in diverse clinical states. Hypertension, by contrast, is now known to accelerate nephron loss in both rats and diabetic humans.

Brenner's group contributes two important basic studies of the pathogenesis of glomerular damage. In the first, Hostetter links glomerular hyperfiltration to initiation and progression of glomerulosclerosis. Hostetter reviews his own and others' work, showing that augmentation of single-nephron glomerular filtration rate occurs in residual glomeruli following loss of renal mass in the rat. He further shows that glomerular hyperfiltration mediated by raised glomerular plasma flow and transcapillary hydraulic pressure leads to progressive glomerular sclerosis, which does not occur when hyperfiltration is prevented. This rat model is then extrapolated to several well-known human disorders such as temporary recovery and then deterioration of renal function in renal cortical necrosis. This suggests that glomerular hyperfiltration may contribute to progressive human nephropathy of diverse etiology.

Baldwin pursues the clinical inference that hypertension is injurious to renal function by studying the effect of superimposed hypertension on nephrotoxic serum nephritis in the rat. There was a clearly apparent enhanced glomerular damage attributable to raised blood pressure perhaps due to transmitted increased arterial pressure. Baldwin's data corroborate the prevailing view that hypertension is unhealthy for kidneys, be they in humans or rats.

This further enlightens us on the mechanisms of renal injury and extends the indictment of hypertension. These new observations allow for a more rational approach to diagnosis and therapy.

M.M.A.

5

Hyperfiltration as a Major Causative Factor in Initiation and Progression of Glomerulosclerosis

THOMAS H. HOSTETTER, HELMUT G. RENNKE,
AND BARRY M. BRENNER

The augmentation of single-nephron glomerular filtration rate (SNGFR) that follows loss of functioning renal mass is generally regarded as a beneficial adaptation in the sense that total filtration by the remnant kidney falls less than would be the case had this augmentation not occurred. However, several lines of evidence have been developed that, when taken together, suggest that single-nephron hyperfiltration may have maladaptive and eventually injurious consequences. For nearly 50 years it has been recognized that removal of approximately three fourths or more of the renal mass in the rat, either by surgical resection, infarction, or a combination of these maneuvers, results in a syndrome of progressive azotemia, proteinuria, and eventual glomerular sclerosis.[1-3]

GLOMERULAR HEMODYNAMICS

The hemodynamic basis for the augmentation in remnant SNGFR following loss of renal mass has recently been delineated using micropuncture methodology. Deen, Maddox, Robertson et al[4] performed studies on adult rats of the Munich-Wistar strain which possess surface glomeruli accessible to direct measurement of glomerular capillary hydraulic pressures. These animals

THOMAS H. HOSTETTER ● Laboratory of Kidney and Electrolyte Physiology, Brigham and Women's Hospital, Boston, Massachusetts.   HELMUT G. RENNKE ● Department of Pathology, Brigham and Women's Hospital, Boston, Massachusetts.   BARRY M. BRENNER ● Department of Medicine, Harvard Medical School; and Renal Division, Brigham and Women's Hospital, Boston, Massachusetts.

were studied two to four weeks following contralateral nephrectomy. At the time of study, remnant kidney weight and total GFR had increased by about 40% over the values in sham operated control rats. SNGFR was also strikingly increased, to a mean value of 45.6 ± 3.1 nl/min (SEM) in the nephrectomized rats compared with 24.9 ± 1.1 nl/min in controls. In order to dissect the mechanism of this increase it is useful to recall that the rate of glomerular ultrafiltration may be expressed as

$$\mathrm{SNGFR} = K_f \cdot \bar{P}_{UF} = k \cdot S \cdot \bar{P}_{UF}$$

where $\bar{P}_{UF}$ is the mean net ultrafiltration pressure (P_{UF} averaged along the length of the capillary) and represents the difference between mean hydraulic and oncotic pressure differences. K_f, the ultrafiltration coefficient, is the product of the effective hydraulic conductivity (k) and total surface area (S) of the glomerular capillaries. It may be seen from this equation that the increase in SNGFR following uninephrectomy could have resulted from an increase in K_f, $\bar{P}_{UF}$, or both. The first of these possibilities, an increase in K_f, was examined by creating an experimental situation in which K_f could be determined in uninephrectomized rats. The necessary condition of filtration pressure disequilibrium was achieved by 2% plasma loading, which permitted calculation of unique values of K_f. K_f averaged 0.078 nl/(sec·mm Hg), a value remarkably similar to that reported by these authors previously for nonnephrectomized rats. To the extent that the average value of K_f determined in this study is identical, however, to that for nonnephrectomized rats, these data suggest that the adaptive increase in SNGFR following uninephrectomy is the result primarily of an increase in $\bar{P}_{UF}$. For constant K_f, changes in $\bar{P}_{UF}$ and SNGFR are determined solely by changes in the mean transcapillary hydraulic pressure difference $\overline{\Delta P}$, systemic protein concentration C_A, and the initial glomerular plasma flow rate Q_A. Changes in Q_A serve to modify the average transcapillary oncotic pressure difference: increases in Q_A tend to reduce this pressure difference and thereby increase SNGFR while the opposite is true for selective decreases in Q_A. In this study uninephrectomy was associated with no difference in C_A relative to nonnephrectomized controls. In contrast, $\overline{\Delta P}$ and Q_A were significantly larger in nephrectomized rats, averaging 40 vs. 34 mm Hg and 136 vs. 76 nl/min respectively. The observed increase in SNGFR was therefore the combined result of these adaptive increments in $\overline{\Delta P}$ and Q_A.

With more extreme degrees of renal ablation, SNGFR tends to increase even further.[5] A direct assessment of the hemodynamic events that cause these more extreme degrees of single-nephron hyperfiltration has recently been completed.[6] One week following right nephrectomy and infarction of approximately five sixths of the left kidney in Munich-Wistar rats, SNGFR and its hemodynamic determinants were assessed in the remnant nephrons and in those of sham operated controls. Values for SNGFR in animals undergoing this extensive degree of renal ablation averaged 62.5 ± 6.4 nl/min, more than twice the mean value of 27.8 ± 3.2 nl/min of control rats. This marked increment in SNGFR one week after extreme ablation was ascribable mainly to two factors. First, Q_A was elevated, on average, to 187 ± 20 nl/min compared with 74 ± 11 nl/min in controls. Second, the mean glomerular transcapillary hydraulic pressure difference, $\overline{\Delta P}$, averaged 44 ± 2 mm Hg, as compared with the control value of 37 ± 1 mm Hg. This greater average value for $\overline{\Delta P}$ resulted despite an increase in proximal tubule hydraulic pressure P_T, since mean glomerular capillary hydraulic pressure $\bar{P}_{GC}$ increased markedly in the remnant glomeruli. Systemic plasma protein concentration C_A was not different between these two groups. Thus, as in the study of Deen et al.,[4] higher average values for $\overline{\Delta P}$ and Q_A were again responsible for the augmented driving force for filtration. The marked increase in Q_A in this study by Hostetter et al.[6] is consistent with the findings of Kaufman, Siegel, and Hayslett,[7] who demonstrated that with graded degrees of ablation mean glomerular blood flow also varies directly with the extent of ablation.

The glomerular ultrafiltration coefficient K_f was calculable as a unique value in these rats with marked reductions in renal mass since they also demonstrated filtration pressure disequilibrium.[6] The mean value of this parameter was 0.063 ± 0.018 nl/(sec·mm Hg), a value not distinguishable from the sham operated controls and similar to those previously reported in normal rats.[8,9] Thus the changes in glomerular hemodynamics following severe reductions in renal mass represent a more extreme expression of the pattern present with lesser degrees of ablation,[4] namely, increased transcapillary hydraulic pressure difference and increased glomerular plasma flow rate without measurable change in K_f.

STRUCTURAL CHANGES IN REMNANT GLOMERULI

Shimamura and Morrison[10] carefully documented the progression of glomerular damage in adult rats subjected to surgical resection of approximately five sixths of their total renal mass. They described an increase in glomerular size within the first three months of nephrectomy. This hypertrophy was accompanied by ultrastructural alterations, including vacuolization of glomerular epithelial cells, deposition of osmophilic droplets within these cells, and "fusion" of their foot processes. By about six months, expansion of mesangial matrix became evident, as did denudation of cells from areas of basement membrane. These ultrastructural alterations heralded progressive hyalinization, and ultimately sclerosis of these remnant glomeruli. Studies employing unilateral nephrectomy and partial infarction of the remaining kidney demonstrated similar light and transmission electron microscopic findings.[3] In addition, immunofluorescence microscopy revealed glomerular deposition of circulating proteins, the most abundant of which was albumin, with lesser amounts of fibrin, immunoglobulin, and complement as well. As in the study by Shimamura and Morrison,[10] all of these changes tended to progress with time. After somewhat more severe reductions in renal mass, Olson et al.[12] observed similar structural disruption but at an apparently accelerated pace since clear abnormalities were present in remnant glomeruli in only one week after the ablative procedure. Glomerular endothelial and epithelial cells were seen to be lifted away from the adjacent basement membrane in a focal manner. Protein reabsorption droplets were visible in the epithelial cells and both mesangial cells and matrix were increased. After two weeks, this pattern of damage became more severe and more widespread among remnant glomeruli. Glomerular damage not only progressed with time but appeared to be directly related to the degree of ablation induced. For example, with unilateral nephrectomy alone a modest degree of glomerular sclerosis occurred.[11] Olson et al.[12] examined this relationship and demonstrated that with greater degrees of ablation a greater proportion of the remnant glomeruli showed progressive sclerosis.

PERMEABILITY CHANGES IN REMNANT GLOMERULI

Not only is there obvious morphologic evidence of glomerular damage but the proteinuria that develops in this model stands as further indication of glomerular injury. The earliest descriptions of the natural history of this model noted the tremendous degree of proteinuria that occurred, with most of the rats subjected to subtotal nephrectomies excreting several hundred milligrams of protein per day as compared with less than 10 mg/day in control animals. This proteinuric response was confirmed by Olson and co-workers,[12] who documented a fourfold increase in protein excretion in rats only one week after unilateral nephrectomy and infarction of approximately five sixths of the remaining kidney. This level of absolute protein excretion is particularly remarkable in view of the fact that total filtration rate of the remnant kidney was less than one sixth of that of control rats. Thus, factored for GFR, excretion of protein was more than 20 times greater in experimental than in control animals. Increased protein excretion has been demonstrated after lesser degrees of ablation of renal mass. For example, unilateral nephrectomy alone leads eventually to some increase in protein excretion, although as with the structural changes, the degree of proteinuria and its rapidity of onset seem to be much less pronounced than with greater degrees of renal ablation.[13]

In an effort to characterize and further quantify this defect in glomerular permselectivity resulting in otherwise normal glomeruli contained in the remnant, the glomerular processing of tracer macromolecules has been studied after severe reduction in renal mass.[12] Glomerular filtration of neutral macromolecules, as assessed by the fractional clearances of neutral dextrans, was not altered for dextrans with molecular radii in the range between 20 and 38 Å. However, for neutral dextrans larger than 38 Å, animals with subtotal nephrectomies displayed significantly increased fractional clearances, indicating some loss of the size-selective properties of the glomerular filtration barrier. When the charge-selective properties of this barrier were probed using both negatively charged dextrans and variously charged molecules of horseradish peroxidase, a clear defect in the ability to exclude negatively charged macromolecules was also apparent. Thus, remnant glomeruli had lost size- and charge-selectivity and these functional defects undoubtedly played a major role in the pathogenesis of the observed proteinuria.

MECHANISM OF THE PROGRESSIVE INJURY
TO REMNANT GLOMERULI

The mechanism underlying the structural and functional derangements following reductions in renal mass has been the focus of several investigations. No evidence for an immunologic process has been uncovered and electron-dense material indicative of immune complexes has been conspicuously absent.[3,8] The evidence for a circulating anti-glomerular basement membrane antibody is conflicting.[3,14] However, the paucity of findings characteristically associated with this form of immune injury, such as linear immunoglobulin deposition along the basement membrane and cellular proliferation, argues against such a mechanism.[3,6,12,15,16]

Since arterial hypertension is a regular accompaniment of severe reduction of renal mass, the possibility that this hypertension is somehow responsible for the progressive glomerulopathy observed in the remnant kidney of the rat has recently been investigated. Systemic arterial pressure was restored to normal levels with antihypertensive drugs in rats previously subjected to large reductions in renal mass.[3] Although this maneuver reduced the extent of injury to remnant glomeruli, the lesions nevertheless persisted and were of the same character as in similarly nephrectomized rats not treated with antihypertensive drugs. Furthermore, the severity and course of the glomerulopathy appear to be more extreme in remnant glomeruli than in those of spontaneously hypertensive rats or rats with other types of hypertension, despite similar or even greater degrees of arterial hypertension.[17] Thus arterial hypertension probably plays a role but does not account fully for the progressive glomerular damage seen in the remnant kidney.

In view of the marked alterations in pressures and flows within the glomerular microcirculation, which, as noted above, underlie the increased SNGFR in remnant glomeruli, it has been suggested that these increased glomerular forces and/or the single-nephron hyperfiltration itself are injurious to the glomerular capillary tuft.[6,10] To test this possibility, an effort was made to blunt the doubling of SNGFR observed in remnant glomeruli of rats one week after unilateral nephrectomy and infarction of about five sixths of the remaining kidney.[6] By severe restriction of dietary protein intake, the increase in SNGFR usually measured after this degree of renal ablation was obliterated. This blunting of the functional hypertrophy was the result of a failure of Q_A or $\overline{\Delta P}$ to increase despite the extensive loss of renal mass. Associated with this near-normalization of SNGFR and its hemodynamic determinants, there was a striking reduction in the structural abnormalities observed in hyperfiltering glomeruli.[6] Additionally, protein excretion was returned to the same daily rate as seen in normal rats. This improvement in the degree of proteinuria resulted from an amelioration of the defect in charge-selectivity described above. Thus this available evidence is consistent with the possibility that single-nephron hyperfiltration (or some hemodynamic determinant thereof) is responsible for the progressive injury observed in remnant glomeruli.

If hemodynamic alterations underlie this glomerulopathy, the question also arises as to how such alterations lead to glomerular destruction. Although no firm conclusions are available, several possibilities suggest themselves. The increased movement of ultrafiltrate across the capillary walls in hyperfiltering glomeruli would be expected to entail an increased transcapillary convective flux of macromolecules as well.[18] The demonstrated changes in the intrinsic permselective properties of the glomerular wall would also result in increased movement of macromolecules through the wall. This increased transglomerular traffic of plasma proteins may ultimately have an injurious effect on some component or components of the glomerulus.[19-21] Indeed, studies of ferritin localization in remnant glomeruli demonstrate a greatly increased deposition of this macro-molecule in the mesangial region as compared with control animals[12] and it is possible that an overloading of this region may be a general mechanism for enhancing matrix deposition, the forerunner of glomerular sclerosis.[20,22,23]

ROLE OF SINGLE-NEPHRON HYPERFILTRATION
IN HUMAN CHRONIC DIFFUSE RENAL INJURY

Clinically, chronic renal insufficiency regularly progresses to end-stage renal failure and several studies indicate that for any given patient the rate of progression is predictable.[24,25] Interestingly, both of these studies indicate that the rate of decline in renal function is idiosyncratic, varying from patient to patient and apparently not related to the underlying cause of the chronic renal insufficiency.

In some instances the factors that initiate the process of renal destruction may persist throughout the entire progression to renal failure and hence be responsible, at least by inference, for the progressive destruction. Often, however, such an initiating factor is not identifiable at the time the disease is detected clinically. Moreover, on occasion an identifiable initiating factor has clearly disappeared, due either to its having been a single, evanescent insult or to effective, specific therapy. Nevertheless, the patient progresses to renal failure. For example, the discrete injury of bilateral cortical necrosis may often demonstrate a temporary period of recovery only to be followed by eventual uremia.[26] Also, a recent report of the nephropathy associated with vesicoureteral reflux has documented the appearance of a progressive glomerulopathic process in the absence of identifiable injurious factors such as hypertension or active urinary infection and even despite surgical correction of the reflux.[27] Thus it seems quite plausible that after some critical reduction in nephron mass that follows an initiating insult, progressive destruction of remnant glomeruli then occurs by a self-perpetuating process that involves one or more final common pathways. Hyperfiltration of residual nephrons might represent such a common pathogenetic mechanism leading to renal failure after any of a variety of initial insults has reduced nephron mass below some critical level.

Several lines of evidence support the possibility that this process may be operative generally and not solely as a response to extreme surgical ablation. As noted above, hyperfiltering nephrons constitute at least a subset of the surviving nephron units in most of the severe diffuse interstitial and glomerular disease models studied to date.[15,28,29] Furthermore, when surgical ablation is superimposed on chronically diseased kidneys, GFR and SNGFR are increased even within the previously diseased kidney, reflecting the capacity of residual nephrons to respond to progressive reduction in renal function.[30,31] Thus single-nephron hyperfiltration seems a likely component of progressive renal disease. In keeping with the suggestion that such hyperfiltration may have deleterious consequences is the observation that when unilateral nephrectomy is performed in diabetic rats their usual pattern of diabetic glomerulopathy progresses at an accelerated pace.[13] This response in diabetic animals presumably to altered renal hemodynamics is reminiscent of the clinical observation that unilateral renal artery stenosis can protect to some degree the stenotic kidney from the diabetic glomerulopathy suffered by its contralateral partner.[32] As with diabetic injury, the glomerulosclerosis induced by renal irradiation is worsened by unilateral nephrectomy, as is the focal sclerosis that follows repeated doses of puromycin aminonucleoside.[22] Yet more striking is the increase in mortality, azotemia, and renal histopathology displayed after uninephrectomy in the animal model of systemic lupus erythematosus, the hybrid of New Zealand black and white mice.[33] Thus, in some way, unilateral nephrectomy, and in all likelihood the hypertrophic responses that follow, appear to be injurious in the presence of diffuse renal injury.

CONCLUSIONS

Augmentation of single-nephron glomerular filtration rate occurs promptly in residual glomeruli after loss of renal mass. Single-nephron hyperfiltration is mediated primarily by increased glomerular plasma flows and transcapillary hydraulic pressure gradients.

Diffuse renal injury induced by nephrotoxic, infectious, and immunologic factors, when severe, generally leads to heterogeneity of SNGFR in remnant nephrons. Changes in the structure of injured glomeruli and, by inference, their filtration properties likely contribute to the alterations in SNGFR. However, changes in glomerular pressure and flows and hence SNGFR may be caused, at least in part, by immune mediators as well as classic vasoactive hormone systems.

The increase in SNGFR after loss of functioning kidney mass may have maladaptive consequences for glomerular architecture and permselective properties. The resultant injury may represent a final common pathway for eventual sclerotic obliteration of residual glomeruli.

REFERENCES

1. Chanutin A, Ferris E: Experimental renal insufficiency produced by partial nephrectomy: 1. Control diet. *Arch Int Med* 49:767, 1932.
2. Morrison AB: Experimental chronic renal insufficiency. *Meth Arch Exp Path* 1:455, 1966.
3. Purkerson ML, Hoffsten PE, Klahr S: Pathogenesis of the glomerulopathy associated with renal infarction in rats. *Kidney Int* 9:407, 1976.
4. Deen WM, Maddox DA, Robertson CR, et al: Dynamics of glomerular ultrafiltration in the rat. VII: Reponse to reduced renal mass. *Am J Physiol* 227:556, 1974.
5. Kaufman JM, DiMeola HJ, Siegel NJ, et al: Compensatory adaptation of structure and function following progessive renal ablation. *Kidney Int* 6:10, 1974.
6. Hostetter TH, Olson JL, Rennke HG, et al: Hyperfiltration in remnant nephrons: A potentially adverse response to renal ablation. *Am J Physiol: Renal Fluid Electro* 241:F85, 1981.
7. Kaufman JM, Siegel NJ, Hayslett JP: Functional and hemodynamic adaptation to progressive renal ablation. *Circ Res* 36:286, 1975.
8. Myers BD, Deen WM, Robertson CR, et al: Dynamics of glomerular ultrafiltration. VIII. Effects of hematocrit. *Circ Res* 36:425, 1975.
9. Tucker BJ, Blantz RC: An analysis of the determinants of nephron filtration rate. *Am J Physiol* 232:F477, 1977A.
10. Shimamura T, Morrison AB: A progressive glomerulosclerosis occurring in partial five-sixths nephrectomy. *Am J Path* 79:95, 1975.
11. Elema JD, Arends A: Focal and segmental glomerular hyalinosis in the rat. *Lab Invest* 33:554, 1975.
12. Olson JL, Hostetter TH, Rennke HG, et al: Altered charge and size selective properties of the glomerular wall: A response to reduced renal mass. *Kidney Int* (in press).
13. Steffes MW, Brown DM, Mauer SM: Diabetic glomerulopathy following unilateral nephrectomy in the rat. *Diabetes* 27:35, 1978.
14. White IN, Grollman A: Autoimmune factors associated with infarction of the kidney. *Nephron* 1:93, 1964.
15. Allison MEM, Wilson CB, Gottschalk CW: Pathophysiology of experimental glomerulonephritis in rats. *J Clin Invest* 53:1402, 1974.
16. Maddox DA, Bennett CM, Deen WM, et al: Determinants of glomerular filtration in experimental glomerulonephritis in the rat. *J Clin Invest* 55:305, 1975.
17. Feld CG, van Liew JB, Galaske RG, et al: Selectivity of renal injury and proteinuria in the spontaneously hypertensive rat. *Kidney Int* 12:332, 1977.
18. Deen WM, Bohrer MP, Brenner BM: Macromolecule transport across glomerular capillaries: Application of the pore theory. *Kidney Int* 16:353, 1979.
19. Couser NG, Stilmant MM: Mesangial lesions and focal sclerosis in the aging rat. *Lab Invest* 33:491, 1975.
20. Velosa JA, Glasser RJ, Nevins TE, et al: Experimental model of focal sclerosis. II. Correlation with immunopathologic changes, macromolecular kihetics, and polyanion loss. *Lab Invest* 36:527, 1977.
21. Davies DJ, Prener DB, Hardwicke J: Urinary proteins and glomerular morphometry in protein overload proteinuria. *Lab Invest* 38:232, 1978.
22. Glasser RJ, Velosa JA, Michael AF: Experimental model of focal sclerosis. I. Relationship to protein excretion in aminonucleoside nephrosis. *Lab Invest* 36:519, 1977.

23. Romen W, Morath R: Diffuse glomerulosclerosis—A dysfunction of mesangium? *Virchows Arch Biol Cell Path* 34:205, 1979.
24. Mitch WE, Walser M, Buffington CA, et al: A simple method for estimating progression of chronic renal failure. *Lancet* 4:1326, 1976.
25. Rutherford WE, Blondin J, Miller JP, et al: Chronic progressive renal disease: Rate of change of serum creatinine. *Kidney Int* 11:62, 1977.
26. Kleinknecht D, Grunfeld JP, Comez PC, et al: Diagnostic procedures and long-term prognosis in bilateral renal cortical necrosis. *Kidney Int* 4:390, 1973.
27. Torres VE, Velosa JA, Holley KE, et al: The progression of vesicoureteral reflux. *Ann Int Med* 92:776, 1980.
28. Bank H, Aynedjian HS: Individual function in experimental phelonephritis. I. Glomerular filtration rate and proximal tubular sodium, potassium and water reabsorption. *J Lab Clin Med* 68:713, 1966.
29. Kramp RA, MacDowell M, Gottschalk CW, et al: A study by microdissection and micropuncture of the structure and the function of the kidneys and the nephrons of rats with chronic renal damage. *Kidney Int* 5:147, 1974.
30. Bricker NS, Klahr S, Rieselbach RE: The functional adaptation of the diseased kidney I. Glomerular filtration rate. *J Clin Invest* 43:1915, 1964.
31. Lubowitz H, Purkerson ML, Sugita M, et al: GFR per nephron and per kidney in chronically diseased (pyelo nephritic) kidney of the rat. *Am J Physiol* 217:853, 1969.
32. Berman J, Rifkin H: Unilateral nodular diabetic glomerulosclerosis (Kimmelsteil-Wilson): Report of a case. *Metabolism* 22:715, 1973.
33. Beyer MM, Steinberg AD, Nilastri AD, et al: Unilateral nephrectomy: Effect on survival in NZB/NZN mice. *Science* 198:511, 1977.

6

Aggravation of Glomerulonephritis by Hypertension

DAVID S. BALDWIN

An immunopathogenetic mechanism, immune complex or antiglomerular basement membrane antibody, is held responsible for most forms of primary glomerular disease in man. Although immunologic mechanisms and the mediators of glomerular damage that they induce may well form the basis initially for most glomerular diseases, certain clinical observations and experimental data suggest that the progression of these diseases is influenced by the operation of nonimmunologic factors as well. The present discussion deals with the role of intrarenal vascular disease and hypertension as mechanisms of glomerular damage.

INTRARENAL VASCULAR DISEASE AND THE PROGRESSION OF GLOMERULONEPHRITIS

Sclerosis of arterioles and prearterioles is a common finding in advanced glomerular disease, long recognized at postmortem in the end-stage kidney and conventionally interpreted as an effect of hypertension. Thus ischemic glomerular sclerosis resulting from intrarenal vascular disease is assumed to play a role in the progression of renal failure during the hypertensive stage of glomerular diseases, and the importance of control of blood pressure has been stressed.[1-5] Malignant hypertension may occur in the course of glomerulonephritis and the associated necrotizing arteriolitis of the renal vessels may justifiably be attributed to the marked elevation of diastolic blood pressure. However, the frequent occurrence of intrarenal vascular sclerosis early in the course of glomerulonephritis prior to the advent of hyperten-

DAVID S. BALDWIN • Department of Medicine, New York University School of Medicine, New York, New York.

55

sion and its relative severity even with modest elevation of blood pressure suggest a particular susceptibility of the renal arterioles to the effects of hypertension in glomerulonephritis, or perhaps that vascular disease may be a primary feature of the disease rather than secondary to hypertension.

Our biopsy studies in the intermediate stages of poststreptococcal glomerulonephritis[6] and in Berger's IgA nephropathy,[7] when renal function is normal or minimally impaired and hypertension mild or absent, have demonstrated a high incidence of arteriolar and prearteriolar sclerosis. Similar observations have been made by ourselves and by Kincaid-Smith[8] in a variety of other glomerular diseases where vascular sclerosis exceeded that which would be anticipated for the age of the patient and for the duration and severity of hypertension. As reported by Kincaid-Smith, the incidence of renal arterial and arteriolar lesions ranged from 54% to 82% in normotensive patients under the age of 40 years with various forms of glomerulonephritis (Table I).

In our studies vascular changes showed a close correlation with glomerular sclerosis, suggesting a cause and effect relationship in which ischemia was responsible for glomerular damage. As shown in Figure 1, 17 of 21 renal biopsy specimens with a statistically increased incidence of glomerular sclerosis for age in patients with poststreptococcal glomerulonephritis also showed arteriolar sclerosis. In 19 specimens without glomerular sclerosis, only five had vascular sclerosis. In Berger's IgA nephropathy, a similar correlation was demonstrated. Sixteen of 20 specimens with statistically increased incidence of glomerular sclerosis showed arteriolar sclerosis as well; of 26 specimens without glomerular sclerosis, only four had vascular lesions.

The frequent presence of ischemic or collapse-type sclerosis of glomeruli rather than disorganization of glomerular structure seemed to lend further support to a causative role for vascular sclerosis in the

Table I. Arterial and Arteriolar Lesions in Normotensive Patients with Glomerulonephritis[a] (Age under 40 years)

Glomerular histology	Vascular lesions
Minor glomerular lesions	44/68(64.7%)
Membranous nephropathy	20/37(54.1%)
Diffuse proliferative glomerulonephritis	91/123(74.0%)
Focal and segmental glomerulonephritis	96/116(82.8%)

[a] From Kincaid-Smith.[8]

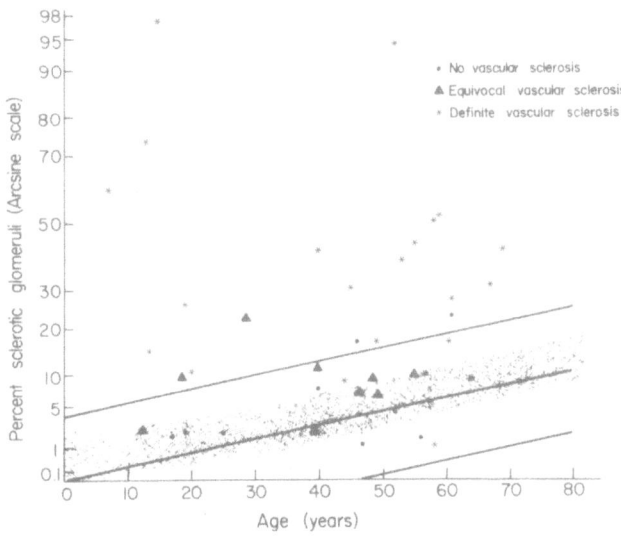

Figure 1. Correlation between glomerular sclerosis and vascular sclerosis in poststreptococcal glomerulonephritis. Percent sclerotic glomeruli in renal biopsy is plotted against age of the patient. The mean (shaded band) and the 95% population confidence limits are shown for the regression of glomerular sclerosis against age in normals (57). Appropriate symbols indicate for each datum whether vascular sclerosis was absent, equivocal, or definitely present. The correlation between glomerular sclerosis and vascular sclerosis is highly significant ($p < 0.002$).

progression of these glomerular diseases.[6,7] The concept of such a mechanism was especially attractive in poststreptococcal glomerulonephritis, where continued immune damage had to be discounted beyond a year or so from onset, since immunoglobulins are generally no longer present in glomeruli beyond this time.[9] Under these circumstances, progressive glomerular sclerosis required the operation of mechanisms other than immunologic, and the clinical-pathologic evidence just cited supported vascular disease and resultant ischemia as one of the likely possibilities.

However, recent hemodynamic and morphologic observations in the remnant kidney and in experimental nephritis suggest that adaptive increases in perfusion following nephron loss or injury may be responsible for further glomerular damage. The emphasis has thus been shifted away from ischemic glomerular sclerosis to hyperperfusion as a possible mechanism for both vascular and glomerular injury.

ADVERSE EFFECT OF HYPERTENSION ON
EXPERIMENTAL GLOMERULONEPHRITIS

The effect of hypertension on the renal arterioles and prearterioles has generally been accepted as the mechanism by which hypertension aggravates the course of glomerulonephritis. Vascular sclerosis is thought to accelerate glomerular sclerosis through ischemia. The "vicious cycle in Bright's disease" as proposed by Wilson and Byrom[9] alludes to this mechanism. However, a number of recent studies of experimental hypertension and of hypertension superimposed on a variety of glomerular diseases provide evidence that glomerular damage may be produced directly by hypertension rather than secondarily through ischemia resulting from occlusive small vessel alterations.

Knowlton et al.[10] in 1946, administering DOCA to rats with nephrotoxic serum nephritis (NSN), produced severe hypertension and a worsening of the glomerular disease; no change in proteinuria was reported. In a series of studies in which NSN was superimposed on clip hypertension or induced in the spontaneous hypertensive rat (SHR), Masayuma and associates[11–13] observed increased severity of hypertension and more persistent proliferative and sclerotic changes in the glomeruli; vascular alterations were not described. Motoki et al.[14] produced hypertension with DOCA and salt-loading in the unilaterally nephrectomized rat with NSN and noted increased glomerular proliferation and sclerosis. Teoduru et al.[15] showed that unilateral nephrectomy or salt-loading in the rabbit with NSN resulted in more severe glomerulonephritis and death in uremia. Blood pressure measurements were not performed in this study, but presumably the salt-loaded rabbits were hypertensive. Increased proteinuria and proliferative-sclerotic glomerular changes have been reported by Tikkanen and associates[16] when DOCA-salt hypertension was superimposed on autologous immune glomerulonephritis (Heymann nephritis) in the rat; vascular sclerosis and necrosis occurred infrequently in this model. In a similar study, using DOCA-salt hypertension in heterologous immune glomerulonephritis (passive Heymann nephritis), Iversen and Ofstad[17] noted more marked glomerular basement membrane thickening, greater proteinuria, and a shortened life span of the experimental animals.

In a study of steroid-induced hypertension in the uninephrectomized rat, Hill and Heptinstall[18] in 1968 were the first to suggest that failure of adequate arteriolar constriction rather than excessive narrowing was responsible for the occurrence of hypertensive lesions that developed in insufficiently hypertrophied vessels and their "unprotected" glomeruli. The following year, in a study of DOCA-salt hypertension in the uninephrectomized rat, Still and Dennison[19] demonstrated that glomeruli could undergo cell swelling and sclerosis that resembled similar changes in arterioles and suggested that hypertension may have a direct effect on the glomerular capillary. The vascular and glomerular damage described by these authors probably was attributable to malignant hypertension, but their proposal that glomerular vessels are affected directly by hypertension and do not suffer secondarily merely as a result of arteriolar narrowing and ischemia introduced a new and important concept.

Azar et al.,[20] in studies of one-kidney "post-salt" hypertension in rats, have recently shown the development of proliferation and sclerosis of glomeruli in association with reduced arteriolar resistance and increases in transcapillary pressure, glomerular blood flow, and single-nephron glomerular filtration rate (SNGFR). They suggest that adaptive decreases in afferent resistance following uninephrectomy override the ability of arterioles to increase their resistance in the presence of superimposed hypertension, thus exposing the glomerular capillaries to damaging increases in hydraulic pressure. In a subsequent study Azar et al.[21] demonstrated that salt-sensitive rats who develop hypertension with both kidneys intact show similar increases in SNGFR due to elevated glomerular blood flow and glomerular transcapillary hydraulic pressure. They propose that the glomerular lesions that develop in these rats are attributable to high glomerular capillary pressures that occur when hypertension and nephrosclerosis are superimposed on a genetically reduced number of adapted nephrons. In related studies, Mauer and associates[22] have examined the effect of clip hypertension on experimental streptozotocin diabetes mellitus in the rat and observed increased mesangial matrix material and heavier deposits of IgG, IgM and C3 in the unclipped "diabetic" kidney. Additional evidence for the possible role of glomerular hemodynamic factors in diabetic glomerulosclerosis was adduced by Azar[23] from the demonstration that glomerular capillary pressure is increased prior to any morphologic changes in pancreatectomized rats with short-term diabetes.

We have undertaken an examination of the effect of superimposed renal artery clip hypertension (CH) on the clinical and morphologic features of NSN in the Sprague-Dawley rat.[24] Our objective was twofold: to determine whether the effects on the renal arterioles of a given elevation of blood pressure were enhanced in the nephritic animal and to determine whether the glomerular abnormalities of NSN would be aggravated by the superimposition of hypertension. To avoid the catastrophic effects of necrotizing vasculitis which would be anticipated with marked elevations of blood pressure and could obscure differences between clip hypertension alone and clip hypertension superimposed on

David S. Baldwin

NSN, animals were selected for comparison with mean systolic blood pressures ranging between 120 and 160 mm Hg. Further, an attempt was made to induce a mild form of NSN in order to facilitate the recognition of any enhancing effects of superimposed hypertension on the severity of glomerular lesions.

In Table II are summarized the clinical data for all animals sacrificed at 3, 4, and 5 months after application of the renal artery clip, which followed injections of nephrotoxic serum by 1 month. Data for control animals and those with NSN alone and CH alone are given for comparison. The mean systolic blood pressures in the two hypertensive groups were almost identical; the similarity in heart weight to body weight ratios lends support to the close correspondence in measured blood pressures in the CH and NSN + CH groups. It will be seen that the superimposition of hypertension on NSN markedly enhances the level of protein excretion at the time of each monthly sacrifice (Table II). The incidence and severity of glomerular and vascular lesions were similarly aggravated by the superimposition of hypertension on NSN (Figures 2–5). While proliferation and tuft necrosis in glomeruli occurred at most in approximately 20% of rats with CH or NSN alone, the incidence exceeded 80% in the later sacrifices of animals when these lesions were combined. Glomerular sclerosis showed a similarly increased incidence and severity in rats with CH superimposed on NSN. Arteriolar medial hypertrophy was not seen at all in NSN, and occurred mildly in occasional rats with CH, while the incidence of severe arteriolar sclerosis reached almost 100% when hypertension was combined with NSN.

Our studies demonstrate that the superimposition of hypertension in the rat with NSN markedly aggravates the glomerular abnormalities and induces changes in the renal arterioles that do not occur in NSN alone or in CH at comparable levels of systolic blood pressure. The results suggest

Table II. Effect of Clip Hypertension on Nephrotoxic Serum Nephritis[a]

	N	BP (mm Hg)	CI (Percent)	UpV (mg/24 hours)
Control	17	102 ± 2	0.27 ± 0.01	2 ± 2
NSN	12	105 ± 2	0.25 ± 0.01	24 ± 12
CH	16	145 ± 3	0.36 ± 0.01	27 ± 11
NSN + CH	15	142 ± 6	0.36 ± 0.03	144 ± 28

[a] NSN: nephrotoxic serum nephritis; CH: clip hypertension; CI: cardiac index (%) = heart weight/ body weight; UpV: proteinuria.

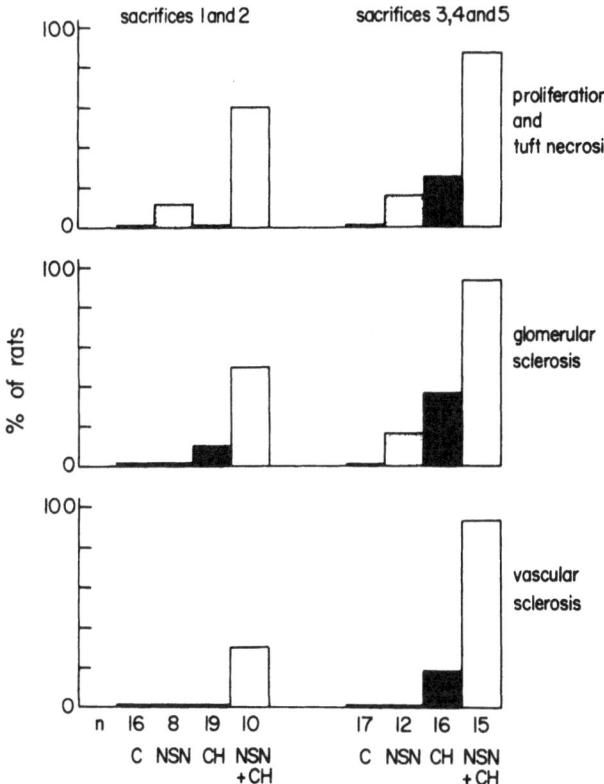

Figure 2. Incidence of glomerular and vascular morphologic lesions in nephrotoxic serum nephritis, in clip hypertension, and in the combination of nephrotoxic serum nephritis with clip hypertension. The superimposition of clip hypertension (CH) on nephrotoxic serum nephritis (NSN) increased the incidence of glomerular proliferation, tuft necrosis, and sclerosis, and resulted in the appearance of vascular sclerosis (arteriolar medial hypertrophy) in almost every instance.

that the intrarenal vessels in experimental nephritis possibly may be abnormal in a way that renders them more susceptible to the effects of increased intraluminal pressure, even though they appear morphologically unaffected by the disease. Similarly, the diseased glomerular capillaries may also be showing an increased susceptibility to damage when subjected to elevations in hydraulic pressure. Alternatively, it may be hypothesized that the glomerulus in experimental nephritis is actually exposed to greater hydraulic pressure than might be anticipated at a given systemic pressure, due to adaptive alterations in renal resistance that occur in disease and that result in a failure of arteriolar constriction to occur in the face of systemic

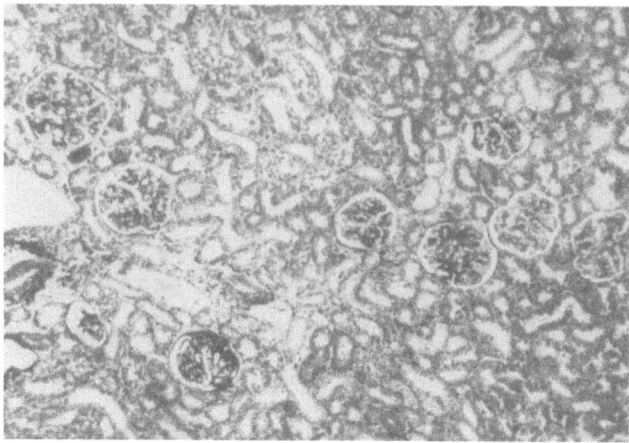

Figure 3. Nephrotoxic serum nephritis. Photomicrograph of rat kidney three months after administration of nephrotoxic serum. Blood pressure, 98 mm Hg. Glomeruli show increased mesangial matrix; a single glomerulus is sclerotic. Several small arteries that are present in the field are normal. Periodic acid-silver methenamine counterstained with hematoxylin and eosin (X 180).

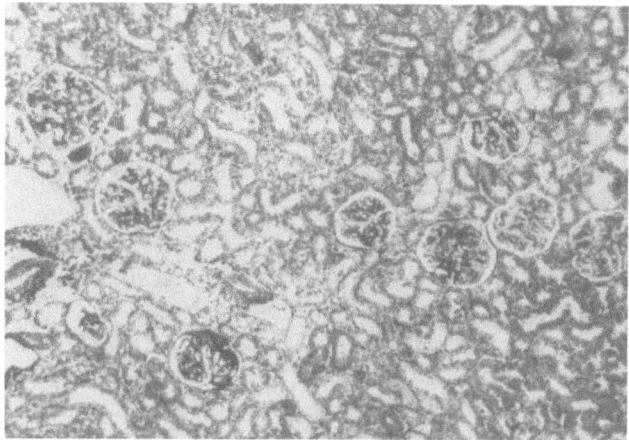

Figure 4. Clip hypertension. Photomicrograph of unclipped right kidney four months after application of clip to left renal artery. Blood pressure, 149 mm Hg. Glomeruli show increased mesangial matrix; a single glomerulus is sclerotic. A normal small artery is shown. Periodic acid-silver methenamine counterstained with hematoxylin and eosin (X 180).

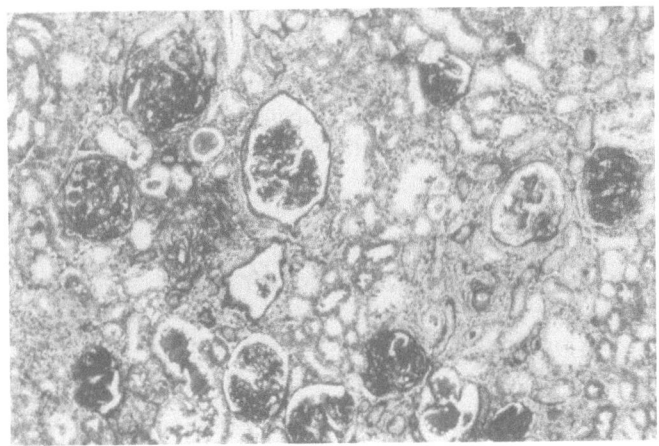

Figure 5. Nephrotoxic serum nephritis with superimposed clip hypertension. Photomicrograph of unclipped right kidney three months after administration of nephrotoxic serum and two months after application of clip to left renal artery. Blood pressure, 140 mm Hg. Glomeruli show widespread sclerosis and severe intra- and extracapillary proliferation. Medial hypertrophy and intimal hyaline are present in prearterioles; there are no necrotizing vascular lesions. Periodic acid-silver methenamine counterstained with hematoxylin and eosin (X 180).

hypertension. This afferent arteriolar "failure" may also be responsible for the markedly increased frequency and severity of small vessel damage that occurs at a given level of systemic pressure when hypertension is combined with glomerulonephritis.

SUMMARY

From our long-term observations in poststreptococcal glomerulonephritis and other glomerular diseases, it appears that nonimmunologically mediated damage is often related to ischemia secondary to intrarenal vascular sclerosis that could be attributed to hypertension. However, an additional basis for glomerular obliteration has emerged from physiologic and morphologic studies on reduced renal mass, post-salt or steroid-induced hypertension, and various forms of hypertension superimposed on experimental nephritis. It appears that nephron loss begets further glomerular damage through adaptive hemodynamic changes that take place in remaining nephrons and that expose the glomerular capillaries to increased hydraulic pressures, flows, and hyperfiltration. When systemic hypertension is superimposed on glomerulonephritis, glomerular damage is further enhanced, possibly through increased transmission of elevated pressures. It may be hypothesized that failure of arteriolar resistance to increase in adapted nephrons is responsible for hypertensive damage in glomerulonehpritis rather than arteriolar narrowing and ischemia, as has been thought conventionally.

REFERENCES

1. Fujise Y, Miyahara M: Comparison of the prognosis of hypertension associated with chronic glomerulonephritis with that of essential hypertension. *Jpn Circ J* 39:793–795, 1975.
2. Hollenberg NK: The kidney in hypertension: Relevance to glomerulonephritis, in Yoshitohi Y, Ueda Y (eds): *Glomerulonephritis*. Baltimore, University Park Press, 1979, pp 423–440.
3. Kajiwara N: Therapy and prognosis of hypertension in chronic nephritis. *Jpn Circ J* 39:779–788, 1975.
4. Kawaguchi Y, Mitarai T, Ueda Y: Clinical aspects of hypertension in advanced chronic glomerulonephritis, in Yoshitoshi Y, Ueda Y (eds): *Glomerulonephritis*. Baltimore, University Park Press, 1979, pp 473–482.
5. Varga I, Beregi E: Clinical and histopathological studies of human renal disease IV. Relationships of renal arterial fibroelastosis, glomerulonephritis and arterial hypertension. *Acta Med Acad Sci Hung* 30:165–175, 1973.
6. Gallo GR, Feiner HD, Steele, JM Jr, et al: Role of intrarenal vascular sclerosis in progression of poststreptococcal glomerulonephritis. *Clin Nephrol* 13:49–57, 1978.
7. Feiner JC, Cabili S, Schacht RG, et al: Intra-renal vascular disease in Berger's IgA nephropathy. Presented at 69th Annual Meeting. US-Canadian Division, International Academy of Pathology, New Orleans, 1980. In *Lab Investigation*, vol 42, 1980, p 166.
8. Kincaid-Smith P: *The Kidney*. Oxford, Blackwell-Scientific Publications, 1975, pp 193–202.
9. Wilson C, Byrom FB: The vicious cycle in chronic Bright's disease. 'Experimental evidence from the hypertensive rat. *Q J Med* 34:65–93, 1941.
10. Knowlton AL, Stoerk H, Seegel BC, et al: Influence of adrenal cortical steroids upon the blood pressure and the rate of progression of experimental nephritis in rats. *Endocrinology* 38:315–324, 1946.
11. Masuyama Y, Nishio I, Motoki K, et al: Hypertension changes in experimental nephritis combined with experimental hypertension. *Contr Nephrol* 6:13–22, 1977.
12. Masuyama Y, Motoki K, Kusuyama Y, et al: Hypertension changes in experimental nephritis combined with experimental hypertension. In Yoshitoshi Y, Ueda Y (eds): *Glomerulonephritis*. Baltimore, University Park Press, 1979, pp 441–454.
13. Motoki K, Kusuyama Y, Ueno Y, et al: Chronic nephrotoxic nephritis in spontaneously hypertensive rats. *Jpn Heart J* 19:662–664, 1978.
14. Motoki K, Kusuyama Y, Jimbo S, et al: Nephrotoxic serum nephritis in DOCA-salt hypertension and SHR. *Jpn Heart J* 20:714, 1979.
15. Teodoru CV, Saifer A, Frankel H: Conditioning factors influencing evolution of experimental glomerulonephritis in rabbits. *Am J Physiol* 196:457–460, 1959.
16. Tikkane I, Fyrquist F, Miettinen A, et al: Autologous immune complex nephritis and

DOCA-NaCl load: A new mode of hypertension. *Acta Pathol Microbiol Scand* 88:241–250, 1980.

17. Iversen BM, Ofstad J: Influence of hypertension on the course of experimental hypertension in rats. Renal Association, London (Feb 28, 1980). *Kidney Int* 18:142, 1980 (abst).

18. Hill GS, Heptinstall RH: Steroid-induced hypertension in the rat. *Am J Pathol* 52:1–20, 1968.

19. Still WJS, Dennison SM: The pathogenesis of the glomerular changes in steroid-induced hypertension. *Lab Invest* 20:249–260, 1969.

20. Azar S, Johnson MA, Hertel B, et al: Single-nephron pressures, flows, and resistances in hypertensive kidneys with nephrosclerosis. *Kidney Int* 12:28–40, 1977.

21. Azar S, Johnson MA, Iwai J, et al: Single-nephron dynamics in "post-salt" rats with chronic hypertension. *J Lab Clin Med* 91:156–16, 1978.

22. Mauer SM, Steffes MW, Azar S, et al: The effects of Goldblatt hypertension on development of the glomerular lesions of diabetes mellitus in the rat. *Diabetes* 27:738–744, 1979.

23. Azar S: Increased glomerular capillary pressure (PGC) in pancreatectomized rats with short-term diabetes. *Clin Res* 26:725A, 1978.

24. Neugarten J, Feiner HD, Schacht RG, et al: Aggravation of experimental glomerulone-phritis by superimposed clip hypertension. *Kidney Int*, in press.

Section III

Genesis and Prevention of Diabetic Nephropathy

New Concepts

It is understandable that, having been the first to report that hemodialysis significantly prolongs the life of diabetics with kidney failure in 1966,[1] our renal program at The Long Island College Hospital has had a continuing interest in the fate of increasing numbers of patients on dialysis with diabetic nephropathy. During 1981—15 years later—approximately 25% of all new hemodialysis patients in large urban centers such as New York and Los Angeles are diabetic. Because uremic diabetics have a significantly more serious prognosis than nondiabetics, the cost in dollars and personnel is substantially higher than for nondiabetics. Following either cadaveric renal transplantation or maintenance hemodialysis, only 50% of patients survive for three years. Considering that more than one billion dollars are expended annually in the United States for uremia therapy,[2] the importance of data in this section suggesting that diabetic nephropathy may be a preventable disease is evident.

Diabetes mellitus is an ubiquitously present metabolic disorder with generalized vasculopathy and resultant multiple endocrine collapse, including the pancreas,[3] pituitary, thyroid, adrenal,[4] and parathyroid function.[5] The creatinine level and parathyroid hormone levels are also lower in diabetic uremics[6] than in their nondiabetic uremic counterparts.

I wish I could serve up, on a silver salver, some glistening problem-solving thought, gleaned from these 16 years of observations of very sick patients. We are closing in fast, but we are not at the finish line. Since Banting and Best discovered insulin in 1921, and then the use of dialysis in 1966, not much changed until recently, with the quest for euglycemia and its further substantiation by the recent report of hemodynamic alterations (hyperglycemic hyperfiltration) in the pathogenesis of diabetic glome-rulopathy reported in the two chapters of this section.

That a normal body constituent may prove toxic in high concentration is emphasized by Levitz, Hirsch, and Friedman, who relate hyperglycemia to microvasculopathy in diabetes. Levitz speculates that with newer techniques of self-monitoring of blood glucose it may be possible for diabetics to sustain euglycemia, preventing degenerative renal and retinal disease.

Next, Hostetter and Brenner extend their hard data into a hypothesis in which it is suggested that glomerular hyperfiltration known to be a constant finding in early diabetes bears "a central responsibility in the initiation of diabetic glomerulopathy..." and subsequently leads to destruction of glomeruli. This fresh thinking opens new investigative paths to the understanding and perhaps ultimate prevention of diabetic nephropathy.

M.M.A.

REFERENCES

1. Avram MM: Use of special hemodialysis methods in diabetic uremia, in *Proceedings of the Conference on Dialysis by the National Dialysis Committee*, New York, National Union Catalogue, 1966, p 15.
2. Avram MM: High prevalence of pancreatic disease in chronic renal failure. *Nephron* 18L:228–231, 1977.
3. Avram MM, Lipner HI, Sadiqali R, et al: Metabolic changes in diabetic uremic patients on hemodialysis. *Trans Am Soc Artif Int Organs* XXII:412–418, 1976.
4. Avram MM, Feinfeld DA, Huatuco AH: Search for the uremic toxin. Decreased motor-nerve conduction velocity and elevated parathyroid hormone in uremia. *N Engl J Med* 298:1000–1003, 1978.
5. Avram MM: Lower parathyroid hormone and creatinine in diabetic uremia, in Avram MM (ed): *Contributions to Nephrology, Vol. 20, Parathyroid Hormone in Kidney Failure*. Basel, London, New York, S. Karger, 1980, pp 4–8.

7

Relationship Between Hyperglycemia and Diabetic Glomerulosclerosis

CELIA S. LEVITZ, SONDRA R. HIRSCH,
AND ELI A. FRIEDMAN

Uremia in diabetics as a result of progressive glomerulosclerosis accounts for one fourth of patients newly accepted in maintenance hemodialysis and renal transplant programs in the United States. Convincing evidence indicates that degenerative vasculopathy in the diabetic eye and glomerulus are a direct result of hyperglycemia and a function of duration of diabetes. Based on animal models of diabetes and clinical observations over the past few years, the thesis that careful control of blood glucose will preempt development of vasculopathy and correct abnormalities of intermediate metabolites and hormonal disturbances is increasingly accepted. Development of simplified methods of self-monitoring of blood glucose and of lightweight battery-powered insulin infusion systems has permitted study of nearly euglycemic diabetics for a year or longer. It can be anticipated that the lessons learned in recent advances in diabetic management will in sum improve well-being and retard development of vasculopathy. Mogenson,[1] for example, has shown that control of hypertension in azotemic diabetics retards deterioration of glomerular filtration at the rate of 9 ml/min/year. Our preliminary experience suggests that, in addition to reduction of blood pressure, morbidity in renal transplanted and uremic diabetics can be further reduced by incorporating self-monitoring of blood glucose into the treatment regimen.

Maintenance of blood glucose concentration between 70 and 150 mg/dl[2]—by definition, euglycemia—must be an early therapeutic objective in the diabetic as the progression of glomerulosclerosis is silent during the first 17 to 20 years of insulin dependence. Insulin-dependent diabetics exhibit a predictable sequence of morphologic and pathophysiologic

CELIA S. LEVITZ, SONDRA R. HIRSCH, AND ELI A. FRIEDMAN • Department of Medicine, Downstate Medical Center, Brooklyn, New York.

changes in the kidney in the years before azotemia develops. Shortly after the appearance of hyperglycemia, a supernormal glomerular filtration rate is associated with large kidneys containing bigger than normal glomeruli. By the fifth year of insulin use, some patients become intermittently proteinuric after exercise, an abnormality that progresses by the tenth to 15th year in about half of the patients to the nephrotic syndrome. Fixed massive proteinuria is followed by renal insufficiency in a mean of 20 years after beginning insulin use. Renal biopsies obtained after the tenth year of insulin dependence disclose atherosclerosis of both afferent and efferent glomerular arteries in the majority of diabetics. Diffuse and nodular intercapillary glomerulosclerosis can be discerned after as little as four years of diabetes and is detectable as early as two years after transplanting a normal kidney into a diabetic.[3] It may be inferred from the gradual pathologic deterioration of diabetic glomeruli that damage attributable to hyperglycemia takes years to evolve and, therefore, that long-term sustained normalization of blood glucose concentration may be necessary to alter the diabetic's course.

That glucose elevation *per se* can cause damage to body proteins and organs has been demonstrated. Post-transcriptional denaturing of plasma proteins (glycosylation) is one direct result of hyperglycemia. Glycosylation of hemoglobin, which proceeds at a rate determined by plasma glucose concentration, alters its oxygen-carrying capacity; the quantitation of glycohemoglobin (HbA_{1c}) is utilized clinically as a measure of mean glucose control over the preceding four to eight weeks, reflecting the life of erythrocytes.[4] Glycosylated albumin concentration also rises proportional to the level of hyperglycemia and may prove to be superior to glycohemoglobin because of the faster turnover of albumin. Peripheral nerves and some tissues, such as the retina, lens, renal papilla, blood vessels, and islets of Langerhans, do not require insulin for glucose penetration. Excess glucose is readily metabolized in nerves to sorbitol, causing cell hypotonicity due to the osmotic activity of excess sorbitol, Schwann cell disruption, and myelin destruction. Aldose reductase converts glucose to sorbitol. Recently, use of altrestatin, an aldose reductase inhibitor, has been shown to reverse sensory nerve deficits.[5] This finding suggests that hyperglycemia can lead to nerve damage, which may be preventable by either interfering with production of a toxic end product (sorbitol) or reducing glucose concentration. Strict glucose control reduces sorbitol levels in peripheral nerves and restores motor nerve conduction velocity in experimentally induced diabetic animals,[6] thus favoring the inference that hyperglycemia is injurious.

More relevant to the premise that diabetic nephropathy is a preventable disease is the observation that the glomerular basement membrane is histologically normal in newly diagnosed insulin-dependent diabetics, a finding against the genetic predisposition theory of diabetic glomerulopathy. Takajakura et al.[7] in studying percutaneous renal biopsies in 23 diabetics after a mean duration of disease of 68 months (range 3 to 156 months) and again after a mean follow-up of 52.6 months (range 24 to 96 months) found that progression of diabetic glomerular lesions was correlated with fasting blood glucose above 150 mg/dl and the need for insulin therapy (5/5 Type I, 2/11 Type II progressed). Insulinopenic patients have slower turnover and faster synthesis of glomerular basement membrane proline, hydroxyproline, and glycine as compared with controls[8] and evidence of basement membrane thickening within three to five years.[9] Glomerular basement membrane thickening is accompanied by glomerular hypertrophy associated with increased mesangial matrix. That hyperglycemia contributes to these pathologic changes may be inferred from the observations that seven mice given repeated infusions of glycosylated plasma proteins had glomerular basement membrane thickening whereas none of four mice given nonglycosylated plasma proteins developed similar lesions.[10]

Microvascular alterations consisting of venular dilation and increased permeability occur within two months of onset of streptozotocin-induced diabetes in hamsters[11] and in the conjunctival venules of diabetic children.[12] Hyperglycemia induces glycosylation of lysine residuals, and since ionic charge and molecular radius affect transcapillary permeability to solutes, glycosylation by itself might affect glomerular membrane restrictability.

Correction of hyperglycemia by islet transplants in induced diabetic rats will cause regression of glomerular lesions bearing some resemblance to human diabetic glomerulosclerosis.[13–15] In hyperglycemic rats mesangial thickening and mesangial deposits of IgG, IgM, and complement can be observed following two months of insulinopenia.[16] Diabetic rats treated with insulin for six months do not develop either enlarged kidneys or glomeruli characteristic of untreated diabetic rats.[17] Following islet transplantation, diabetic rats have a reduction in glomerular mesangial space and widening of capillary lumena as well as a decrease in the member of endothelial cells, thus reverting to the appearance of nondiabetic kidneys.[18] Control of hyperglycemia by diet in genetically diabetic db/db mice will prevent development of glomerular mesangial lesions.[19]

Human studies have also demonstrated a favorable effect of tight control of blood glucose on glomerular function. Abnormally high urinary albumin excretion decreased significantly within one to three days in seven diabetics given a continuous subcutaneous insulin infusion while there was no change in excretion of the tubular protein β_2-microglobulin.[20] Supporting the deleterious effect on the kidney of a hyperglycemic environment is the observation that 85% of kidneys transplanted into diabetics show glomerular arteriolar degenerative changes in graft biopsies obtained two to four years after transplantation.[3] Of great significance to the "hyperglycemia causes glomerulopathy" argument are the small number of cases in which diabetic renal allograft recipients maintained euglycemic escape the "inevitability" of recurrent diabetic glomerulopathy. For example, no evidence of recurrent diabetic glomerulopathy was found in a 32-year-old Type I diabetic who died of sepsis 50 months following a segmental pancreatic transplant, which retained islet function, and 46 months after receiving a renal transplant.[21]

Reversibility by euglycemia of numerous extrarenal diabetic metabolic and histopathologic changes has been illustrated in more than 50 reports. White blood cell adherence to glasswool, fibrinogen survival, chrominum 51 labeled red blood cell survival, and platelet hyperaggregation all improve with normalization of blood glucose. Triglycerides,[22] amino acids,[22] and growth hormone[23] levels in blood all return to normal once glucose concentration is corrected. Preliminary evidence suggests that retinopathy as judged by the number of microaneurysms developing per year detected by fluorescein angiography improves with better control of blood glucose.[24] In one report, florid proliferative retinopathy with vitreous hemorrhage regressed during continuous insulin infusion by a wearable pump. Sensory nerve conduction has improved with the obtainment of euglycemia.[25]

TREATING UREMIC DIABETES

Subsequent to Avram's demonstration that maintenance hemodialysis was possible in diabetes,[26] several workers attempted long-term dialytic therapy with mortality rates as high as 78% in one year. Recognition of the important role of hypertension control has increased survival on hemodialysis to 50% for three years. Diabetic cadaveric renal graft recipients also have a three-year survival of 50%, which is about 20% below that of nondiabetics. Insulin-dependent dialysis patients and transplant recipients have mortality rates that are two to four times as high as nondiabetics in most large series. Hyperglycemia uniformly found in transplant and dialysis diabetic patients (Table I) must contribute to morbidity and mortality. Diabetic renal transplant recipients receive high doses of adrenal corticosteroids, which frustrate efforts at glucose regulation. Blood glucose levels of 300–1,000 mg/dl are common in diabetic recipients. Hyperglycemia causes decreased chemotaxis, diapedesis, and adherence of leukocytes,[27] predisposing to fatal fungal, protozoal, and viral

Table I. Blood Glucose in Insulin-Requiring Hemodialysis Patients

Patient	Age	Sex	Insulin dose	Duration of diabetes (years)	Blood glucose concentration (mg/dl)
V.P.	26	F	18 U	15	156–57
W.M.	43	F	26 U	28	362–35
J.C.	44	M	65 U	21	495–192
G.S.	32	F	25 U[a]	23	232–127
M.F.	27	F	25 U	22	556–81
F.A.	33	M	15 U	19	714–232

[a] Patient was receiving this dose prior to the start of dialysis; insulin administration was discontinued before dialysis treatment began.

infections. Vascular access problems in hemodialyzed uremic diabetes might be compounded by the platelet abnormalities, decreased fibrinolysis, and decreased prostacylin levels found in hyperglycemic diabetics.

ROLE OF PRESSURE IN NEPHROLOGY

Increased blood flow in a functioning transplanted kidney could accelerate diabetic glomerulopathy. In experiments involving renal artery clipping or uninephrectomy in diabetic rats, the unclipped (or remaining) kidney demonstrated accelerated mesangial matrix thickening and localization of IgG, IgM, and complement.[28,29] Consistent with this view is a report of a diabetic with unilateral renal artery stenosis who demonstrated marked diabetic glomerulopathy in the kidney exposed to hypertension whereas the kidney with the stenotic artery revealed little change.[30] The role of vascular pressure in the development of diabetic vasculopathy is also implied by the protective effect of carotid insufficiency on the course of diabetic retinopathy.[31]

The foregoing is consistent with the opinion of Pirart,[32] who reviewed the course of 4,400 diabetics and concluded: "The only factors consistently related to the presence (and severity of retinopathy) of all three specific complications (including nephropathy) were the intensity and duration of diabetes." Studies in experimentally induced diabetic rats show the reversibility by normalization of blood glucose level of increased kidney size, glomerular volume, and capillary surface area, as well as a return to normal of increased glomerular filtration rate, functional proteinuria, and decreased mesangial clearance of IgG, IgM, and C3. It remains to be proved that human diabetics made euglycemic will behave similarly, but the case is compelling.

DIABETIC NEPHROPATHY IN THE 1980S

How should the nephrologist of the 1980s approach the diabetic? Consider the lesson learned about the effect of glucose control on mortality in peritoneal dialysis. Oreopoulos,[33] who pioneered the use of peritoneal dialysis in diabetics using conventional insulin therapy, reported a 44% one-year and 20% two-year survival. By adding insulin to the dialysate, Flynn[34] was able to maintain blood glucose below 200 mg/dl with greatly improved survival. Confirmatory reports of enhanced survival in both hemo- and peritoneally dialyzed diabetics in whom tight control is achieved can be anticipated. Segmental pancreatic and islet cell transplantation are in the investigational stage as euglycemia-inducing treatment.

SELF-MONITORING OF GLUCOSE

We have demonstrated the usefulness of self-monitoring of blood glucose in the management of diabetes in an in-hospital transplant service. Conventionally treated transplant recipients' daily blood glucose levels ranged from <50 mg/dl to >400 mg/dl while hospitalized post-transplant. Using a twice-daily insulin regimen employing intermediate (NPH) and short-acting (regular) insulin and fingersticks as described below, blood glucose was maintained between 80 and 240 mg/dl throughout hospitalization in 21 consecutive diabetic recipients except after pulse doses of methyl prednisolone.

Self-monitoring of blood glucose is efficacious in-hospital for transplant recipients. What of the long-term out-of-hospital need for glucose regulation? Long-term euglycemia in insulin-dependent nonuremic young diabetics induces reversion to normal plasma amino acids and lipids; normalization of counter regulatory hormones, including growth hormone, catecholamines, and glucagon; improvement in peripheral neuropathy; increased perfusion of the lower extremity; and a decrease in skin thickness. Preliminary evidence hints at improvement in microvasculopathy as judged by less proteinuria and interruption in progression of proliferative retinopathy.

Uremic diabetics, however, may be expected to show less dramatic benefits of established euglycemia. The diabetic presenting to a nephrologist/renal transplant physician team suffers cumulative effects of 20 years of poorly controlled metabolic disease. Almost all have retinopathy and neuropathy, and half have evidence of coronary artery disease. Is it reasonable to expect that control of hyperglycemia is worth the effort in such patients? To determine the degree of control usually effected in uremic diabetics, we studied nine renal transplant recipients over 24 hours and found that none had blood glucose maintenance within the desired 70–150 mg/dl range (Table II). Seven of nine recipients (78%) had at least one glucose value above 300 mg/dl while one had a hypoglycemic reaction during which his blood glucose level fell to 31 mg/dl. From this pilot study we concluded that poor glucose control is common in renal recipients and might contribute to their inferior prognosis. To assess the feasibility of long-term self-regulation of blood glucose, a group of nine patients on home self-monitoring of blood glucose including six renal transplant recipients followed for seven months, three hemodialysis patients, and two uremic patients (serum creatinine >4 <8 mg/dl), is now under study.

Blood glucose monitoring is accomplished by employing a simple automatic lancet (Autolet, Vister Scientific Inc., Highland, New York), disposable needles (Monolet, Sherwood Medical Industries, Deland, Florida), and a glucose reagent strip (Chemstrip, Biodynamics Industries, Deland, Florida). Patients puncture the lateral margin of a terminal phalanx and express one drop of whole blood, which is directed to fall on the reagent-containing area of the strip. After exactly 60 seconds of contact

Table II. Blood Glucose in Insulin-Requiring Renal Transplant Recipients

Patient	Age	Sex	Insulin dose	Duration of diabetes (years)	Blood glucose centration (mg/dl)
R.K.	35	M	50 U	26	350–181
N.N.	42	M	103 U	7	540–48
B.R.	48	M	80 U	27	306–57
B.J.	51	M	50 U	7	612–280
A.P.	51	F	20 U	8 mo	975–279
R.B.	37	M	57 U	22	152–31
N.A.	37	M	92 U	4	314–78
I.B.	48	M	65 U	5[a]	300–105
E.L.	51	M	20 U	1.5[a]	224–96

[a] Steroid-induced diabetes.

with the reagent strip, which contains horseradish peroxidase and glucose oxidase, the blood is cleared with a cotton ball. A tan, green, or blue color reaction develops with o-toluidine and tetramethylbenzidine in two adjacent areas of the strip. One minute later for blood glucose levels below 240 mg/dl and two minutes later for levels above 240 mg/dl, the strip is compared with a color chart that defines glucose values of 20, 40, 80, 120, 240, 400, and 800 mg/dl. Intermediate values are approximated. An advantage of the chemstrip is that developed colors remain stable for at least two weeks, allowing objective verification of the patient's at-home interpretation. Patients are instructed to mount each strip in a daily log, thus facilitating periodic verification of glucose determinations by one of the investigators. Blood glucose measurements are performed fasting, prelunch, predinner, and before retiring.

To date we have observed that patients will continue blood glucose monitoring for at least seven months (six patients), showing a motivation equivalent for Jovanovic et al.'s[35] pregnant diabetic patients. As shown in Table III, home monitoring facilitated tighter blood glucose control in our renal transplant (RT) and hemodialysis (HD) patients, with all maintaining a blood glucose concentration below 180 mg/dl much of the time. Table IV shows the course of HgA_{1c} during the study. It is readily apparent that we are dealing with patients with multisystem disease and not just "hyperglycemia." Patient R.K. was able to lower his HgA_{1c} from 12.9 to 7.7% but operative

Table III. Response of Renal Transplant Patients to Home Blood Glucose Monitoring

Patient	Treatment	Age	Prednisone dose (mg)	Insulin (total units)		Glucose range	
				Pre	SMGB[e]	Pre	SMBG[e]
A.K.	RT	35	15	90	90	181–350	100–180
R.B.	RT	48	25	59	59	31–152	100–180
H.A.	RT	37	20	57	57	96–314	80–80
B.J.	RT	51	25	50	36	280–612	120–120
E.C.[a]	RT	41	22.5	20	21	96–224	110–120
L.C.	HD	54		42	58	160–375[c]	80–180
H.P.[b]	HD	54		25	15	78–162[d]	80–120
J.C.	HD	44		65	58	192–495	150–180

[a] Steroid-induced diabetes for 18 months.
[b] Subsequently able to come off insulin.
[c] Prior to dialysis when Cr_{cl} 15 ml/min.
[d] Prior to dialysis when Cr_{cl} 2 ml/min.
[e] SMBG: self-monitoring blood glucose .

Table IV. Glyco-Hemoglobin Level in Renal Transplant Recipients

Patient	Treatment	Pre SMBG[a]	HgA$_{1c}$							
			1 mo	2 mo	3 mo	4 mo	5 mo	6 mo	7 mo	8 mo
R.K.[b]	RT	12.9	7.7		11.3[c]		9.4	13.2[d]		12.9
R.B.[b]	RT	9.0						7.0	7.8	
H.A.	RT	9.3		7.9	6.8					
E.C.	RT	7.9	6.5		7.0					
F.A.[a]	RT				8.7	7.3			8.8	
B.J.	RT	10.5	6.8		11.4[e]				9.7	
H.P.	HD	9.1	6.8	Insulin	discontinued					
L.C.	HD	12.9		11.4		9.0	8.1	10.7[f]		
J.C.	HD	10.8		9.4	12.2[g]					
R.G.	Uremia				9.1	10.3[h]				

[a] Home blood glucose monitoring.
[b] (C peptide <1).
[c] Hospitalized for below-knee amputation and unable to work.
[d] Vitrectomy and unable to read test strips.
[e] Below-knee amputation, noncompliant.
[f] Hemodialysis in another unit.
[g] Problems with hemodialysis.
[h] Unsuccessful cadaveric renal transplant.

interventions, including below-knee amputation (macrovascular disease) and vitrectomy (prior hemorrhage), temporarily prevented adherence to the control regimen, with a subsequent rise in HgA$_{1c}$ concentration. B.J. also lost control when hospitalized for a below-knee amputation secondary to a foot ulcer (neuropathy).

We have detailed the background leading to our study of the practicality of establishing tight glucose control in insulin-dependent diabetic renal transplant recipients. In-hospital, self-monitoring of glucose has enhanced the degree of control achieved in the immediate post-transplanted period. Out-of-hospital patients have proved compliant for as long as seven months, except during major stresses such as leg amputation or vitrectomy. Refinement in our approach proffering additional support to patients confronted by surgery may encourage more continuous following of the control regimen. To judge whether the effort is worthwhile, the morbidity of self-monitored and conventionally treated patients will have to be evaluated over several years. Improved morbidity, reduced mortality, and prevention of recurrent glomerulosclerosis in the renal allograft will serve as sufficient objective markers of the efficacy of striving for euglycemia.

78   Celia S. Levitz et al.

REFERENCES

1. Mogenson CE: Diabetes and hypertension. *Lancet* 1:308, 1979.
2. Service FJ, Molnar GD, Rosevear JW: Mean amplitude for glycemic excursion. A measure of diabetic instability. *Diabetes* 19:644, 1970.
3. Mauer SM: Development of diabetic vascular lesion in normal kidneys transplanted into patients with diabetes. *N Engl J Med* 295:916, 1976.
4. Koenig RJ, Peterson CM, Jones RH, et al: Correlation of glucose regulation and hemoglobin A_{1c} in diabetes mellitus. *N Engl J Med* 295:471, 1979.
5. Culebras A, Alio J, Herrera J, et al: Effect of an aldolase reductase inhibitor on diabetic peripheral neuropathy. Preliminary Reports. *Arch Neurol* 38:133, 1981.
6. Gabbay KH: Hyperglycemia, polyol metabolism, and complication of diabetes mellitus. *Ann Rev Med* 26:521, 1975.
7. Takajakura E, LaKamoto S, Goshido E, et al: Onset and progression of diabetic glomerulosclerosis. A prospective study based on serial renal biopsies. *Diabetes* 24:1, 1975.
8. Price RG, Spiers RG: Studies on the metabolism of the renal glomerular basement membrane. Turnover measurements in the rat with the use of radio labed amino acid. *J Biol Chem* 252:8597, 1977.
9. Osterby R: Quanitative electron microscopic studies of glomerulus in diabetes mellitus, in Ditzel J, Lewis DH (eds): *Microcirculatory Approach to Current Therapeutic Problems: Lung in Shock, Organ Transplantation, Diabetic Microangiopathy.* Basel, New York, Karger, 1971, p 142.
10. McVerry BA, Fisher C, Hopp A, et al: Production of pseudo diabetic glomerular changes in mice after repeated injections of glucos ylated proteins. *Lancet* 1:738, 1980.
11. Joyner WL, Mayhan WG, Johnson RL, et al: Microvascular alterations develop in Syrian hamsters after induction of diabetes mellitus by streptozotocin. *Diabetes* 30:93, 1981.
12. Ditzel J, Duckers J: The bulbar conjunctival vascular bed in diabetic children. *Acta Paediatr* 46:535, 1957.
13. Weber CJ, Silva FG, Hardy MA, et al: Effects of islet transplantation on renal function and morphology of short and long term diabetic rats. *Transplant Proc* 11:549, 1979.
14. Mauer SM, Steffes MW, Sutherland DER, et al: Studies of the rate of regression of the glomerular lesions in diabetic rats treated with pancreatic islet transplantation. *Diabetes* 24:280, 1975.
15. Silva FG, Weber CJ, Pirani CH, et al: Effects of islet transplantation of glomerular basement membrane thickness and proteinuria in diabetic Lewis rats. *Diabetes* 28:426, 1978.
16. Mauer SM, Sutherland DER, Steffes MW, et al: Pancretic islet transplantation effects on the glomerular lesions of experimental diabetes in the rats. *Diabetes* 23:748, 1974.
17. Rasch R: Prevention of diabetic glomerulopathy in streptozotocin diabetic rats by insulin treatment. *Diabetologia* 16:125, 1979.
18. Bretzel RG, Breidenbach C, Mofmann J, et al: Islet transplantation in experimental diabetes of the rat. Rate of regression in diabetic kidney lesions after iosgenic islet transplantation: Quantitative measurements. *Horm Metab Res* 11:200, 1979.
19. Leo SM, Bressler R: Prevention of diabetic nephropathy by diet control in the db/db mouse. *Diabetes* 30:106, 1981.
20. Champion MC, Shepard GAA, Rodger NW, et al: Continuous subcutaneous infusion of insulin in the management of diabetes mellitus. *Diabetes* 29:206, 1980.
21. Gliedman ML, Tellis VA, Soberman R, et al: Long term effect of pancreatic transplant function in patients with advanced JODM. *Diabetes Care* 1:1, 1978.

22. Tamborlane WV, Sherwin R, Gene M, et al: Restoration of normal lipid and amino acid metabolism in diabetic patients treated with a portable insulin infusion pump. *Lancet* 1:1258–1261, 1979.

23. Tamborlane WV, Koursto V, Mendler R, et al: Normalization of the growth hormone and catecholamine response to exercise in juvenile-onset diabetic subjects treated with a portable insulin infusion pump, *Diabetes* 28:785–788, 1979.

24. Exchwege E, Job D, Guy OL, et al: Delayed progression of diabetic retinopathy by divided insulin administration: A future follow-up. *Diabetologia* 16:13, 1979.

25. Irsigler K, Kritz H, Najemnik C, et al: Reversal of florid diabetic retinopathy. *Lancet* 1068, 1979.

26. Avram MM, Slater PA, Fein PA, et al: Comparative survival of 673 patients with chronic uremia treated with renal transplantation and maintenance hemodialysis. *Trans Am Soc Artif Intern Organs* 25:391, 1979.

27. Peterson CM, Jones RL: Hematologic alterations in diabetes mellitus. *Amer J Med* 70:339, 1981.

28. Mauer SM, Steffes MW, Agar S, et al: The effects of Goldblatt hypertension on the development of glomerular lesions of diabetes mellitus in the rat. *Diabetes* 27:738, 1978.

29. Steffes MW, Brown DM, Mauer SM: Diabetic glomerulopathy following unilateral nephrectomy in the rat. *Diabetes* 27:25, 1978.

30. Berkman J, Rifkin H: Unilateral nodular diabetic glomerulosclerosis (Kimmerstel-Wilson): Report of a case. *Metab Clin Exp* 22:715, 1973.

31. Behrindt T, Duane TD: Unilateral complications in diabetic retinopathy. *Trans Am Acad Ophth Otol* 74:28, 1970.

32. Pirart J: Diabetes Mellitus and its degenerative complications: A prospective study of 4400 patients observed between 1947 and 1973. *Diabetes Care* 1:(part I)168–188, (part II) 252–263, 1978.

33. Rubin J, Oreopoulos DG, Blair RBG, et al: Chronic peritoneal dialysis in the management of diabetes with terminal renal failure. *Nephron* 19:265, 1977.

34. Flynn CT, Mibbana J, Dohrman B: Advantages of continuous ambulatory peritoneal dialysis to the diabetic with renal failure. *Proc EDTA* 16:184, 1979.

35. Jovanovic L, Peterson CM, Savena BB, et al: Feasibility of maintaining normal glucose profiles in insulin dependent pregnant diabetic women. *Am J Med* 68:105, 1980.

8

The Role of Hemodynamic Alterations in the Pathogenesis of Diabetic Glomerulopathy

THOMAS H. HOSTETTER AND BARRY M. BRENNER

Although nephrotic-range proteinuria and progressive azotemia are unequivocal indications of disordered glomerular function in patients with long-standing insulin-dependent diabetes mellitus, it is apparent that alterations in glomerular function also occur at an early stage of this disease in humans and experimental animals. Stalder and Schmid[1] reported more than 20 years ago that the glomerular filtration rate (GFR) is elevated above normal in diabetic children and young adults, a finding confirmed by Ditzel and Schwartz[2] and extensively investigated in recent years by Mogensen.[3,4] Mogensen described a 40% increment in GFR in 11 newly diagnosed juvenile diabetic patients when compared with values in 31 normal subjects of similar age.[3] This remarkable hyperfiltration was shown to be related to the patient's metabolic status since reduction of blood sugar levels over several days to weeks by standard insulin therapy tended to return GFR to normal or near-normal levels. Indeed, recent studies by Christiansen et al.[5] have demonstrated that with reduction in blood glucose levels to normal in diabetics by continuous insulin infusion, GFR also declines from elevated to near-normal values in a matter of hours.

A number of clinical studies have been performed, largely by these and other Danish investigators, in an attempt to dissect the particular component or components of the diabetic state responsible for these early elevations in glomerular filtration rate. One factor that has been incrimi-

THOMAS H. HOSTETTER ● Laboratory of Kidney and Electrolyte Physiology, Brigham and Women's Hospital, Boston, Massachusetts. BARRY M. BRENNER ● Department of Medicine, Harvard Medical School; and Renal Division, Brigham and Women's Hospital, Boston, Massachusetts.

nated is hyperglycemia *per se*. Indeed, acute elevations of GFR occur in response to glucose infusion in normal subjects.[6-8] While the structural hypertrophy observed in kidneys of diabetic humans and animals, best documented by Osterby and Gundersen[9] and Seyer-Hansen et al.,[10] has also been proposed to contribute to the augmented GFR, this process would be unlikely to explain the relatively rapid changes in GFR that occur with insulin therapy. Augmented levels of glucagon and growth hormone are usual accompaniments of diabetic hyperglycemia and each of these hormones is capable of inducing a rise in GFR in normal individuals at plasma levels comparable to those found in the hyperglycemic diabetic patient.[11-14] However, increments in GFR achieved by these hormones are substantially less than the usual increment observed in the early insulin-dependent diabetic patient. Finally, changes in circulating and tissue levels of classic vasoactive hormones such as angiotensin II, catecholamines, and prostaglandins have been demonstrated in a variety of circumstances in diabetes.[15-17] Also, changes in vasoresponsiveness to angiotensin II and catecholamines have been demonstrated in several extrarenal vascular beds in diabetic patients and animals.[18,19] Whether changes in the levels of these hormones or the vascular response to them contribute to the hyperfiltration is as yet unknown. In any case, a variety of factors present in the diabetic state may contribute to hyperfiltration and no single factor appears to account fully for this phenomenon.

Though insights into the stimuli responsible for diabetic hyperfiltration have been forthcoming from such clinical studies, the intrarenal basis for the elevated GFR cannot be established definitively within the constraints of these human studies. GFR is determined by four factors.[20] First, glomerular plasma flow influences the mean net ultrafiltration pressure and is directly related to single-nephron GFR (SNGFR). Recent studies indicate that renal plasma flow does indeed increase in patients with early diabetes.[21] A second determinant of GFR is systemic oncotic pressure, which appears to be normal as estimated from plasma protein concentration in the circumstance of glomerular hyperfiltration in early diabetes.[3] A third determinant of GFR is the glomerular transcapillary hydraulic pressure difference, which has not yet been measured in humans and therefore cannot be evaluated. The last determinant of GFR is the glomerular ultrafiltration coefficient, which represents the product of glomerular capillary hydraulic permeability and available surface area for filtration. Measures of total glomerular capillary surface area are increased in early human and chemically induced diabetes in animals.[9,10] On this basis it has been conjectured that the hyperfiltration results, at least in part, from the increased glomerular surface area.

Recent studies conducted in our laboratory have provided a detailed description of the glomerular hemodynamic basis for the hyperfiltration in early diabetes.[22] Animals were made diabetic by intravenous injection of streptozotocin and were maintained at a moderate level of hyperglycemia by daily low-dose insulin administration. The resultant plasma glucose concentration in these diabetic rats averaged 375 mg/dl as compared with 115 mg/dl in control rats. Animals were studied after only one to two months of diabetes, at a time when structural lesions were not yet apparent. This degree of hyperglycemia was associated with increases of both whole kidney and superficial cortical SNGFR of about 40%. Thus the hyperfiltration observed in early human diabetes can be reproduced in animals with chemically induced diabetes.

Micropuncture studies demonstrated that the increase in SNGFR in this animal model was attributable to two factors. First, the plasma flow rate in single glomeruli was increased due to pronounced intrarenal vasodilatation of both the afferent and efferent arterioles. Second, the glomerular transcapillary hydraulic pressure gradient was increased and also contributed to the hyperfiltration. Of note, changes in the glomerular ultrafiltration coefficient did not contribute to the observed increase in SNGFR and, as in the clinical studies, there was no measurable fall in plasma protein concentration to account for increased filtration. Therefore, the higher values for GFR and SNGFR in diabetic rats were the result of the increased glomerular pressures and flows made possible by the acquired renal vasodilatation, a series of findings recently confirmed by others.[23,24]

We hypothesize that these early changes in intrarenal hemodynamics are a central causative factor in the initiation and progression of diabetic glomerulopathy. Support for this hypothesis derives from studies of animals with single-nephron hyperfiltration induced by renal ablation.[25,26] We removed approximately 90% of the functioning renal mass in nondiabetic rats by surgical ablation and infarction. One week after this maneuver the SNGFR values of the residual nephrons had more than doubled, due to marked increases in the same two determinants of SNGFR that accounted for the hyperfiltration observed in moderately hyper-glycemic diabetic rats. First, glomerular plasma flow rate was strikingly increased as a result of vasodilatation of both afferent and efferent arterioles. Second, the glomerular transcapillary hydraulic pressure gradient was increased. Additionally, the pronounced hyperfiltration in remnant nephrons was accompanied by clear evidence of glomerular structural damage. Specifically, morphologic studies demonstrated areas of detachment of glomerular epithelial cells from the underlying basement membrane as well as expansion of the mesangial area and the presence of dense droplets representing trapped plasma proteins in the glomeruli and proximal tubule epithelial cells. The functional correlate of these protein reabsorption droplets was a fourfold increase in protein excretion by these remnant kidneys. The pathophysiologic mechanism responsible for this proteinuria proved to be an impairment in both the size-selective and charge-selective barriers to macromolecule filtration that normally characterize the glomerular capillary wall. Thus both structure and permselective function were altered in the presence of extreme single-nephron hyperfiltration of one week's duration. Not only did proteinuria occur due to the disruption of glomerular capillary permselectivity, but this increased transglomerular movement of proteins resulted in their deposition in the mesangial regions of the glomerulus as well. This deposition was demonstrable by immunofluorescence microscopy but was also easily documented by the finding of enhanced accumulation of electron-dense ferritin particles in the mesangium after systemic injection of this tracer. Several workers have suggested that excessive mesangial deposition of circulating macromolecules might serve to increase the number of mesangial cells and to promote mesangial matrix deposition, forerunners of the glomerular sclerosis ultimately displayed by rats with this degree of renal ablation.[27,28]

Based on this correlation of readily apparent glomerular abnormalities and single-nephron hyperfiltration at this one-week interval after reduction in renal mass, we next sought to determine whether the increment in SNGFR (or its hemodynamic determinants) might be responsible for the eventual structural disruption observed.[25,26] We therefore studied a third group of rats with equivalent loss of renal mass in which the increment in SNGFR was blunted by placing the animals on a low-protein diet. This maneuver vitiated the increase in SNGFR observed in the rats fed a normal diet, by preventing the adaptive increases in glomerular plasma flow and the transcapillary hydraulic pressure gradient. Glomerular structural abnormalities of the type described above were also largely prevented in this group. Furthermore, urinary protein excretion was reduced to normal rates, due to the preservation of the normal permselective properties of the glomerular capillary wall. Finally, accumulation of circulating macromolecules by the glomerular mesangium was demonstrably attenuated in these animals and matrix formation was not increased. From these studies we have concluded that single-nephron hyperfiltration, or some hemodynamic determinant thereof, is a major cause of the observed glomerular injury and eventual sclerosis.

Thus it appears that irrespective of the nature of the initial destructive process that critically reduces renal mass, relatively spared glomeruli eventually undergo progressive damage that is largely independent of the nature of the initial injury and dependent only on some critical loss of renal mass. This general hypothesis may help to explain the clinical observation that patients with a wide variety of renal diseases regularly demonstrate a predictable progression from mild renal insufficiency to eventual overt renal failure.[29,30] Moreover, such progression has been documented even after the initiating insult has disappeared and other sustained damaging influences such as systemic hypertension are absent.[31,32] Thus a final common pathway of raised renal pressures and flows may underlie the ultimate sclerotic destruction of those glomeruli that survive an initial renal insult.

The pathogenetic importance of intrarenal hemodynamic alterations in diabetic glomerulopathy also receives support from a variety of observations made by others over the last decade. Steffes, Brown, and Mauer[33] compared the progression of mesangial expansion in streptozotocin-induced diabetic rats with or without unilateral nephrectomy. They found that the degree of mesangial deposition of circulating proteins, and mesangial widening, was far more marked in the diabetic animals with superimposed unilateral nephrectomy. Though intrarenal hemodynamics were not measured in this study, it is reasonable to assume that values for SNGFR, glomerular plasma flow rate, and glomerular hydraulic pressure were elevated above normal in the remnant kidneys of these diabetic rats as a result of contralateral nephrectomy.[34] Hence the authors' conclusion that "altered microcirculatory dynamics influence the rate of development of diabetic complications"[33] appears likely to be correct. Further studies by these same investigators using the streptozotocin model of diabetes in rats have defined the effects on the diabetic glomerular lesion of a unilateral renal artery clip, the so-called two-kidney Goldblatt hypertensive model.[35] Both diabetic and normal animals became hypertensive with this maneuver. Unclipped normotensive diabetic rats developed characteristic glomerular lesions equally in both kidneys. However, in diabetic rats with a unilateral renal artery clip, a distinct asymmetry in the development of these glomerular lesions was found in that the unclipped kidneys, exposed to the elevated systemic arterial pressure, showed more severe glomerular injury than did normotensive diabetic rats. Moreover, the clipped kidneys in the same diabetic animals showed lesser degrees of glomerulopathy than did the normotensive diabetic rats. This disparity between the two kidneys was present despite identical procedures for producing diabetes in the two diabetic groups, and despite equivalent degrees of hyperglycemia in normotensive and hypertensive animals. These studies clearly indicate that local, intrarenal alterations in hemodynamics can influence the glomerular structural changes characteristic of experimental diabetes. The clinical counterpart to these findings has also been reported[36] based on autopsy findings in a patient with diabetes and unilateral renal artery stenosis. Kimmelstiel–Wilson lesions were confined to the kidney with the patent renal artery while its contralateral partner with the tight stenosis had no such lesions. Finally, human diabetics with essential hypertension are believed to have more rapid progression of their renal insufficiency than do normotensive diabetics and recent studies by Mogensen indicate that treatment of the hypertension in these patients slows the progression to renal failure.[4] Taken together these clinical observations and experimental studies strongly suggest that renal hemodynamics exert a key influence on the initiation and progression of diabetic glomerulopathy.

We therefore suggest that the process leading to overt diabetic glomerulopathy is consistent with the general principle that sustained single-nephron hyperfiltration (or some hemodynamic determinant thereof) is ultimately detrimental to the glomerulus. Initiation of the glomerulopathic process in the diabetic derives from any or all of the following factors that are likely to eventuate in a pattern of sustained increases in glomerular pressures and flows: hyperglycemia-induced extracellular fluid volume expansion, structural hypertrophy of the kidney, and altered glucoregulatory or vasoregulatory hormone action. These hemodynamic alterations serve to increase SNGFR, which, in turn, augments the glomerular transcapillary convective flux of plasma proteins. These long-term changes in glomerular pressures and flows would also be expected to alter the permselective properties of the glomerulus and further increase protein filtration. Albuminuria is a direct result of this enhanced protein filtration and is demonstrable by ultrasensitive analytical techniques even at the onset of diabetes.[37-39] But perhaps of greater long-range import, this increased transglomerular traffic of proteins leads to their accumulation in the mesangium, thereby serving as a stimulus to proliferation of mesangial cells and matrix, with eventual glomerulosclerosis. Additional evidence is accumulating that altered renal hemodynamics may also exert direct effects on the mesangium.[40] Thus the renal hemodynamic alterations intrinsic to less than optimal metabolic control of diabetes would themselves *initiate* the process of glomerulosclerosis. With functional attrition of such sclerotic glomeruli, less severely afflicted glomeruli would undergo compensatory hyperfiltration, thereby closing a positive feedback loop favoring *progressive* glomerular injury and eventual loss of renal function.

The available data suggest that this process may be interrupted in its earliest or initiation phase. Indeed, Rasch[41,42] has prevented the glomerular structural changes characteristic of diabetes in rats by rigorously establishing euglycemia with exogenous insulin at the very onset of diabetes. At later stages, euglycemia achieved through pancreatic islet cell transplantation reverses many but not all of the structural changes in glomeruli of diabetic rats.[43,44] Though sufficient data are not yet available, it is reasonable to assume that the achievement of normal glucose metabolism is accompanied by a normalization of renal hemodynamics and we suggest that this latter effect accounts for the beneficial influence of such treatment on renal structure and function. In the late phases of progression, however, when GFR is frankly reduced and proteinuria is massive and nonselective, it seems unlikely that rigorous metabolic control alone will reverse the final common pathway leading to end-stage diabetic nephropathy. Hence it follows that the prevention of diabetic nephropathy will require that optimal insulin therapy to achieve euglycemia be initiated at the earliest stages in the disorder. To the extent that this may remain impractical, other maneuvers for preventing sustained glomerular hyperfiltration might prove beneficial, such as diuretics to reduce extracellular fluid volume, antihypertensive drugs, and possibly specific antagonists of hormone-induced renal vasodilation.

ACKNOWLEDGMENTS. This work was supported by a Clinical Investigator Award (AM00767) to Dr. Hostetter and grants from the Juvenile Diabetes Foundation and USPHS (AM19467). We are grateful to Ms. Lee Riley for secretarial assistance.

REFERENCES

1. Stalder G, Schmid R: Severe functional disorders of glomerular capillaries and renal hemodynamics in treated diabetes mellitus during childhood. *Ann Paediat* 193:129–138, 1959.
2. Ditzel J, Schwartz M: Abnromally increased glomerular filtration rate in short-term insulin-treated diabetic subjects. *Diabetes* 16:264–267, 1967.
3. Mogensen CE: Kidney function and glomerular permeability to macromolecules in early juvenile diabetes. *Scand J Clin Lab Invest* 28:91–100, 1971.
4. Mogensen CE: Renal function changes in diabetes. *Diabetes* 25:872–879, 1976.
5. Christiansen JS, Frandsen M, Parving H-H: The effect of intravenous insulin infusion on kidney function in insulin-dependent diabetes mellitus. *Diabetologia* 20:199–204, 1981.
6. Mogensen CE: Glomerular filtration rate and renal plasma flow in normal and diabetic man during elevation of blood sugar levels. *Scand J Clin Lab Invest* 28:177–182, 1971.
7. Brochtner-Mortensen J: The glomerular filtration rate during moderate hyperglycemia in normal man. *Acta Med Scand* 194:31–37, 1973.
8. Christiansen JS, Frandsen M, Parving H-H: Effect of intravenous glucose infusion on renal function in normal man and in insulin dependent diabetes. *Diabetologia* 21:368–373, 1981.
9. Osterby R, Gundersen HJG: Glomerular size and structure in diabetes mellitus. I. Early abnormalities. *Diabetologia* 11:225–229, 1975.
10. Seyer-Hansen K, Hansen J, Gundersen HJG: Renal hypertrophy in experimental diabetes. *Diabetologia* 18:501–505, 1980.

11. Unger RH: Diabetes and the alpha cell. *Diabetes* 25:136–151, 1976.
12. Lundbaek K: Growth hormone's role in diabetic microangiography. *Diabetes* 25(suppl. 2): 845–849, 1976.
13. Parving H-H, Christiansen JS, Noer I, et al: The effect of glucagon infusion on kidney function in short-term insulin-dependent juvenile diabetes. *Diabetologia* 19:350–354, 1980.
14. Corvilain J, Abramow M: Some effects of human growth hormone on renal hemodynamics and on tubular phosphate transport in man. *J Clin Invest* 41:1230–1235, 1962.
15. Christlieb AR: Renin, angiotensin, and norepinephrine in alloxan diabetes. *Diabetes* 23:962–970, 1974.
16. Christensen NJ: Plasma norepinephrine and epinephrine in untreated diabetics, during fasting and after insulin administration. *Diabetes* 23:1–8, 1974.
17. Johnson M, Reece AH, Harrison HE: An imbalance in arichadonic acid metabolism in diabetes. *Adv Prostaglandin Thromboxane Res* 8:1283–1286, 1980.
18. Altura BM, Halevy S, Turlapaty PDMV: Vascular smooth muscle in diabetes and its influence on the reactivity of blood vessels. *Adv Microcirc* 8:118–150, 1979.
19. Christlieb AR, Janica HU, Kraus B, et al: Vascular reactivity to angiotensin II and to norepinephrine in diabetic subjects. *Diabetes* 25:268–274, 1976.
20. Brenner BM, Humes HD: Mechanics of glomerular ultrafiltration. *N Engl J Med* 297:148–154, 1977.
21. Christiansen JS, Gammelgard J, Frandsen M, et al: Increased kidney size, glomerular filtration rate, and renal plasma flow in short term insulin-dependent diabetics. *Diabetologia* 20:451–456, 1981.
22. Hostetter TH, Troy JL, Brenner BM: Glomerular hemodynamics in experimental diabetes. *Kidney Int* 19:410–415, 1981.
23. Michels LD, Keane WF, Davidman M: Glomerular function and albuminuria in alloxan diabetes. The effects of insulin. *Clin Res* 28:455A, 1980.
24. Jensen PK, Christiansen JS, Steven K, et al: Renal hemodynamics in diabetic rats. *Diabetologia* 19:286, 1980.
25. Hostetter TH, Olson JL, Rennke HG, et al: Hyperfiltration in remnant nephrons: A potentially adverse response to renal ablation. *Am J Physiol* (in press).
26. Olson JL, Hostetter TH, Rennke HG, et al: Altered charge and size selective properties of the glomerular wall: A response to reduced renal mass. *Kidney Int* (in press).
27. Couser NG, Stilmant MM: Mesangial lesions and focal sclerosis in the aging rat. *Lab Invest* 33:491–501, 1975.
28. Velosa JA, Glasser RJ, Nevins TE, et al: Experimental model of focal sclerosis. II. Correlation with immunopathologic changes, macromolecular kinetics, and polyanion loss. *Lab Invest* 36:527–534, 1977.
29. Mitch WE, Walser M, Buffington CA, et al: A simple method for estimating progression of chronic renal failure. *Lancet* 4:1326–1328, 1976.
30. Rutherford WE, Blondin J, Miller JP, et al: Chronic progressive renal disease: Rate of change of serum creatinine. *Kidney Int* 11:62–70, 1977.
31. Kleinknecht D, Grunfeld JP, Comez PC, et al: Diagnostic procedures and long-term prognosis in bilateral renal cortical necrosis. *Kidney Int* 4:390–400, 1973.
32. Torres VE, Velosa JA, Holley KE, et al: The progression of vesicoureteral reflux. *Ann Int Med* 92:776–784, 1980.
33. Steffes MW, Brown DM, Mauer SM: Diabetic glomerulopathy following unilateral nephrectomy in the rat. *Diabetes* 27:35–41, 1978.

34. Deen WM, Maddox DA, Robertson CR, et al: Dynamics of glomerular ultrafiltration in the rat. VII: Response to reduced renal mass. *Am J Physiol* 227:556–562, 1974.
35. Mauer SM, Steffes MW, Azar S, et al: The effects of Goldblatt hypertension on development of the glomerular lesions of diabetes mellitus in the rat. *Diabetes* 27:738–744, 1978.
36. Berkman J, Rifkin H: Unilateral nodular diabetic glomerulosclerosis (Kimmelstiel–Wilson): Report of a case. *Metabolism* 22:715–722, 1973.
37. Viberti GC, Pickup JC, Jarett RJ, et al: Effect of control of blood glucose on urinary excretion of albumin and β_2 microgluculin in insulin-dependent diabetes. *N Engl J Med* 300:638–641, 1979.
38. Mogensen CE: Urinary albumin excretion in early and long-term juvenile diabetes. *Scand J Clin Lab Invest* 28:183–193, 1971.
39. Rasch R: Prevention of diabetic glomerulopathy in streptozotocin diabetic rats by insulin treatment: Albumin excretion. *Diabetologia* 18:413–416, 1980.
40. Raij L, Keane WF, Osswald H, et al: Mesangial function in ureteral obstruction in the rat. *J Clin Invest* 64:1204–1212, 1979.
41. Rasch R: Prevention of diabetic glomerulopathy in streptozotocin diabetic rats by insulin treatment: kidney size and glomerular volume. *Diabetologia* 16:125–128, 1979.
42. Rasch R: Prevention of diabetic glomerulopathy in streptozotocin diabetic rats by insulin treatment: Glomerular basement membrane thickness. *Diabetologia* 16:319–324, 1979.
43. Steffes MW, Brown DM, Basgen JM, et al: Amelioration of mesangial volume and surface alterations following islet transplantation in diabetic rats. *Diabetes* 29:509–515, 1980.
44. Steffes MW, Brown DM, Basgen JM, et al: Glomerular basement membrane thickness following islet transplantation in the diabetic rat. *Lab Invest* 41:116–118, 1979.

Section IV

Use and Misuse of Pharmacologic Agents in Kidney Disease

Active nephrology services are familiar with the high frequency of admissions resulting from complications of drug therapy. In one study, for example, 45% of all cases of acute renal failure were caused by toxic reactions to antibiotics. While it is reasonable to tolerate the still unavoidable deleterious side effects of cytotoxic drugs in order to sustain a kidney transplant, clinicians become uneasy about administering potent drugs whose value has not been substantiated. Both reports in this section are concerned with the desire to balance therapeutic effect against deleterious untoward reaction.

Physicians expect much of the medications they use. Digitalis can dramatically alter heart failure, insulin affects keto-acidosis, and antibiotics, infection. In renal diseases the benefit of drugs is less clear and even controversial because of the lack of good prospective studies.

As a closing to our state-of-the-art attempts at preventing renal failure, Hayslett interprets the maze of conflicting reports weighing "evidence that a pharmacologic agent can alter the rate of progression of a glomerular lesion . . . " For lipoid nephrosis, systematic necrotizing arteritis, and Wegener's granulomatosis, the verdict is that drugs are efficacious. On the other hand, for lupus glomerulopathy and other glomerulopathies, their worth is "ill defined and uncertain."

Adding to the problem of renal failure is the misuse of drugs such as analgesics and aminoglycosides, or simply too much of most medications with a falling filtration rate.

In a broader context, Maher has collected and digested a vast literature of substances exhibiting nephrotoxicity. We would be wise to heed Maher's caution that " . . . the contribution of toxin exposure to decreased renal function is easily overlooked and misinterpreted as nontoxic disease." It may also be underestimated and certainly under-reported. What must be learned from this section is a great respect for the pharmacologic tools we use. Meaning to do good is not sufficient reason to employ a regimen of dubious efficacy.

M.M.A.

9

Prevention of Glomerular Damage with Pharmacologic Agents

JOHN P. HAYSLETT

Histopathologic lesions in the glomerulus may result in increased protein excretion and/or a reduction in glomerular filtration rate, depending on the type and severity of the pattern of injury. In the absence of necrosis and replacement of normal structure with sclerosis it is usually assumed that there is a potential for reversibility. During the past 30 years a variety of pharmacologic agents have been employed clinically in the hope of hastening recovery by inducing resolution of the injury reaction or preventing progressive glomerular sclerosis with further decline in renal function. Since most forms of acquired glomerulopathy are presumably due to immunologic processes, therapeutic modalities have often been employed on the basis of their known or assumed action to alter immunologic responses, or their action to reduce inflammation or inhibit intravascular clotting. Despite this long experience, however, the pharmacologic basis for treating various patterns of glomerular injury remains empirical. Selection of individual pharmacologic agents for their effect on reversing or stabilizing different types of glomerular lesions is usually based on empirical clinical evidence that the cause of changes in renal function of treated patients is or is not more favorable than observed in nontreated patients. In some instances serial renal biopsies have been performed that provide information on changes in the underlying renal histopathologic lesion during the course of treatment.

In this analysis we summarize the evidence for the beneficial effect of pharmacologic agents on reversing or preventing progression of injury reactions in the glomerulus. Although a reduction in the degree of proteinuria is usually taken as a favorable sign, and may benefit the patient, there is no evidence that this effect alters the natural course of

JOHN P. HAYSLETT • Section of Nephrology, and Department of Internal Medicine, Yale University School of Medicine, New Haven, Connecticut.

disease. Our discussion, therefore, does not include disease entities such as lipoid nephrosis where there is a clear evidence that glucocorticoids and some cytotoxic agents are capable of reversing heavy proteinuria and/or reducing the frequency of clinical relapse.[1,2]

Therapeutic agents used to treat glomerulopathies include synthetic glucocorticoid substances. These agents have been administered chronically in daily doses eight to 20 times higher than physiologic production rate or as "pulse therapy" in which doses approximately 200 times higher than physiologic levels are administered intermittently for periods of up to several weeks. A second category of therapeutic agents that has been extensively employed includes "cytotoxic" drugs. These pharmacologic agents, originally introduced to treat malignant processes or to prevent organ transplant rejection, include alkylating drugs, such as cyclophosphamide and chlorambucil, and antipurines, such as azathioprine and 6-mercaptopurine. Last, anticoagulants such as heparin and dipyridamole, an antithrombotic agent that reduces platelet adhesiveness, have been used to inhibit intravascular coagulation.[3]

The efficacy of a particular pharmacologic agent in treating patients with clinical and histopathologic signs of glomerular disease is usually correlated with different categories of glomerular disease. Classification of glomerular disease remains imprecise since the etiology and pathogenesis of only a few types are understood. For practical purposes, therefore, criteria for classification include (1) histopathologic features by light microscopy and (2) associated clinical features, as shown in Table I. Subclassification is often made on the basis of histologic changes found by electromicroscopy and immunofluorescent studies of renal biopsy material.

Analysis of the effect of pharmacologic agents in reversing or

Table I. Classification of Glomerulonephropathies

1. Histopathology
   Epithelial cell involvement
      Epithelial cell disease
      Focal segmental glomerulosclerosis
   Membranous glomerulonephropathy
   Glomerular inflammatory disease
   Chronic glomerulonephritis
2. Associated clinical features
   Hemolysis, thrombocytopenia–hemolytic–uremic syndrome
   Pulmonary hemorrhage and crescentic lesions—Goodpasture's syndrome
   Anti-DNA antibodies, antinuclear antibodies—lupus nephropathy
   Lesions of necrotizing arteritis in respiratory tract—Wegener's granulomatosis

preventing progression of glomerular injury reactions is complicated by two major factors. First, the imprecise and probably inaccurate classification of specific disease entities results in an undesired degree of heterogeneity in patient populations. Second, most disease entities of clinical interest are characterized by a marked variation in clinical course and rate of progression of the histopathologic lesion. Appropriate safeguards to account for this latter factor have been taken only infrequently in most reported clinical trials. Uncontrolled and inadequately controlled clinical trials do not provide scientific evidence, in the usual sense, and can only be used as offering "suggestive" evidence that an individual therapeutic modality is capable of altering the natural course of a glomerular lesion.

Evidence that a pharmacologic agent can alter the rate of clinical progression of a glomerular lesion is provided by the effect of glucocorticoids on the course of idiopathic membranous nephropathy. In a prospective, randomized study of 72 adult patients with idiopathic membraneous nephropathy, treatment with prednisone in a dose of 100 to 150 mg every other day, depending on body weight, was shown to reduce the rate of deterioration of glomerular filtration rate compared with subjects treated with placebo during an average period of observation of 23 months.[4] As shown in Table II, only one of 34 treated patients progressed to renal failure (serum creatinine more than 5 mg/dl) or death by the end of follow-up, compared with 10 of 38 patients given placebo. Treatment with predisone, however, had no increased benefit over placebo in reducing protein excretion during the observation period.

Despite lack of comparable prospective studies in other types of glomerular injury, recent evidence suggests that cytotoxic agents are useful in modifying diseases due to systemic necrotizing arteritis. For example, Fauci and associates[5] reported a retrospective analysis of 17 patients with evidence of severe systemic vasculitis, including renal involvement in 13, treated with glucocorticoids and cyclophosphamide or azathioprine. Although detailed information on initial renal function was not provided, complete clinical remission, and often angiographic improvement, occurred in the 14 surviving patients. Apparent dramatic

Table II. Collaborative Study of the Adult Idiopathic Nephrotic Syndrome[a]

	Control	Prednisone Rx
Doubling of serum C_r	10/38	1/34 $p < 0.02$
Remission of proteinuria	5/38	9/34 $p =$ n.s.

[a] N Engl J Med 301:1301–1306, 1979; mean follow-up—24 months.

improvement has also been reported in patients with Wegener's granulomatosis treated with glucocorticoids in combination with cytotoxic
drugs. In the largest reported series 21 patients with this diagnosis were
treated with cyclophosphamide and prednisone.[6] Of 14 patients with
clinical and/or biopsy findings of renal involvement, renal function (on the
basis of serum creatinine values) remained normal in six, worsened in
four, and improved markedly in four. Not surprisingly, a lack of response
usually was found in patients with severe renal failure at onset of
treatment with cyclophosphamide. It is of interest that the use of cytotoxic
agents has also been associated with a high rate of improvement of
extrarenal lesions, including lesions in the upper respiratory tract and
pulmonary sites.[7] Although these studies were not controlled and the
course of patients treated with cytotoxic agents over the past decade
should not be compared with previously reported series, the generally
poor response of these disorders to glucocorticoids used alone is strongly
suggestive that cytotoxic drugs are effective in suppressing the inflammatory reaction that characterizes systemic arteriti s.

Lupus nephropathy is a major course of morbidity and mortality in
patients with systemic lupus erythomatosus (SLE), and is established as an
immune complex disorder. Although there has been no prospective study
comparing glucocorticoids with a non-steroid-treated group, treatment
with prednisone, in a realtively high daily dose in patients with moderately
severe lupus glomerulonephritis, was demonstrated markedly to improve
the glomerular lesion by light microscopy and to preserve renal function.[8]
The effect of cytotoxic agents in lupus glomerulonephropathy remains
undetermined. Results of two of the larger controlled studies are
equivocal, but are briefly summarized. In a report by Decker et al.[9] a
comparison of groups of about ten patients each treated with either
cyclophosphamide, azathioprine, or prednisone demonstrated a slight
benefit of each cytotoxic agent as compared with prednisone alone. In this
study patients were not randomized on the basis of the renal lesion and
some patients appear in both treatment groups. In the controlled study by
Donadio, Holley, Ferguson et al.[10] comparison of prednisone treatment
with treatment consisting of prednisone plus cyclophosphamide in 50
patients with a diffuse glomerulonephritis showed that the proportion of
patients alive after four years with stable or improved renal function was
similar in the two groups. The authors reported, however, that a higher
incidence and average rate of clinical recurrence of nephritis occurred in
the group initially treated with only steroids than in the group initially
given both therapeutic agents. It should be noted that although follow-up
averaged four years, cyclophosphamide was administered for only six
months. Treatment with cytotoxic agents, in combination with steriods, has

also been associated with substantial improvement in the underlying renal lesion. In a study of 31 patients with moderately severe glomerulonephritis and subendothelial electron-dense deposits, treatment with low-dose prednisone and azathioprine, for an average of 40 months, resulted in a marked histologic and clinical improvement in two thirds of patients, including reduction of glomerular inflammation, disappearance of subendothelial deposits and, concurrently, clinical improvement.[11]

Numerous reports, based on uncontrolled therapeutic trials, attest to the apparent efficacy of specific pharmacologic agents in the treatment of many types of glomerular disorders; these agents include daily and "pulse" steroid therapy, cytotoxic drugs, and anticoagulants in the treatment of crescentic glomerulonephritis, hemolytic–uremic syndrome, membranoproliferative glomerulonephritis, and similar clinical disorders. Although pilot studies of this type are often helpful in identifying potentially useful forms of treatment, the study of glomerular disease has unfortunately not included subsequent well-designed, controlled clinical trials. Usually untreated comparison groups are represented by a previously observed series of patients from the same institution or reported series of patients by other authors. It seems clear, however, that such comparisons are not valid since marked differences in the natural course and the course of treated patients with the same types of glomerular lesions have been clearly demonstrated to occur in the same and different institutions. In addition, changes in diagnostic criteria, supportive therapy, referral populations,and other variables influence rates of morbidity and mortality. For example, the high death rate of 80% to 90% in patients with diffuse lupus glomerulonephritis, reported in the early 1960s,[12] was not observed in the subsequent decade.[11,13,14] Another example concerns the glomerular lesion of crescentic glomerulonephritis. Most clinicians regard the presence of extensive crescent formation, especially if 50% or more of the glomerular population is involved, as an ominous prognostic sign that is associated with rapid loss of renal function.[15,16] Although histopathologic evidence for immune complex or anti-GBM nephritis has been reported in most series, Stilmant et al.[17] reported that 35% of 46 patients in their series with acute crescentic glomerulonephritis lacked evidence for an immune-mediated process. Moreover, nearly 30% of these patients exhibited signs of pulmonary hemorrhage as well as a crescentic glomerular lesion, hallmark features of Goodpasture's syndrome, and the correlation between percent of crescents, initial severity of disease, and ultimate outcome was poor. These data, along with recent reports of clinical improvement in more than one half of patients with crescentic glomerulonephritis,[17,18] suggest substantial heterogeneity in patient populations characterized by this clinicopathologic disease entity and highlight the practical difficulty and pitfalls of attempting to evaluate therapeutic modalities in the absence of randomized prospective clinical trials.

The task of discussing the prevention of glomerular damage with pharmacologic agents is severely limited by the available data. Prospective well-designed clinical trials are urgently needed to determine, on an empirical basis, whether acquired glomerular lesions can be modified by treatment. These trials must take into account the features of the histopathologic lesion, the chronic nature of most types of glomerulone-phritis, and the broad spectrum of clinical course, even in apparently well-defined disease entities. Until these goals are met, clinical decisions regarding management of patients with glomerular lesions will remain ill defined and uncertain.

REFERENCES

1. Siegel NJ, Goldberg B, Krassner LS, et al: Long-term followup of children with steroid-responsive nephrotic syndrome. *J Pediat* 81:251–258, 1972.
2. Barratt TM, Soothill JF: Controlled trial of cyclophosyphamide in steroid-sensitive relapsing nephrotic syndrome of children. *Lancet* 2:479–482, 1970.
3. Arieff AI, Piggera WF: Rapidly progressive glomerulonephritis treated with antico-agulants. *Arch Inter Med* 129:77–84, 1972.
4. Collaborative Study of the Adult Idiopathic Nephrotic Syndrome: A controlled study of short-term predinsone treatment in adults with membranous nephropathy. *N Engl J Med* 301:1301–1306, 1979.
5. Fauci AS, Katz P, Haynes BF, et al: Cyclophosphamide therapy of severe necrotizing vasculities. *N Engl J Med* 301:235–238, 1979.
6. NIH conference, Wolff SM (moderator): Wegener's granulomatosis. *Ann Intern Med* 81:513–525, 1979.
7. Novack SN, Pearson CM: Cyclophosphamide therapy in Wegener's granulomatosis. *N Engl J Med* 284:938–942, 1971.
8. Donadio JV, Holley KE, Wagoner RD, et al: Treatment of lupus nephritis with prednisone and combined prednisone and azathioprine. *Ann Intern Med* 77:829–835, 1972.
9. Decker JL, Kluppel JH, Plotz PN, et al: Cyclophosphamide or azathioprine in lupus glomerulonephritis. *Ann Intern Med* 83:606–615, 1975.
10. Donadio JV, Holley KE, Ferguson RN, et al: Treatment of diffuse proliferative lupus nephritis with prednisone and combined predinsone and cyclophosphamide. *N Engl J Med* 299:1151–1155, 1978.
11. Hecht B, Siegel NJ, Adler M, et al: Prognostic indices of lupus nephritis. *Medicine* 55:163–181, 1976.
12. Pollak VE, Pirani CL, Kark RM: Effect of large doses of prednisone on the renal lesions and life span of patients with lupus glomerulonephritis. *J Lab Clin Med* 57:495–511, 1961.
13. Mahajan SK, Ordonez NC, Feitelson PJ, et al: Lupus nephropathy without clinical renal involvement. *Medicine* 56:493–501, 1977.
14. Appel GB, Silva FG, Pirani CL, et al: Renal involvement in systemic lupus erythematosus (SLE). *Medicine* 57:371–410, 1978.

15. Beirne GJ, Wagnlid JP, Zimmerman SW, et al: Idiopathic crescentic glomerulonephritis. *Medicine* 56:349–381, 1977.

16. Whiteworth VA, Morel-Maroger L, Megnon F, et al: The significance of extracapillary proliferation. Clinicopathological review of 60 patients. *Nephron* 16:1–19, 1976.

17. Stilmant NM, Bolton WK, Sturgill BC, et al: Crescentic glomerulonephritis without immune deposits: Clinicopathologic features. *Kidney Inter* 15:184–195, 1979.

18. Bolton WK, Couser WC: Intravenous pulse methyleprednisolone therapy of acute crescentic rapidly progressive glomerulonephritis. *Am J Med* 66:995–502, 1979.

10

Prognosis and Prevention of Renal Failure Induced by Toxins

JOHN F. MAHER

Deleterious functional effects caused by nephrotoxins can result when such noxious agents induce renal failure *de novo*, either acutely or chronically, or when preexisting impairment of renal function is aggravated by toxin exposure. Severe acute renal failure can usually be recognized easily. Moreover, the association with acute toxin exposure is often apparent, although its role may not be appreciated in patients with coexistent problems such as septicemia and shock. Chronic nephrotoxicity and toxicity superimposed on chronic renal impairment are frequently more difficult to diagnose.

Although the contribution of nephrotoxicity to the prevalence of irreversible renal failure cannot be defined precisely, toxins do account for 20% of acute renal failure and analgesic nephropathy causes 3% of end-stage renal disease.[1] Under certain circumstances, these percentages are much higher. For example, a higher fraction of renal failure is caused by toxins in children, the elderly, Australians, and those with certain underlying diseases such as diabetes mellitus.

Acute renal failure is generally considered a reversible lesion from which full recovery can be anticipated. Some toxins, however, induce irreversible acute renal failure. Examples include methyl CCNU[2] and amphotericin B[3]. After recovery from toxic tubular necrosis, renal function returns to normal and remains so indefinitely in most patients.[4] Whether chronic interstitial fibrosis is preceded by acute partially reversible renal

JOHN F. MAHER ● Division of Nephrology, Uniformed Services University of the Health Sciences School of Medicine, Bethesda, Maryland. The opinions or assertions contained herein are the private views of the author and should not be construed as official or as necessarily reflecting the views of the Uniformed Services University of the Health Sciences or Department of Defense. There are no objections to its presentation and/or publication.

failure in an important fraction of patients remains to be established. Exposure to toxins known to induce chronic disease is a more frequently recognized antecedent of end-stage renal disease than is an episode of acute renal failure in the remote past. On the other hand, acceleration of the progression of renal failure by acute exposure to such toxins as organic iodides is observed frequently

Obviously, nephrotoxicity does not have an identifiable universal prognosis since this segment of nephrology covers many syndromes of varied causes. Accordingly, the outlook for renal functional loss and its prevention cannot be addressed *in toto*, but only in reference to specific circumstances. Moreover, the data base is not precise since diagnostic inaccuracy includes some cases inappropriately and excludes others erroneously and, as in other areas of clinical nephrology, much of the reported data is uncontrolled and anecdotal.

Many factors affect the prognosis in specific forms of toxic nephropathy. Some are subtle, generally not recognized, and rarely measured in clinical studies. These include such determinants of drug metabolism as microsomal cytochrome P 450 oxygenases, which biotransform furan compounds into toxic chemically active metabolites within the kidney,[5] and the genetically determined rate of acetylation of such drugs as procainamide. More easily quantified factors that determine the prognosis of nephrotoxin exposure are those listed in Table I.

The nature of the renal injury varies according to the toxin. Table II outlines the types of lesions that may be encountered and lists illustrative toxins. It should be noted that the dose, duration of exposure, and type of chemical compound can influence the resultant lesion. Accordingly, acute exposure to a highly toxic dose of inorganic mercury causes oliguric renal failure whereas lower doses—for example, in the organic form—cause

Table I. Factors Affecting the Prognosis of Nephrotoxin Exposure

1. The nature of the resultant renal injury
2. Chemical properties of the toxin
3. Antecedent renal or extrarenal lesions
4. The effects of age on vasculature and pharmacokinetics
5. Hemodynamics and hydration
6. Mechanisms of renal elimination
7. Concurrent exposure to other toxins
8. Preexisting hypersensitivity
9. The dose and route of administration
10. The duration and continuity of exposure
11. The interval from the onset of toxicity to cessation of exposure
12. The capability of removing the toxin

Table II. Clinical Spectrum of Nephrotoxicity

Nephrotoxic syndromes	Illustrative causes
Renal ischemia	Indomethacin, naproxen
Acute renal vasculitis	Sulfonamides
Necrotizing glomerulonephritis	Petroleum fuels, bacitracin
Extracapillary glomerulonephritis	Substituted benzidines
Lipoid nephrosis	Oxazoladines
Membranous glomerulonephritis	D-penicillamine, gold
Tubular injury	
a. Tubular acidosis	Amphotericin B
b. Fanconi syndrome	Heavy metals
c. Nephrogenic diabetes insipidus	Lithium, demeclocycline
d. Acute renal failure	Aminoglycosides, iodides
Reversible interstitial nephritis	Penicillins, rifampin
Progressive interstitial nephritis	Methyl CCNU
Nephrocalcinosis	Vitamin D
Intrinsic acute urinary obstruction	Uricosurics, methotrexate
Papillary necrosis	Analgesics
Periureteral fibrosis	Methysergide, radiation
Uroepithelial carcinoma	Analgesics, aniline dyes
Renal cysts	Biphenyl

milder proximal tubular injury that manifests the Fanconi syndrome. When chronic exposure to a metallotoxin such as mercury causes prolonged injury to the proximal tubular cells, the resultant release of renal tubular epithelial antigens may induce immune complex membranous glomerulonephritis with nephrotic syndrome and slow progression to renal failure.

The influence of the chemical form of a solute on its toxicity is overtly exemplified by the greater safety of heavy metals when administered in organic rather than inorganic form. Other examples of varied toxicity among a specific class of drugs include the higher incidence of acute interstitial nephritis with the semisynthetics, ampicillin and methicillin, than with penicillin, and the dependence of sulfonamide toxicity on the solubility of the particular congener. Aminoglycosides also exhibit nephrotoxicity of varying severity, related in part to their affinity for proximal tubular epithelium. The relative nephrotoxicity of aminoglycoside congeners[6] is shown in Table III.

Included among the toxic renal lesions are several that should reverse spontaneously on withdrawal of the offending agent or with drug therapy. The acute decline in renal function that occurs in selected patients when blockade of prostaglandin synthetase results from nonsteroidal anti-inflammatory agents is typically reversible when the drug is stopped.[7]

Table III. Relative Nephrotoxicity of Aminoglycosides

Neomycin (most toxic)
Gentamycin
Kanamycin
Amikacin
Sisomycin
Tobramycin
Netilmicin
Streptomycin (least toxic)

Whether prolonged exposure causes ischemic damage in susceptible patients is not known. Occasionally, exposure to such drugs causes interstitial nephritis and nephrotic syndrome, possibly by unrelated mechanisms.[8] Unexplained decrements in renal function in patients taking such drugs calls for their cessation.

Severe necrotizing glomerular lesions, whether associated with toxin exposure or not, may progress to renal failure despite the use of prednisone, immunosuppressive drugs, and other treatments such as plasmapheresis. Nevertheless, a review of published cases suggests that improvement of toxic glomerular lesions, with or without therapeutic intervention, may be more likely to occur than in spontaneous glomerulo-nephritides.

Direct tubular toxins cause necrosis of varying severity correlating roughly with the dose. Mild lesions manifest only transport defects such as tubular acidosis (amphotericin) or impaired water conservation (lithium). With persistent exposure or higher doses, nonoliguric acute renal failure can occur, while even greater doses induce more severe lesions and oliguria. Whereas continued exposure to the toxin does not preclude spontaneous recovery in animals, the experience with patients is often more persistent or even irreversible acute renal failure when exposure continues after the onset of oliguria. Monitoring of specific aspects of renal function is important in such patients so that early detection of functional abnormalities and prompt cessation of the drugs or lowering of the dose can prevent more severe irreversible changes.

Hypersensitivity acute interstitial nephritis also can follow a variable course mainfesting predominantly tubular functional abnormalities with only modest renal failure. Conversely, acute oliguria may accompany intense interstitial inflammation and edema. The interval to spontaneous recovery is unpredictable in a given case, but may be accelerated by prednisone therapy.[9] A progressive form of acute interstitial nephritis may begin after treatment of malignancy with methyl CCNU.[2] This irreversible

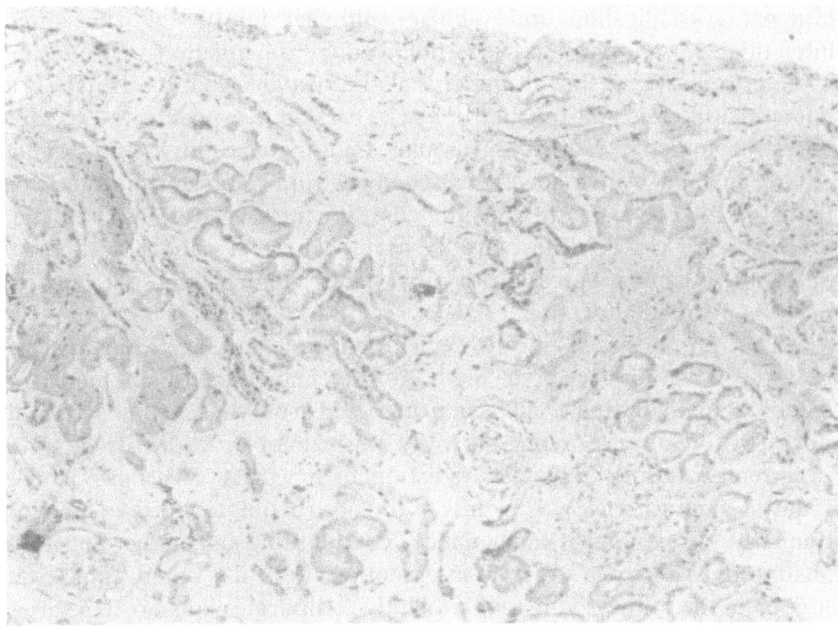

Figure 1. Low-power H and E stained section of renal cortex demonstrates marked tubular atrophy and relatively acellular interstitial reaction in a case of methyl CCNU nephrotoxicity.

lesion is characterized by severe tubular atrophy and interstitial fibrosis with little cellular reaction (Figure 1) somewhat reminiscent of the findings of radiation nephritis except for the absence of vascular abnormalities. Since toxicity appears to correlate with cumulative dose but does not become manifest for several months thereafter, the dose should be monitored carefully and limited.

Chronic interstitial nephritis can follow tubular injury, for example, from lead or cadmium, crystalline deposits, such as from vitamin D induced hypercalcemia, or papillary necrosis after analgesic abuse. Discontinuation of exposure is not easily accomplished with analgesic abusers because of poor compliance and may not decrease the body burden in the case of lead intoxication unless chelation is employed.[10] Accordingly, improvement occurs slowly, if at all, and correlates inversely with the extent of interstitial fibrosis and the increase in plasma creatinine concentration. Prevention requires awareness of the association of renal failure with such toxins, early detection, and actual cessation of exposure before advanced disease occurs.

In the case of crystalline injury, it has been shown that after initial lumenal crystallization and tubular epithelial injury, the subsequent interstitial crystallization can be followed by an inflammatory reaction leading to disappearance of the crystals but progression, nevertheless, to interstitial fibrosis and renal atrophy.[11] Years after exposure to excessive doses of ionizing radiation, vascular endothelial injury and tubular epithelial damage are followed by ischemic atrophy and chronic interstitial fibrosis with a relentlessly downhill clinical course even though radiation exposure has ceased. These are examples where cessation of exposure does not prevent progression to renal failure. Rather, high-dose toxicity must be avoided altogether.

The prognosis of intrinsic obstruction to urinary drainage, for example, from uric acid or methotrexate, may depend on increasing solubility by hydration or altering urinary pH,[12] or when a stone or papilla obstructs, on physical removal, while extrinsic obstruction secondary to periureteral fibrosis following radiation or a variety of drugs[13] usually requires surgical release or bypass of the obstruction to improve function. Similarly, uroepithelial malignancy complicating analgesic abuse or analine dyes requires urologic intervention.[14] On the other hand, cystic lesions of the kidney, which infrequently complicate exposure to a variety of chemicals,[15] are not amenable to treatment and can only be prevented by the awareness to avoid such exposures.

The variable incidence and severity of renal lesions in response to nephrotoxin exposure are in part related to the preexisting health of the individual. For example, severe renal ischemia following exposure to aspirin, indomethacin, or other nonsteroidal anti-inflammatory drugs occurs in those who depend on high levels of the vasodilator prostaglandin E to maintain renal blood flow despite excessive angiotensin-mediated vasoconstriction resulting from such causes as systemic lupus erythematosus or cardiac failure.[7] Inhibition of prostaglandin synthetase under this circumstance blocks the compensatory vasodilation and thereby induces reversible renal ischemia.

Preexisting impairment of the normal extrarenal elimination pathway allows increased delivery of such toxins as cholecystographic agents to the kidney.[16] The extent of extrarenal elimination determines, in part, the dose delivered to the kidney and thereby the severity of the resultant lesion. With arteriographic or pyelographic dyes normally eliminated by the kidney, the severity of antecedent renal insufficiency determines the persistence of the iodide in circulation and increases the risk of nephrotoxicity.[17] Although the dose eliminated by the kidney is no greater than in health, the dose per functioning nephron is increased. The persistence of organomercurials in blood allows more metabolism to the inorganic, more toxic radical but such a phenomenon has not been demonstrated for organic iodides. It is not clear why iodide toxicity is more likely in patients with diabetes mellitus or myeloma, nor why such acute oliguria often persists. Obviously, the organic iodides must be used prudently in such patients and avoided altogether, if possible.

Resistance to some types of nephrotoxic injury, such as the glycerol hemoglobinuric model, characterizes the recovery phase of acute renal failure. On the other hand, the growing or regenerating kidney has increased susceptibility to a given dose of other potential toxins, for example, radiation, and reduction of renal mass augments the toxicity that results from a given dose of inorganic mercury. To prevent renal injury, these factors should be recalled before exposing a patient to the potential toxins.

Both the young and the elderly are especially vulnerable to nephrotoxic injury. The young are more susceptible because of growing kidneys and an increased risk of overdosage of drugs and toxins. The elderly are especially vulnerable because of inapparent decrements in elimination kinetics and of vascular disease predisposing to ischemia. Physicians must be especially careful in quantifying dosages for these two age extremes.

When elimination of a toxic solute depends primarily on the kidney, the specific mechanism of excretion determines, in part, the potential risk. Inhibition of the secretory pathway of a toxin can decrease the concentration within the cell, lowering the toxic potential,[18] whereas renal ischemia, by decreasing filtration, increases the plasma concentration delivered to the secretory pathway. On the other hand, when toxic solutes are reabsorbable, intracellular concentrations can be increased by augmented reabsorption during ischemia or dehydration. This provides a rationale for the use of osmotic diuretics to prevent renal injury on exposure to certain toxins.

On exposure to a given dose of a nephrotoxin, hemodynamic factors affect the severity of the functional change. Clinical and laboratory observations have repeatedly suggested that extracellular fluid volume depletion increases the likelihood of inducing renal failure, whereas prolonged saline loading protects renal function either by decreasing renin or by tubular factors.[19] Despite uncertainty about the mechanism, it is apparent that overt renal failure can be prevented by saline loading before exposure to certain potential toxins.

The state of hydration obviously influences vulnerability to intrarenal or urinary precipitation of such toxins as methotrexate or sulfonamides, such metabolites as oxalate, or those solutes excreted in excess because of the toxin's effect such as uric acid. Dehydration also increases the concentration of toxins in the renal medulla, which may explain the recognized concurrence of laxative abuse and analgesic nephropathy.[20] Irritation of the uroepithelium (e.g., cyclophosphamide hemorrhagic cystitis) is also less likely with forced diuresis. Intratubular obstruction by hemoglobinuric or myoglobinuric casts should be diminished by forced diuresis but, *post facto*, potent diuretics can be harmful by stimulating renin. In general, prophylaxis of nephrotoxicity is more likely achieved by hydrating the patient than by artificially increasing the urine volume.

Clinically, acute antibiotic nephrotoxicity often follows exposure to several toxins simultaneously, but synergism is not proved easily.[21] Because nephrotoxicity frequently occurs when hemodynamic abnormalities of heart failure, dehydration, or infection preexist, the contribution of a specific agent is not readily discerned. Gentamicin combined with a cephalosporin, however, causes a higher incidence of renal lesions than when combined with methicillin. When possible, such toxic combinations should be avoided or used only briefly until the best single agent is identified.

Not only does concurrent nephrotoxin exposure or use of furosemide (a stimulator of renin and a determinant of transport) increase cephalosporin toxicity but prior hypersensitivity to cephalosporins or penicillins raises the risk as well. Moreover, repeated exposure to phenytoin has caused recurrent episodes of acute interstitial nephritis with recovery after each episode, even though presensitization would predict a more extensive and less reversible lesion.[23] When a potential nephroallergen cannot be avoided, such patients should be monitored carefully, particularly if vulnerability is increased.

Except for cephaloridine, excessive doses of the cephalosporins are required to induce toxicity unless the drug elimination is impaired. A dose/toxicity relationship has also been established for aminoglycoside and polymyxin antibiotics, amphotericin, *cis*-platinum, lithium, analgesics, and several other drugs. Because the margin of safety of some of these drugs is quite narrow, dosage must be carefully titrated against blood levels or modified when the earliest signs of toxicity appear. Hypersensitivity interstitial nephritis due to methicillin also occurs more frequently, however, at high doses than at low doses. The route of administration also determines the toxic potential since some toxins, neomycin, for example, are absorbed poorly from the gastrointestinal tract.

When delayed elimination of drugs such as gentamicin increases toxicity, it correlates with the trough rather than the peak plasma concentration, but relates even more closely to the renal cortical concentration of the toxin.[24] The typical onset of toxicity after ten days of treatment is consistent with gradual accumulation of the aminoglycoside in the renal cortex from which elimination occurs slowly. When the same total dose of gentamicin is given in short rather than long dosing intervals, renal failure is more likely, which dissociates nephrotoxicity and the peak plasma concentration.[25] It is therefore safer to increase the dosing interval than to decrease the single dose.

For certain toxins, the duration and continuity of exposure influence the likelihood of nephrotoxicity. The chronic toxicity of mixed analgesics, gold, or lithium requires months or years to develop and interruption of exposure during the early stages induces at least partial healing. Conversely, the interstitial nephritis associated with such drugs as rifampin typically occurs after interrupted therapy, suggesting sensitization and a serum sickness-like abnormality.[26] In further contrast, radiation nephritis correlates with the peak exposure and is decreased by fractionation of the dose.[27]

Acute aminoglycoside nephrotoxicity often begins insidiously with enzymuria, saluresis, and proteinuria that may be completely reversible. Depending on the dose and other factors, 10% to 30% of patients develop measurable renal insufficiency after 14 days of treatment.[28] When gentamicin therapy has been discontinued before azotemia occurs, mild renal insufficiency may still follow, but the prognosis is usually quite good. Even 24 hours after the onset of azotemia, stopping the drug may abort the acute renal failure, which often is nonoliguric. Continuing gentamicin after renal failure has begun leads to accumulation of the drug in plasma and in the kidney and severe, prolonged oliguria with a mortality rate that may approach 50% (Figure 2). Such a vicious cycle causing severe renal failure can be prevented by careful clinical monitoring and prompt cessation of the drug at the first signs of toxicity.

Papillary necrosis, interstitial nephritis, and chronic renal failure correlate with the cumulative analgesic dose. Early recognition can abort overt toxicity and diagnosis before the late stages allows discontinuation of the drugs early enough for improvement in renal function and increased renal mass to occur.[29] With more advanced lesions, renal function may stabilize on cessation of analgesics or progress more slowly than anticipated.[30] Abstinence can be monitored by urinary excretion of N-acetyl-para-aminophenol, but is difficult to achieve.

The continuing dose-dependent and potentially reversible renal damage of analgesic nephropathy contrasts with radiation and methyl CCNU nephritis. Because of the long interval between exposure and toxicity, the progressive interstitial fibrosis cannot be prevented, reversed, or delayed after excessive exposure. Similarly, although glomerulone-phritis has been associated with hydrocarbon exposure,[31] once this lesion has commenced it progresses without continued exposure.

From the dose/toxicity relationship it appears that the severity and

110

John F. Maher

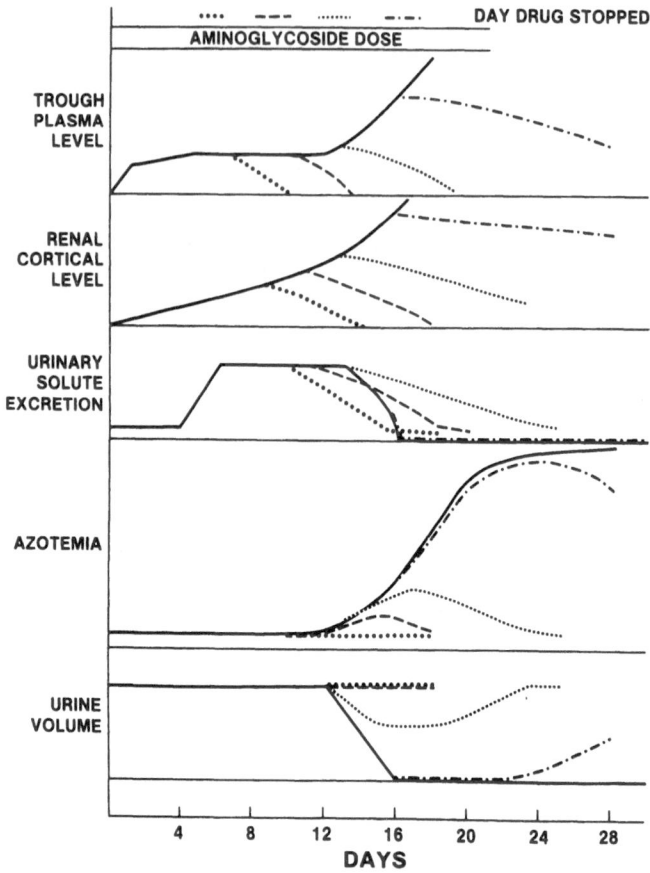

Figure 2. The effect of duration of aminoglycoside exposure on manifestations of nephrotoxicity is illustrated.

duration of nephrotoxic lesions might be lessened by augmented elimination of the toxin, but such a hypothesis has not been proved for most toxins. We have treated, by early dialysis, a patient who inadvertently was overdosed with neomycin parenterally and recovered uneventfully without evidence of ototoxicity or nephrotoxicity. Our anecdote and other reports[32] do not demonstrate that nephrotoxicity was prevented, however, since there were no comparable untreated patients. Similarly, early dialysis after organic iodide, or halogenated hydrocarbon, or ethylene glycol poisoning has not been shown to prevent or lessen oliguria despite some encouraging anecdotal experiences.[33] On the other hand, lowering excessive plasma concentrations of uric acid by dialysis can reverse acute nephrotoxicity.[34] With heavy metal intoxication or acute hypercalcemia, early dialysis may improve well-being and possibly the survival rate, but tissue deposits are affected only minimally and renal failure usually persists nevertheless. It is apparent, therefore, that for nephrotoxic lesions, removal of the offending agent after the injury has occurred induces reversibility only infrequently and slowly, if at all.

Because nephrotoxins induce a variety of clinical nephrologic syndromes, the prognosis is quite diverse. Nephrotoxic acute renal failure usually has a better prognosis for survival than ischemic injury but may have a higher incidence of such late sequelae as interstitial fibrosis. When chronic renal failure results from exposure to toxins, the prognosis may be better than it is with nontoxic causes because progression can sometimes be delayed or reversed by cessation of exposure. The course of chronic renal failure due to natural causes, although unpredictable, progresses downhill in a given patient at an orderly, diagnosis specific, rate.[35] When deterioration accelerates, a variety of correctable factors should be sought. These include hemodynamic insults, infection, obstruction, and nephrotoxin exposure. The outlook can be improved by early detection of nephrotoxic lesions, greater awareness of the hazards of environmental toxins, especially for patients who have increased susceptibility, careful monitoring of dosage, and, when possible, total avoidance of nephrotoxins.

REFERENCES

1. Maher JF: Toxic and irradiation nephropathies, in Earley LE, Gottschalk CW (eds): *Strauss and Welt's Diseases of the Kidney*. Boston, Little, Brown and Co, 1978, pp 1431–1474.
2. Harmon WE, Cohen HJ, Schneeberger EE, et al: Chronic renal failure in children treated with methyl CCNU. *N Engl J Med* 300:1200–1203, 1979.
3. Takacs FJ, Tomkiewicz AM, Merrill JP: Amphotericin B nephrotoxicity with irreversible renal failure. *Ann Intern Med* 59:716–720, 1963.
4. Lewers DT, Mathew TH, Maher JF, et al: Long-term follow-up of renal function and histology after acute tubular necrosis. *Ann Intern Med* 73:523–529, 1970.
5. Mitchell JR, McMurtry RJ, Statham CN, et al: Molecular basis for several drug induced nephropathies. *Am J Med* 62:518–526, 1977.
6. Luft FC, Block R, Sloan RS, et al: Comparative nephrotoxicity of aminoglycoside antibiotics in rats. *J Infect Dis* 138:541–545, 1978.
7. Kimberly RP, Bowden RE, Keiser HR, et al: Reduction of renal function by newer nonsteroidal anti-inflammatory drugs. *Am J Med* 64:804–807, 1978.
8. Gary NE, Dodelson R, Eisinger RP: Indomethacin-associated acute renal failure. *Am J Med* 69:135–136, 1980.
9. Lawrence JR: Clinical use of corticosteroids in renal disease. *Drugs* 8:438–447, 1974.
10. Emmerson BT: Chronic lead nephropathy. The diagnostic use of calcium EDTA and the association with gout. *Aust Ann Med* 12:310–324, 1963.

11. Farebrother DA, Hatfield P, Simmonds HA, et al: Experimental crystal nephropathy (one year study in the pig). *Clin Nephrol* 4:243–250, 1975.
12. Pitman SW, Frei E, III: Weekly methotrexate-calcium leucovorin rescue: Effect of alkalinization on nephrotoxicity; pharmacokinetics in the CNS; and use in CNS non-Hodgkin's lymphoma. *Cancer Treat Rep* 61:695–701, 1977.
13. Curtis JR: Drug induced renal disease. *Drugs* 18:377–391, 1979.
14. Gonwa TA, Corbett WT, Schey HM, et al: Analgesic associated nephropathy and transitional cell carcinoma of the urinary tract. *Ann Intern Med* 93:249–252, 1980.
15. Evan AP, Gardner KD, Jr: Nephron obstruction in nordihydroguaiaretic acid-induced renal cystic disease. *Kidney Int* 15:7–19, 1979.
16. Setter JG, Maher JF, Schreiner GE: Acute renal failure following cholecystography. *JAMA* 184:102–110, 1963.
17. Byrd L, Sherman RL: Radiocontrast-induced acute renal failure: A clinical and pathophysiologic review. *Medicine* 58:270–279, 1979.
18. Tune BM, Wu KY, Longerbeam DF, et al: Transport and toxicity of cephaloridine in the kidney. Effect of furosemide p-aminohippurate and saline diuresis. *J Pharmacol Exp Ther* 202:472–478, 1977.
19. Bidani A, Churchill D, Fleischmann L: Sodium-chloride induced protection in nephrotoxic acute renal failure: Independence from renin. *Kidney Int* 16:481–490, 1979.
20. Wainscoat JS, Finn R: Possible role of laxatives in analgesic nephropathy. *Br Med J* 4:697–698, 1974.
21. Barza M: The nephrotoxicity of cephalosporins: An overview. *J Infect Dis* 137:S60–S73, 1978.
22. Wade JC, Smith CR, Petty BG, et al: Cephalothin plus an aminoglycoside is more nephrotoxic than methicillin plus an aminoglycoside. *Lancet* 2:604–606, 1978.
23. Agarwal BN, Cabebe FG, Hoffman BI: Diphenylhydantoin-induced acute renal failure. *Nephron* 18:249–251, 1977.
24. Cronin RE: Aminoglycoside nephrotoxicity: Pathogenesis and prevention. *Clin Nephrol* 11:251–256, 1979.
25. Bennett WM, Plamp CE, Gilbert DN, et al: The influence of dosage regimen on experimental gentamicin nephrotoxicity: Dissociation of peak serum levels from renal failure. *J Infect Dis* 140:576–580, 1979.
26. Mattson K, Riska H, Forsstrom J, et al: Acute renal failure following rifampicin administration. *Scand J Respir Dis* 55:291–297, 1974.
27. Phillips TL, Ross BS: A quantitative technique for measuring renal damage after irradiation. *Radiology* 109:457–462, 1973.
28. Milman N: Renal failure associated with gentamicin therapy. *Acta Med Scand* 196:87–91, 1974.
29. Dubach UC, Levy PS, Rosner B, et al: Relation between regular intake of phenacetin-containing analgesics and laboratory evidence for urorenal disorders in a working female population of Switzerland. *Lancet* 1:539–543, 1975.
30. Nanra RS, Fairley KF, Kincaid-Smith P: Recovery of function in patients with analgesic nephropathy. *Aust Ann Med* 19:195–196, 1970.
31. Finn R, Fennerty AG, Ahmad R: Hydrocarbon exposure and glomerulonephritis. *Clin Nephrol* 14:173–175, 1980.
32. Ho PWL, Pien FD, Kominami N: Massive amikacin "overdosage." *Ann Intern Med* 91:227–228, 1979.

33. Winchester JF, Gelfand MC, Knepshield JH, et al: Dialysis and hemoperfusion of poisons and drugs—update. *Trans Am Soc Artif Intern Organs* 23:762–842, 1977.
34. Maher JF, Rath CE, Schreiner GE: Hyperuricemia complicating leukemia: Treatment with allopurinol and dialysis. *Arch Intern Med* 123:198–200, 1969.
35. Maher JF, Bryan CW, Ahearn DJ: Prognosis of chronic renal failure II. Factors affecting survival. *Arch Intern Med* 135:273–278, 1975.

Section V

New Insights into Complications of Uremia

Elucidation of the complexities of the pathophysiology of uremia is more than an exercise in puzzle-solving. With each new, hard-won fact about why uremic patients are sick comes a clue to relief of symptoms, and sometimes to prevention of complications. Consider how understanding of the vitamin D/parathyroid hormone/calcium relationship has provided a rationale for planning prevention or retardation of complications of uremia. There are still incompletely clarified aspects to the kidney patient's sick bones. An approach to developing further answers is given in this section. Included with the unwinding bone story is our first perception of the importance of autonomic neuropathy in renal insufficiency. This aspect of the uremic patient is virtually unknown. It can be anticipated that quantification of the severity of autonomic defects will prompt wise clinicians to construct corrective treatments.

Massry found that about one half of predialysis and dialysis patients have clinically apparent autonomic neuropathy. Management of the treated uremic patient requires attention to abnormalities of autonomic function. The degree of anemia did not correlate with the presence of severity of neurologic malfunction. We know far too little of the extent to which subtle neurologic deficiencies may contribute to uremic morbidity.

Letteri, after classifying renal bone disease into three types by histomorphometry of double tetracycline labeled iliac bone biopsies, suggests that specific therapy can be tailored to each patient's biopsy findings. Once toxins that inhibit normal bone matrix formation or calcification are identified, it should prove possible to retard their action, preserving bone integrity.

Bone disease remains one of the least treatable complications of uremia, as described elsewhere in this volume. Therefore, Letteri's interesting concepts for retarding progression of osteodystrophy become even more significant.

M.M.A.

11

Functional Abnormalities of the Autonomic Nervous System in Uremic and Dialysis Patients

SHAUL G. MASSRY AND VITO M. CAMPESE

Abnormalities in the function of the autonomic nervous system are encountered in patients with uremia.[1-8] These are listed in Table I.

Hennessy and Siemsen[1] were the first to report a reduction in the number of functioning eccrine sweat glands in three uremic patients with somatic neuropathy. Goldberger et al.[2] described an abnormal heart rate and blood pressure response during the Valsalva maneuver in 23 of 29 patients with chronic renal failure. They also showed a reduction in the volume of sweat and its chloride concentration in 13 of 18 patients studied. Soriano and Eisinger[3] measured, by continuous electrocardiographic recording, the R-R interval during the strain and release phases of the Valsalva maneuver. They found a normal increase in heart rate in all patients during the strain phase, but a failure to develop the expected bradycardia during the release phase of the maneuver in 12 of 18 patients. Pickering et al.[4] found reduced baroreflex sensitivity to the administration of phenylephrine in 31 patients on long-term hemodialysis. These investigators also suggested that hemodialysis improves baroreflex sensitivity over the long term, but does not have any consistent immediate effect. Lazarus et al.[5] found that the slope of the line relating R-R intervals to systolic blood pressure during infusion of angiotensin II was lower in uremic patients on maintenance hemodialysis than in normal subjects.

SHAUL G. MASSRY ● Division of Nephrology, Department of Medicine, University of Southern California School of Medicine, Los Angeles, California.   VITO M. CAMPESE ● Division of Nephrology, Department of Medicine, University of Southern California School of Medicine, Los Angeles, California. This work was supported by contract NO1-AM-7-2225 with the Chronic Uremia Programs, a grant GCRG-RR-43 from the General Clinical Research Center Program of the Division of Research Resources, NIH, and a contract with the Department of Health of the State of California.

Table I. Abnormalities in Autonomic Nervous System Function in Uremia

---

Defective sweat gland function
Abnormal response to the Valsalva maneuver
Reduced baroreceptor sensitivity
Non-volume-responsive hypotension during hemodialysis
Abnormal response to sustained hand-grip exercise
Abnormal amyl nitrite inhalation test

This abnormality was also more pronounced in patients with hypertension than in those with normal blood pressure. They concluded that uremic patients have a blunted baroreceptor response to pharmacologically induced changes in blood pressure. Kersh et al.[6] studied eight patients with chronic uremia who had suffered frequent hypotensive episodes during hemodialysis. Only two of these patients had normal Valsalva maneuver and a normal compensatory rise in systemic vascular resistance and in heart rate during hypotensive episodes while on hemodialysis. The remaining six patients manifested an abnormal blood pressure response during the Valsalva maneuver and a fall in total systemic vascular resistance and fixed heart rate during hemodialysis-induced hypotension. The hypotension in these six patients did not improve with volume expansion, but did respond to the administration of norepinephrine. Ewing and Winney[7] evaluated 24 patients on maintenance hemodialysis and found that 50% had abnormal Valsalva ratio and 45% had abnormal blood pressure and heart rate response to sustained hand-grip exercise. There was no significant correlation between the blood pressure response to hand-grip exercise and the Valsalva ratio; however, there was a close correlation between the heart rate response to hand-grip exercise and the Valsalva ratio ($r = 0.61$, $p < 0.01$). Lilley et al.[8] found reduced heart rate response to amyl nitrite inhalation in uremic patients with frequent intradialysis hypotension in comparision with patients with rare episodes of intradialysis hypotension. In contrast, both groups of patients had normal blood pressure response to cold-pressor test. Furthermore, they found that patients with abnormal amyl nitrite test had, on the average, higher levels of blood pressure and greater serum concentration of dopamine-beta-hydroxylase. These investigators concluded that patients with frequent hemodialysis hypotension may have a lesion in the baroreceptors, cardiopulmonary receptors, or visceral afferent nerves, and not in the efferent pathway. Furthermore, they suggested that the elevated baseline blood pressure in patients with hemodialysis hypotension may be neurogenic in origin and similar to the hypertension that follows baroreceptor deafferentation in experimental animals.

The mechanisms responsible for the dysfunction of the autonomic nervous system are not fully elucidated and may be multifactorial. The various pathogenetic possibilities are listed in Table II.

Our presentation describes the results of studies designed to examine the possible mechanisms responsible for the dysfunction of the autonomic nervous system in uremic patients and those treated with maintenance hemodialysis.

POPULATION STUDIED

A total of 112 subjects, including 60 normal volunteers, 37 patients with chronic uremia, and 15 patients with chronic illness but normal renal function were studied for evaluation of autonomic nervous system function. Patients with diabetes mellitus or congestive heart failure and those receiving medication that might affect the autonomic nervous system were excluded from the study. Other studies were carried out on an additional ten patients with essential hypertension for the evaluation of pressor response to norepinephrine infusion and an additional 16 patients on maintenance hemodialysis for the examination of the effect of dialysis procedure on blood levels of catecholamines. The nature of the research was explained to all participants and an informed consent was obtained prior to the study.

Among the normals there were 41 males and 19 females with their ages ranging between 18 and 52 (34 ± 1.1) years. They were selected from the medical and paramedical personnel of the Los Angeles County–University of Southern California Medical Center. The 37 uremic patients were made up of two groups: (1) The first group consisted of 21 patients with creatinine clearance of less than 8 ml/min who were not treated with dialysis and will be referred to hereafter as "predialysis" patients. Among them were 12 males and 9 females aged between 19 and 62 (40 ± 3.2) years. These patients were ambulatory before admission to the hospital for

Table II. Possible Factors Involved in the Pathogenesis of
Autonomic Nervous System Dysfunction of Uremia

Anemia
Chronic illness state
Lesions in various segments of the baroreceptor arc
Abnormalities in plasma levels of catecholamines
Abnormal responsiveness of target organs to plasma catecholamines

evaluation and preparation for dialysis. (2) In the second group were 16 patients treated with chronic maintenance hemodialysis for 0.5–10 (4.5 ± 0.88) years. They received four to five hours of hemodialysis thrice weekly. Among them were 11 males and 5 females aged 21–60 (38 ± 3.1) years. All patients were at home and came to the Center three times a week for dialysis. The studies on the patients were carried out on the day when they did not receive dialysis therapy.

The cause of the renal failure in the 37 patients were chronic glomerulonephritis in 11, malignant hypertension in 7, obstructive uropathy in four, pyelonephritis in three, polycystic kidney disease in two, interstitial nephritis in one, and medullary cystic disease in one patient, and the cause was unknown in 8 patients. All the patients with chronic uremia received a diet containing 40–60 g of protein and 100 mEq of sodium per day and all antihypertensive medications were discontinued at least two weeks prior to the study.

The 15 patients with chronic illness and normal renal function were all males and their ages ranged between 22 and 63 (43 ± 3.3) years. Eleven were recruited from the medical outpatient clinic and four were at the hospital at the time of the study. Creatinine clearance was 85 to 160 (113 ± 57) ml/min and hematocrit was 19.0 to 44.7 (39.6 ± 1.87%). Four patients had rheumatoid arthritis, five had Hodgkin's disease, two had chronic obstructive pulmonary disease, one had sarcoidosis, one had gout, one had scleromyxedema, and one had chronic peptic ulcer.

METHODS

The following parameters were evaluated: (1) mean blood pressure (MBP), heart rate, plasma levels of norepinephrine (NE) and epinephrine (E), and plasma renin activity (PRA) after resting supine for one hour, after hand-grip exercise, after 10 minutes of upright posture, and after an additional 50 minutes of ambulation; (2) Valsalva ratio during the Valsalva maneuver, which is estimated by the ratio between the longest R-R interval during the release phase of the maneuver and the shortest R-R interval during the strain phase of the maneuver; and (3) blood pressure response to infusion of 20, 50, and 100 ng/kg/min of NE. This test was done in five predialysis and six dialysis patients, ten normal subjects, and ten patients with essential hypertension and normal renal function.

The details of the various tests and methodologies employed in our studies have been reported by us elsewhere.[9]

RESULTS

Basal Levels of MBP, Pulse Rate, Plasma NE and E, and PRA

The data for these parameters in all subjects are given in Table III. Predialysis and dialysis patients had significantly ($p < 0.01$) higher levels of MBP and pulse rate than normal subjects and patients with chronic illness and normal renal function. Plasma levels of NE and E were significantly ($p < 0.01$) elevated only in predialysis patients. The normal plasma levels of NE in the dialysis patients were not due to losses of NE during the dialysis procedure. In 16 patients studied before and after the dialysis procedure, the plasma levels of NE were 25 ± 5.2 and 27 ± 3.6 ng/dl respectively.

Valsalva Ratio

The Valsalva ratio was significantly lower ($p < 0.01$) in both the predialysis [1.51 ± 0.08 (SE)] and dialysis patients (1.62 ± 0.09) than control subjects (2.1 ± 0.05) and those with chronic illness (2.0 ± 0.13) (Figure 1). The ratio was not different among the predialysis and the dialysis patients. Even though there was considerable overlap between groups, almost half of the predialysis (52%) and of the dialysis (44%) patients had values of Valsalva ratio lower than the lowest value seen in normal subjects or in those with chronic illness. The difference in the Valsalva ratio was mainly due to significantly different falls in pulse rate (as determined by R-R intervals) during the release phase of the Valsalva maneuver (Figure 2).

Tables IV and V depict the relationship between the Valsalva ratio and

Table III. Basal Values After One Hour Supine

	Normals	Predialysis	Dialysis	Chronic illness
Mean blood pressure, mm Hg	81 ± 0.9	100 ± 4.0^a	95 ± 3.7^a	86 ± 2.9
Pulse rate, beats/min	64 ± 1.1	80 ± 3.3^a	79 ± 3.2^a	67 ± 2.2
Plasma NE, ng/dl	21 ± 0.9	35 ± 3.6^a	24 ± 2.7	21 ± 2.7
Plasma E, ng/dl	2.5 ± 0.23	3.3 ± 0.55^a	2.1 ± 0.37	2.1 ± 0.38
PRA, ng/ml/hr	1.3 ± 0.13	3.4 ± 0.58^b	3.2 ± 0.61^b	1.6 ± 0.22

$^a p < 0.01$ compared with values in normal subjects.
$^b p < 0.05$.

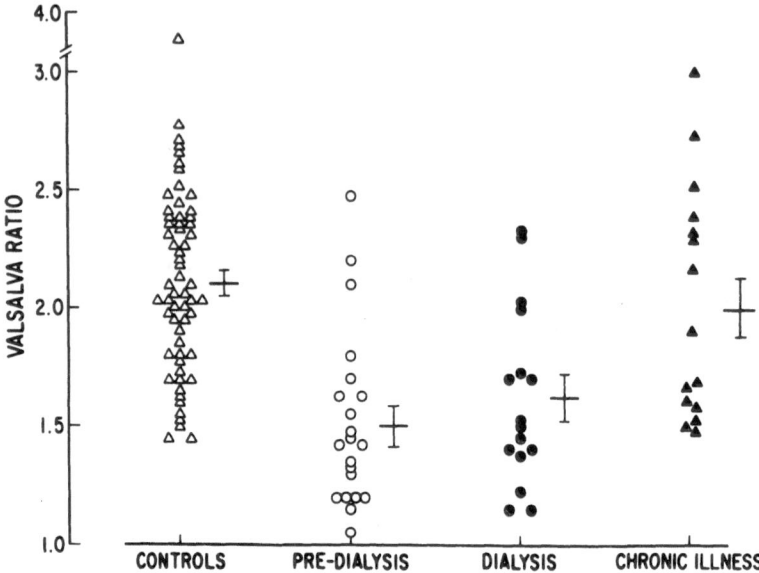

Figure 1. The Valsalva ratio, that is, the ratio between the longest R-R interval during the release phase and the shortest R-R interval during the strain phase of the Valsalva maneuver, in 60 normal subjects, 21 predialysis patients, 16 patients on maintenance hemodialysis, and 15 patients with chronic illnesses but with normal renal function. The brackets denote mean ± SEM. (By permission from Campese et al.[9])

Table IV. Relationship Between Valsalva Ratio and
Hematocrit in Uremic Patients

	Valsalva ratio	Hematocrit percent
I. Predialysis		
a. Low Valsalva		
Range	1.14–1.42	15.8–37.3
Mean ± SE	1.25–0.04	22.5 ± 2.6
b. Normal Valsalva		
Range	1.46–2.46	18.8–29.1
Mean ± SE	1.80 ± 0.11	22.8 ± 1.5
p value	<0.01	n.s.
II. Dialysis		
a. Low Valsalva		
Range	1.14–1.45	16.8–32.9
Mean ± SE	1.31 ± 0.05	23.9 ± 2.4
b. Normal Valsalva		
Range	1.51–2.32	19.4–38.8
Mean ± SE	1.87 ± 0.1	24.9 ± 2.5
p value	<0.01	n.s.

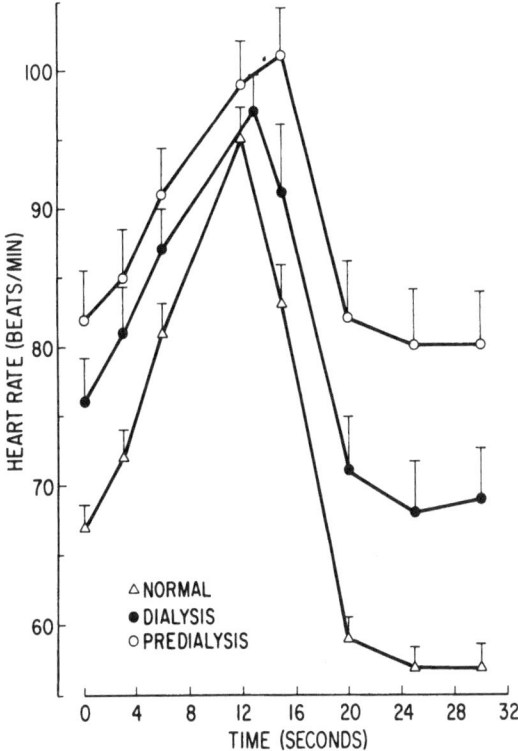

Figure 2. Heart rate before and during the Valsalva maneuver in normal subjects and predialysis and dialysis patients. During the release phase, heart rate was significantly lower ($p<0.01$) in normal subjects than in the two groups of uremic patients and lower in dialysis ($p < 0.05$) than in predialysis patients. Data are presented as mean ± SEM. (By permission from Campese et al.[9])

Table V. Relationship Between Valsalva Ratio and Blood Pressure

	Mean blood pressure mm Hg	Valsalva ratio
I. Predialysis		
a. Normotensive	84 ± 4.4	1.54 ± 0.17
$n = 8$		
b. Hypertensive	113 ± 4.6	1.50 ± 0.08
$n = 13$		
p value	$p < 0.01$	n.s.
II. Dialysis		
a. Normotensive	88 ± 4.4	1.67 ± 0.11
$n = 10$		
b. Hypertensive	108 ± 2.1	1.53 ± 0.18
$n = 6$		
p value	$p < 0.01$	n.s.

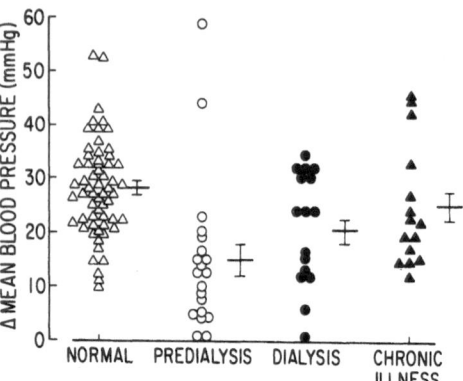

Figure 3. Changes in mean blood pressure in normal subjects, in predialysis and dialysis patients, and in patients with chronic illnesses but with normal renal function in response to sustained hand-grip exercise at one third of maximum voluntary contraction. The increments in mean blood pressure were significantly lower ($p < 0.01$) in the two groups of uremic patients. The brackets denote mean ± SEM. (By permission from Campese et al.[9])

hematocrit or mean blood pressure in both the predialysis and dialysis patients. It is evident that the abnormalities in the Valsalva ratio were not related to the anemia of uremia or the presence or absence of elevated mean blood pressure.

Hand-Grip Exercise

During hand-grip exercise, MBP increased significantly in all subjects but the magnitude of the increment was significantly less ($p < 0.01$) in the predialysis and dialysis patients than in normal subjects and in patients with chronic illness (Figure 3). In 7 of 20 (35%) predialysis patients and in two of 16 (13%) dialysis patients the change in blood pressure was lower than the lowest value observed in normal subjects. Similarly, the increments in heart rate was significantly greater in normal subjects ($p <$

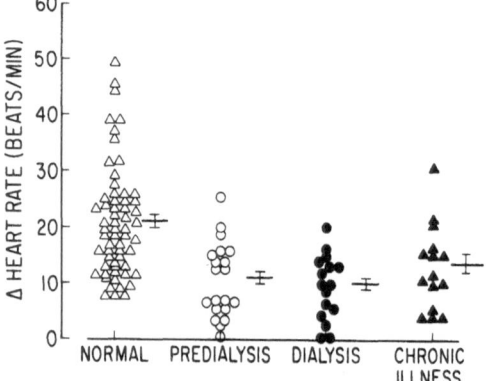

Figure 4. Changes in heart rate in normal subjects, in predialysis and dialysis patients, and in patients with chronic illnesses but with normal renal function in response to sustained hand-grip exercise at one third of maximum voluntary contraction. The increment in heart rate was significantly lower ($p < 0.01$) in the two groups of uremic patients. The brackets denote mean ± SEM. (By permission from Campese et al.[9])

0.01) than in the predialysis and dialysis patients (Figure 4). In 16 of 36 (44%) uremic patients, the increment in heart rate was lower than the lowest value observed in normal subjects. Only in four of 15 patients (27%) with chronic illness, the change in heart rate was below the normal range. It is of interest that eight of 11 predialysis (73%) and five of seven dialysis (71%) patients who had low Valsalva ratio also had abnormal heart rate response to hand-grip exercise (Table VI).

Effects of Upright Posture and Ambulation

There was a modest fall in MBP after standing and ambulation in normal subjects and those with chronic illness, but the change was significant only in the normal controls. Dialysis patients did not have a decrease in blood pressure during these maneuvers. However, a marked and significant ($p < 0.01$) decrease in MBP occurred in the predialysis patients; it fell by 15 ± 3.5 and 15 ± 2.8 mm Hg after 10 and 60 minutes of ambulation, respectively. The concentration of plasma NE increased significantly in all four groups. However, the magnitude of rise in plasma NE after 60 minutes of ambulation in the predialysis patients (60 ± 7.4 ng/dl) was significantly ($p < 0.01$) higher than that in normal subjects (28 ± 2.0 ng/dl) dialysis patients (30 ± 4.9 ng/dl) and those with chronic illness (37 ± 5.0 ng/dl), The increments in heart rate after orthostasis were not different among the four groups of subjects. Both plasma E and PRA increased significantly with orthostasis in all subjects and the magnitudes of the increments were not different among the four groups studied (Figure 5).

Table VI. Relationship Between Results of Valsalva and Hand-Grip Tests in Uremic Patients

	Low heart rate	
	No.	Percent
Total population		
Normal Valsalva (19)	5	26
Low Valsalva (18)	13	72
Predialysis		
Normal Valsalva (10)	3	30
Low Valsalva (11)	8	73
Dialysis		
Normal Valsalva (9)	2	22
Low Valsalva (7)	5	71

Shaul G. Massry and Vito M. Campese

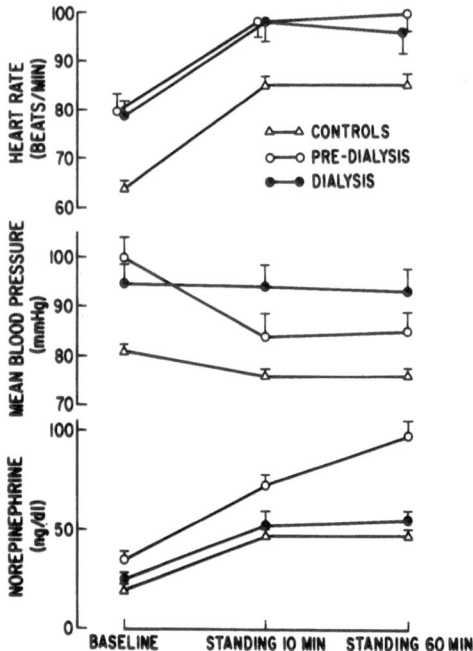

Figure 5. Effect of standing for 10 and 60 minutes on heart rate, mean blood pressure, and plasma norepinephrine in normal subjects, and in predialysis and dialysis patients. Data are presented as mean ± SEM.

Effect of NE Infusion

There was a dose response relationship between the changes in both MBP and heart rate and the amount of NE infused (Figure 6). In the predialysis patients the changes in MBP with 20, 50, and 100 ng/kg/min of NE were significantly ($p < 0.05$) lower than those observed in normal subjects and in those with essential hypertension and normal renal function. The changes in the latter group were significantly ($p < 0.01$) greater than in normals. The changes in MBP in the dialysis patients were not different than in normal subjects. Similarly, the decrements in heart rate were significantly smaller ($p < 0.05$) in the predialysis patients than in dialysis patients, normal subjects, and those with essential hypertension. There was no significant difference in the changes in heart rate between the dialysis patients and normal subjects.

DISCUSSION

The results of our studies demonstrate that a large number of predialysis and dialysis patients have dysfunction of the autonomic nervous system. These included abnormal Valsalva ratio, abnormal response to hand-grip exercise, and abnormal fall in blood pressure during

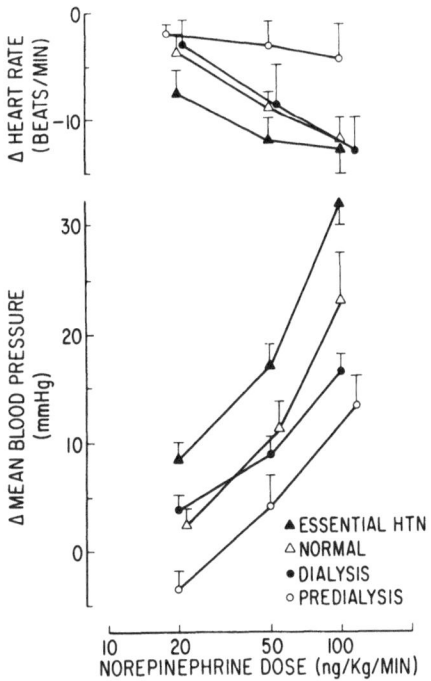

Figure 6. Changes in mean blood pressure and heart rate during norepinephrine infusion at progressive doses of 20, 50, 100 ng/kg/min in ten normal subjects, and five of the predialysis and six of the dialysis patients included in Table III, and in ten patients with essential hypertension and normal renal function. Each infusion rate was given for ten minutes. The changes in MBP and heart rate were significantly ($p<0.01$) lower in dialysis but not in predialysis patients than in normal subjects. (By permission from Campese et al.[9])

orthostasis. The disturbances appear to be related to uremia *per se* or to some of its consequences rather than to the state of chronic illness since patients with other chronic disease, but normal renal function, did not have such abnormalities. Our results also show that these abnormalities are not related to the anemia of uremia or to the presence or absence of elevated MBP.

Two findings in our data indicate that some of these abnormalities are more extensive in the predialysis patients. First, the abnormal response of blood pressure during the hand-grip exercise was more frequent among the predialysis patients. Second, the majority of the predialysis patients (67%) displayed orthostatic hypotension whereas the response to upright posture in the dialysis patients was not different from normal subjects.

The abnormality in heart rate response during the Valsalva maneuver was more pronounced during the release phase of the test in both the predialysis and dialysis patients. During this phase an increase in systemic arterial pressure occurs that is sensed by the baroreceptors in the aortic arch and carotid arteries, subsequently leading to reflex bradycardia.[10,11] The increase in blood pressure is the result of an increase in cardiac output secondary to enhanced venous return and of increased peripheral vascular resistance produced by augmented sympathetic tone.[10-13] The abnormal response in heart rate during the release phase could be due to failure of the blood pressure to rise secondary to an inappropriate change in peripheral vascular resistance, derangement in the vagal pathway, and/or disturbance in cardiac function. Indeed, dialysis patients display blunted arterial pressure overshoot during the release phase of the test.[6] The more pronounced abnormality in heart rate response during the release phase of the Valsalva in the predialysis patients could be, at least partially, attributable to greater impairment in arterial pressure response during this phase. This impairment could be secondary to resistance to the action of norepinephrine on blood vessels.

Certain data suggest that the change in heart rate during hand-grip exercise is due to parasympathetic inhibition (vagus release),[14] and the rise in MBP due to increased peripheral resistance, secondary to enhanced sympathetic activity.[14] The observation in our study that the majority of the patients who displayed an abnormal response of heart rate during the hand-grip exercise also have an abnormal Valsalva ratio is consistent with the notion that a disturbance in the vagus pathways is present in uremic patients. Furthermore, the demonstration that 35% of the predialysis patients, but only 13% of the dialysis patients, had abnormal pressor response (despite similar incidence of deranged heart rate response) suggests that a disturbance in sympathetic activity is more predominant in the predialysis patients; this proposal is consistent with the finding of peripheral resistance to NE infusion in the predialysis patients.

The maintenance of arterial pressure during orthostasis is dependent on the ability to augment peripheral vascular resistance.[15,16] Our data clearly demonstrate that the majority of the predialysis patients displayed marked postural hypotension (ΔMBP > 12 mm Hg) while the changes in blood pressure were not different from normal subjects in the dialysis patients. The reason for this difference is most probably target organ resistance to NE present only in the predialysis patients. Our data do not necessarily imply that orthostatic hypotension due to autonomic nerve dysfunction is not encountered in dialysis patients but would suggest that such a problem is not frequent. It is our opinion that if orthostatic hypotension is noticed in a dialysis patient, a vigorous search for causes other than uremic dysfunction of the autonomic nervous system should be undertaken.

SUMMARY

The results of our studies could be summarized as follows:

1. Dysfunction of autonomic nervous system is common in uremia.
2. About 50% of both predialysis and dialysis patients have reduced

Valsalva ratio and most of these (70%) also have smaller increments in heart rate in response to hand-grip exercise.

3. About 40% of predialysis patients have smaller increments in MBP in response to hand-grip exercise while only 2 of 16 dialysis patients have such a defect.

4. In response to orthostasis, the predialysis patients displayed a marked drop in MBP, an exaggerated rise in plasma NE, and a rise in heart rate similar to normal subjects but inappropriate for the changes in MBP and plasma NE. In contrast, the response to orthostasis in the dialysis patients was not different from normal subjects.

5. Predialysis patients have higher plasma NE levels and smaller increments in MBP in response to NE infusion than dialysis patients.

CONCLUSIONS

Our data permit the following conclusions.

1. Disturbances in autonomic nervous system function are common in uremia and are more extensive in predialysis than in dialysis patients.

2. The mechanisms underlying these disturbances are multifactorial and include lesions of the various components of the baroreceptor reflex arc, derangements in the parasympathetic nervous system, abnormalities in cardiac function, and reduced end-organ response to NE. The last abnormality may play a major role in the predialysis patients.

3. The anemia of uremia and the state of chronic illness are not critical determinants of the autonomic nervous system dysfunction in uremia.

ACKNOWLEDGMENTS. The authors wish to thank Ms. Jamie Jimenez, Ms. Joann Little, and Mrs. Caroline Baray for their excellent secretarial assistance.

REFERENCES

1. Hennessy WJ, Siemsen, AW: Autonomic neuropathy in chronic renal failure. Clin Res 16:385, 1968.
2. Goldberger S, Thompson A, Guha A, et al: Autonomic nervous dysfunction in chronic renal failure. Clin Res 19:531, 1971.
3. Soriano G, Eisinger RP: Abnormal response to the Valsalva maneuver in patients on chronic hemodialysis. Nephron 9:251–256, 1972.
4. Pickering TG, Gribbin B, Oliver DO: Baroreflex sensitivity in patients on long-term hemodialysis. Clin Sci 43:645–657, 1972.
5. Lazarus JM, Hampers CL, Lowrie EG, et al: Baroreceptor activity in normotensive and hypertensive uremic patients. Circulation 47:1015–1021, 1973.

6. Kersh ES, Kronfield SJ, Unger A, et al: Autonomic insufficiency in uremia as a cause of hemodialysis-induced hypotension. *N Engl J Med* 290:650–653, 1974.

7. Ewing DJ, Winney R: Autonomic function in patients with chronic renal failure on intermittent haemodialysis. *Nephron* 15:424–429, 1975.

8. Lilley JJ, Golden J, Stone RA: Adrenergic regulation of blood pressure in chronic renal failure. *J Clin Invest* 57:1190–1200, 1976.

9. Campese VM, Romoff MS, Levitan D, et al: Mechanisms of autonomic nervous system dysfunction in uremia. *Kidney Int* 20:246–253.

10. Sarnoff SJ, Hardenbergh E, Whittenberger JL: Mechanism of the arterial pressure response to the Valsalva test: The basis for its use as an indicator of the intactness of the sympathetic outflow. *Am J Physiol* 154:316–327, 1948.

11. Elisberg EI, Miller G, Weinberg SLM, et al: The effect of the Valsalva maneuver on the circulation. II. *Am Heart J* 45:227–236, 1953.

12. Lee D de J, Matthews MB, Sharpey-Schafer EP: The effect of the Valsalva maneuver on the systemic and pulmonary arterial pressure in man. *Br Heart J* 16:311–316, 1954.

13. Bunnell IL, Greene DG, Kunz WW: Influence of tetraethylammonium chloride on the circulatory responses to the Valsalva maneuver. *J Appl Phys* 4:345–350, 1951.

14. Freyschuss U: Cardiovascular adjustment to somatomotor activation. *Acta Physiol Scan* suppl:342, 1970.

15. Ibrahim MM, Tarazi RC, Dustan HP: Orthostatic hypotension: Mechanisms and management. *Am Heart J* 90:513–520, 1975.

16. Hickler RB, Hoskins RG, Hamlin JT: The clinical evaluation of faulty orthostatic mechanisms. *Med Clin N Am* 44:1237–1250, 1960.

12

The Pathogenesis, Treatment, and Possible Prevention of Uremic Bone Disease

JOSEPH M. LETTERI

CLASSIFICATION OF UREMIC BONE DISEASE

Uremic bone disease can be classified into three major types based on histomorphometric analysis of double tetracycline labeling of iliac crest bone obtained by trephine (Table I). Type I consists of patients with high-turnover bone disease. Type II consists of patients with high-turnover bone disease in which the major manifestation of the abnormal mineral metabolism associated with uremia is metastatic calcification. Type III consists of patients with low turnover bone disease.

In Type I high-turnover bone disease, marked increases in parathyroid hormone and serum alkaline phosphatase are associated with a low serum calcium. The bone histology typically demonstrates an increase in bone resorption manifested by enhanced osteoclastic activity, fibrosis of the marrow, and some increase in the osteoid seam width. Bone mass, as estimated by trabecular bone volume, is usually decreased in this group of patients. Radial bone densitometry, total body calcium, and bone radiographs reveal a heterogeneous population in that increased, normal, and decreased bone mass have all been observed. Thus the response of various portions of the skeleton may be heterogeneous in patients with uremic bone disease. Trabecular bone may be responding in a fashion different from cortical bone and should be considered in our understanding of the bone lesions observed in this group.

In a subtype of patients with high-turnover bone disease, the major

JOSEPH M. LETTERI • Division of Renal Diseases, Department of Medicine, Nassau County Medical Center; and Department of Medicine, State University of New York at Stony Brook, Stony Brook, New York.

Table I. Mineral and Skeletal Defects in Uremia

	High-turnover bone disease	Metastatic calcification	Low-turnover bone disease
$[CA^{++} \times PO_4^-]$	↑	↑↑	N
PTH	↑↑	↑↑	N↓
Alkaline phosphatase	↑	↑	N↑
Bone resorption	↑↑	↑	?N
Bone formation	?↑	?↑	↓
Marrow fibrosis	N↑	N↑	N
Osteoid	↑	↑	↑↑

manifestation of the abnormal mineral metabolism is the presence of extensive metastatic calcification (Type II). This massive increase in extraskeletal calcification is seen almost exclusively in adult patients with long-standing chronic renal disease and is rarely seen in children. Periarticular calcification, and ischemic syndromes involving small and large vessels leading to occlusive disease of the coronary arteries and large and small peripheral vessels, have been described. In addition, unusual pulmonary syndromes and bizarre cardiac arrhythmias have been noted in some patients with extensive metastatic calcification due to deposits of calcium in the cardiac and pulmonary systems.

Chemically, this group of patients is characterized by rather large increases in parathyroid hormone blood levels. The alkaline phosphatase is usually very increased. Bone biopsy of the iliac crest reveals a marked increase in osteoclastic activity. There are enhanced bone resorption and bone fibrosis. The percentage of the bone lined by osteoid is increased. Trabecular bone mass is generally calculated to be diminished but there is obvious metastatic calcification on radiograph examination. Generally, total body calcium is increased or normal, suggesting that there is redistribution of bone calcium into soft tissues in this group of patients.

The third type of bone disease described with uremia is classified as low-turnover bone disease because it appears that the bone remodeling processes are depressed (Table I). In this subset of patients the calcium : phosphorus product is normal; parathyroid hormone levels are not increased but very often are normal to low. Alkaline phosphatase is generally normal but may be increased in patients with fluoride-induced low-turnover bone disease. Bone resorption does not appear to be increased; the bone formation rate is markedly decreased. There is very little marrow fibrosis on examination of the iliac crest and the osteoid volume of bone is markedly increased. It is presumed that the low-turnover bone disease is related to the accumulation of factors that interfere with bone formation and collagen synthesis and nutritional deficiency of vitamin D.

PATHOGENESIS OF UREMIC BONE DISEASE

Table II lists the factors implicated in uremia that alter calcium and phosphorus metabolism.[1-3] These include altered vitamin D metabolism, an absolute calcium deficiency, excess parathyroid hormone, skeletal resistance to the calcemic response to parathyroid hormone, metabolic acidosis associated with uremia, and uremic factors inhibiting collagen synthesis and bone formation.

ABNORMAL VITAMIN D METABOLISM IN UREMIA

A true deficiency of $1,25\text{-}(OH)_2D_3$ has been implicated in the pathogenesis of uremic bone disease associated with advanced renal failure (Table III). Decreased plasma levels of $1,25\text{-}(OH)_2D_3$ are usually observed late in the course of renal disease, particularly when creatinine clearance is below 20 ml/min, and have been attributed to decreasing renal functioning tissue. However, early in renal failure, that is, creatinine clearance in excess of 50 ml/min, $1,25\text{-}(OH)_2D_3$ levels may actually be increased. Table IV lists the modulators of 1α-hydroxylase activity necessary for the conversion of $25\text{-}OHD_3$ to $1,25\text{-}(OH)_2D_3$. Note that an increase in 1α-hydroxylase activity has been noted with hypocalcemia, increased parathyroid hormone blood levels, hypophosphatemia, hyperkalemia, and increased prolactin and estrogen levels. It is presumed that the high levels of $1,25\text{-}(OH)_2D_3$ in blood in early renal failure are related to the increased parathyroid hormone levels noted in early renal failure.

The 1α-hydroxylase activity appears to be depressed under certain conditions that can be associated with uremia, namely, acidosis, occasionally the hypercalcemia and hyperphosphatemia noted in renal

Table II. Factors Implicated in Uremia That Alter Mineral
Metabolism and the Skeleton

Abnormal vitamin D metabolism
Calcium deficiency
Parathyroid hormone
Acidosis
Uremic factors inhibiting collagen synthesis and bone formation

Table III. Plasma Levels of Vitamin D Metabolism in Renal Failure

25-OHD$_3$	Usually normal but may be decreased in nephrotic patients
1,25-(OH)$_2$D$_3$	Increase in early renal failure, normal to low levels in late renal failure
24,25-(OH)$_2$D$_3$	Decreased

failure, and, very commonly, increased circulating levels of thyrocalcitonin. All of these factors could be contributing to depression of lα-hydroxylase in late renal failure and result in low levels of 1,25-(OH)$_2$D$_3$ in the blood of patients with uremia. Thus the levels of 1,25-(OH)$_2$D$_3$ in uremia reflect both the loss of structural renal tissue and the influence of factors modulating the residual activity of the enzyme in diseased nephrons. On the one hand, parathyroid hormone, hypercalcemia, and phosphate deficiency may be enhancing the lα-hydroxylase activity and be opposed by such factors as acidosis, hyperphosphatemia, and elevated thyrocalcitonin levels in uremia. Therefore it is not surprising that the 1,25-(OH)$_2$D$_3$ levels do fluctuate in renal failure, are elevated in early renal failure, and decrease as renal failure progresses.

High-turnover bone disease is believed to be a reflection of enhanced parathyroid hormone blood levels acting on a bone that is relatively resistant to the calcemic properties of endogenous parathyroid hormone. The mechanisms responsible for the increased parathyroid hormone

Table IV. Modulators of
1α-Hydroxylase Activity in
the Conversion of 25-OHD$_3$
to 1,25-(OH)$_2$D$_3$

I. Increasing activity
  A. Hypocalcemia
  B. Increased parathyroid hormone
  C. Hypophosphatemia
  D. Increased potassium
  E. Increased prolactin
  F. Increased estrogens
II. Decreasing activity
  A. Acidosis
  B. Hypercalcemia
  C. Hyperphosphatemia
  D. Thyrocalcitonin

levels and the diminished calcemic response to the circulating parathyroid hormone have not been clearly elicited. Two major theories have been advanced to explain the enhanced parathyroid hormone secretion and the diminished calcemic responsiveness of the skeleton in the face of the high parathyroid hormone levels. Diminished calcemic response of the skeleton to parathyroid hormone must be postulated because most patients with advanced renal failure continue to manifest decreases in ionizable calcium in the face of increased circulating parathyroid hormone levels. If the skeleton was responding appropriately to the increased parathyroid levels, serum ionized calcium should return to normal as the skeleton releases calcium.

$1,25\text{-}(OH)_2D_3$ is necessary for an appropriate calcemic skeletal response to parathyroid hormone. In tissue culture the rat embryonal bone response to various concentrations of parathyroid hormone is depressed in uremic sera. Some of the responsiveness of normal bone is restored by the addition of $1,25\text{-}(OH)_2D_3$ and $24,25\text{-}(OH)_2D_3$ to uremic plasma. Thus it appears that the calcemic response to parathyroid hormone can be partially restored in uremia by the addition of pharmacologic quantities of $1,25\text{-}(OH)_2D_3$ and $24,25\text{-}(OH)_2D_3$. The lack of a calcemic response to circulating parathyroid hormone in uremia is sustaining the continuous parathyroid hormone secretion due to the lack of elevation of serum calcium.

In addition to the various $1,25\text{-}(OH)_2D_3$ levels noted above, normal levels of circulating $25\text{-}OHD_3$ have been observed in the vast majority of patients with uremia (Table III). However, approximately 8–10% of patients entering a dialysis program may have absolute deficiency of circulating $25\text{-}OHD_3$. In addition, nephrotic patients excrete protein-bound $25\text{-}OHD_3$ in the urine. There are low levels of $25\text{-}OHD_3$ in some patients with nephrotic syndrome. Many of the patients with nephrotic syndrome have a bony lesion consistent with high-turnover bone disease. Administration of $25\ OHD_3$ to these patients improves the bone and reverses the abnormal calcium metabolism.[4–5] Thus a deficiency of $25\text{-}OHD_3$ due to loss with massive proteinuria or occasionally in patients who have severely restricted diets could be a factor in the genesis of bone disease and potentially be a preventable component of uremic bone disease. Administration of $1,25\text{-}(OH)_2D_3$ and $25\text{-}OHD_3$ early in renal failure and in nephrotic patients may reverse the negative calcium balance observed in these patients, restore the calcemic responsiveness of bone to parathyroid hormone, and reverse the high-turnover bone disease. In this subset of patients calcium deficiency can be prevented by the addition of one gram of elemental calcium to the diet to maintain near-zero calcium balance.

PARATHYROID GLAND HYPERPLASIA

Parathyroid gland hyperplasia is a common event in established renal failure. The proportional reduction in dietary phosphate relative to changes in filtration rate in uremic patients and dogs is associated with lowering of parathyroid hormone blood levels.[3] Phosphate retention early in renal failure occurs and may be an important factor in the genesis of secondary hyperparathyroidism and result in a high calcium : phosphorus product and metastatic calcification. The administration of aluminum hydroxide gels early in renal failure appears to diminish the high parathyroid hormone levels in many patients and reduces the incidence of metastatic calcification if the calcium : phosphorus product can be maintained below 50. However, in patients with massive metastatic calcification, parathyroidectomy, and severe restriction of the phosphate content of the diet are required to reverse the calcifications around joints. It would appear prudent to control the blood phosphorus in patients with early renal failure by aluminimum hydroxide gels to limit the parathyroid hyperplasia commonly seen in renal failure.

METABOLIC ACIDOSIS

The skeleton acts as an intracellular buffer system by three major mechanisms (Table V). Dissolution of bone by acidosis has been described. Hydroxyapatite crystals act as a buffer releasing calcium, mono-hydrogen phosphate, and dihydrogen phosphate into the circulation when hydrogen ions are added to bone. Another mechanism involving the reaction between hydrogen ion and extra-apatitic carbonate results in the release of calcium and bicarbonate into the circulation. And finally, monohydrogen phosphate may substitute for carbonate in the bone crystal with the release of bicarbonate into the systemic circulation. The chemical composition of uremic bone reflects these reactivities and is characterized by a decrease in bone carbonate and by an increase in the bone magnesium

Table V. Hydrogen Ion and Skeletal Carbonates

Skeleton acts as an intracellular buffer system:
1. Dissolution of bone
   $$H^+ + \text{hydroxyapatite} \rightarrow Ca^{++}, HPO_4^=, H_2PO_4$$
2. Buffering by extra-apatitic $CaCO_3$
   $$H^+ + CaCO_3 \rightarrow HCO_3^- + Ca^{++}$$
3. Substitution of $HPO_4^=$ for CO_3 in bone crystal reaction release of HCO_3^-

and the monohydrogen phosphate content (Table VI). The sodium content of bone is not changed in the uremic state in humans. The high magnesium content of bone is positively correlated with the percent of the total bone occupied by osteoid, suggesting that high bone magnesium may play a role in the mineralization defect noted in some patients with uremia. High bone magnesium has been implicated as a factor in the maturation of amorphous calcium salts into hydroxyapatite crystals.

The metabolic acidosis associated with uremia has been implicated as a factor in the genesis of uremic bone disease. Induction of metabolic acidosis in nonazotemic animals and patients is associated with negative calcium balance and a high bone turnover rate, which are partially corrected by either removal of the acidifying regimine or correction of the acidosis by sodium bicarbonate. Thus acidosis could be contributing to the uremic bone disease. Recent evidence suggests that a hyperchloremic metabolic acidosis occurs early in the course of renal failure. This modest positive hydrogen ion balance early in renal disease could be influencing bone metabolism. The treatment of metabolic acidosis not associated with uremia in children improves growth in acidotic children and appears to prevent the dissolution of bone. Thus it would seem prudent to correct metabolic acidosis in early renal failure and to treat it aggressively throughout the course of renal disease.

THERAPY OF UREMIC BONE DISEASE

Table VII lists the recommended strategies for the prevention of mineral skeletal defects in uremia. The object of therapy should be to

Table VI. Bone Mineral Composition in Uremia—Principal Bone Mineral Constituents (mmol/g ash)[a,b]

		Ca	PO$_4$	CO$_3$	Ca/P
Controls	(36)	9.59(0.09)	5.47(0.12)	1.43(0.03)	1.75
Group I[c]	(16)	9.63(0.13)	5.45(0.18)	1.42(0.10)	1.76
Group II[c]	(16)	9.58(0.10)	5.71(0.20)	1.16(0.13)	1.70
Group III[c]	(12)	9.59(0.13)	5.75(0.19)	1.08(0.12)	1.68

[a] Calculated dry weight values.

[b] Mean values (2 SEM); Underlined numbers signify $p < 0.0001$; Group II significantly different from Group III.

[c] Group I—uremia < 1 year; Group II—uremia > 1 year; Group III—hemodialyzed.

Table VII. Recommended Strategies
for Prevention of Mineral and
Skeletal Defects in Uremia

- 1 gram dietary calcium
- Maintain $[Ca \times P]$ at 40–50
- Maintain calcium at 9–10 mg%
- Maintain P_I at 4–5 mg/%
- Maintain serum HCO_3 at 18–22 mEq/ liters

supply the essential nutrients to maintain growth and bone remodeling. All patients with renal failure should ingest a diet containing one gram of elemental calcium. The calcium phosphorus product should be maintained between 40 and 50; the serum calcium should be maintained at 9–10 mg/dl by appropriate therapy with vitamin D metabolites or by adding calcium to the diet. The serum inorganic phosphorus should be maintained at 4–5 mg/dl by appropriate use of antacids. The serum bicarbonate should be maintained at 18–22 mEq/liter by the appropriate and judicious use of sodium bicarbonate. Avoidance of hypercalcemia and alkalosis is necessary to prevent metastatic calcification.

Treatment of patients with high-turnover bone disease has been quite successful.[1-5] In response to the administration of 25-OHD$_3$ and 1,25-(OH)$_2$D$_3$, the high turnover rate of bone decreases toward normal, resulting in a more normal appearing skeleton (Table VIII). Following treatment with either of these agents, the clinical incidence of fractures diminishes and there is amelioration of the bone pain in many of these patients. Concomitant with the administration of vitamin D metabolites, a marked increase in mobility and muscle strength is often noted. Chemically, alkaline phosphatase rises, which is then followed by a fall, and parathyroid hormone levels decrease approximately 50% in association

Table VIII. Effects of Vitamin D Metabolites on Mineral
and Skeletal Defects in Uremia

	High-turnover bone	Low-turnover bone
$[Ca^{++} \times PO_4^-]$	↑	↑↑
PTH	↓	No change
Alkaline phosphatase	↑ then ↓	No change
Bone resorption	?↓	No change
Bone formation	↑	No change
Marrow fibrosis	↓	
Osteoid	↓	No change

with an increase in serum calcium and phosphorus. Bone histology improves. Marrow fibrosis and osteoclastic activity decrease. In some studies a further decrease in trabecular bone mass has been noted. Bone formation and bone resorption are both depressed but it appears that bone resorption relative to bone formation is increased, resulting in a calculated decrease in bone mass. Interestingly, total body calcium increases in these patients on therapy.

Following parathyroidectomy there is marked improvement in some patients with metastatic calcification. The incidence of fractures usually decreases and the bone heals more quickly following parathyroidectomy. Bone mass may increase after parathyroidectomy. Occasionally, the pruritic and ischemic syndromes improve but the vascular deposits persist for many months to years after parathyroidectomy in this group.

The treatment of low-turnover bone disease with vitamin D has not been effective. In Table VIII the effects of vitamin D metabolites on low- and high-turnover bone disease are summarized. In high-turnover bone disease the calcium:phosphorus product rises, the parathyroid hormone tends to fall, alkaline phosphatase first increases then falls, bone resorption decreases, bone formation is increased, marrow fibrosis decreases, and the percentage of the bone lined by osteoid is decreased. In low-turnover bone the calcium: phosphorus product rises abruptly with therapy and is not associated with healing of the bone. There is no change in the parathyroid hormone or alkaline phosphatase blood levels. Bone resorption, bone formation, and marrow fibrosis do not change. There is no increase in bone mineralization. Thus it appears that factors inhibiting collagen synthesis and bone formation could be contributing to the altered

Table IX. Endogenous and Exogenous Toxins
That May Contribute to the Altered Mineral
Metabolism and Skeletal Defects in
Low-Turnover Bone Disease

Exogenous toxins
  Heparin
  Fluoride
  Aluminum
Endogenous toxins
  Inhibitors of parathyroid hormone effects on bone metabolism
  Pyrophosphates
  1α-Hydroxylase inhibitors
  Collagen synthesis inhibitors
  Magnesium
  ? Other trace metals; ? zinc; ? strontium, aluminum

---

mineral and skeletal defects noted in low-turnover bone disease. Table IX lists the endogenous and exogenous toxins that have been implicated as factors in the genesis of the defects. Heparin, fluoride, and aluminum are prominent contaminants or administered to patients on dialysis and also could be contributing to low-turnover bone disease noted in some patients. The endogenous toxins such as pyrophosphates, 1α-hydroxylase inhibitors, inhibitors of parathyroid hormone effects on bone, certain collagen synthesis inhibitors, as well as magnesium and other trace metals, have been implicated in the pathogenesis of the defect and should be considered as potential factors that could be altered early in disease to prevent the skeletal deficit.

SUMMARY

By analyzing the biochemical and histomorphometric characteristics of bone, the mineral and skeletal defects in uremia can be classified into three major catagories: high-turnover bone disease, high-turnover bone disease with metastatic calcification, and low-turnover bone disease. The pathobiology of the skeletal and mineral defects involves many factors, including abnormalities of vitamin D metabolism, parathryoid hormone, metabolic acidosis, and alterations in bone and collagen synthesis and metabolism. Therapy of uremic bone disease requires careful analysis of the histomorphometric characteristics of the bone obtained by trephine and biochemical assessment of mineral metabolism before effective therapy can be initiated. Prevention, on the other hand, may require the elimination of many factors that contribute to alteration of collagen synthesis and bone formation. Further investigation is required before prevention of the skeletal and mineral defects of uremia can be accomplished.

REFERENCES

1. Coburn JW, Massry SG (eds): Uses and actions of $1,25(OH)_2D_3$ in uremia. *Contrib Nephrol* 18:1–217, 1980.
2. Healy MD et al: Effects of long-term therapy with $1,25(OH)_2D_3$ in patients with moderate renal failure. *Arch Intern Med* 140:1030, 1980.
3. Massry SG, Coburn JW: Divalent ion metabolism and renal osteodystrophy, in Massry SG, Sellers AL (eds): *Clinical Aspects of Uremia and Dialysis.* Springfield, Ill, Charles C Thomas, 1976, pp 304–399.
4. Massry SG, Goldstein DA: Is calcitriol ($1,25(OH)_2D_3$) harmful to renal function? *JAMA* 242:1875, 1979.
5. Massry SG, Goldstein DA, Malluche HH: Current status of the use of $1,25(OH)_2D_3$ in the management of renal osteodystrophy. *Kidney Int* 18:409, 1980.

Section VI

Uremia Therapy and the Long-Term Dialysis Patient

Natural History and Clinical, Psychological, and Economic Characteristics of the Over-Decade Frontier

Chronic uremia is mainly treated by dialysis or transplantation. It is helpful, on occasion, to step back in order to survey the roads behind and ahead. In early 1982 more than 130,000 people are alive because of regular hemodialysis treatments. How sick are these machine-sustained humans? To answer this question, a task force approach was used to assess a unique group of long-term hemodialysis survivors. Key divisions of a university teaching service familiar wtih dialysis patients were asked to take a fresh look at the problem of renal failure in the context of dialysis as a partial solution. What follows represents a form of multivariate analysis. The long-term dialysis patient has accomplished a miracle in staying alive. From what follows, it may be anticipated that even longer survivals will be the rule so long as hypertension and bone disease are well treated.

Scribner, whose epochal first report[1] opened the modern era of kidney treatment, begins the patients' analysis by first reviewing the early years of his Seattle program and notes that one of his first three patients is alive today, 22 years after initiating dialysis and 13 years after receiving a kidney transplant from his mother. According to Scribner, the serious risk of accelerated atherosclerosis in hemodialysis patients may be minimized by controlling hypertension.

Avram and his colleagues provide a careful dissection of key variables altering the pathobiology of treated uremic patients. Employing the unique device of having the same group of long surviving patients studied by key medical subspecialty divisions at The Long Island College Hospital, Avram was then able to reconstruct a composite picture of his long successful patients. Based on continuing biochemical studies of dialysis patients, some now in their 18th year of treatment, Avram identified hypertension and excess parathyroid hormone levels as significant life-limiting factors to

141

be avoided. A comparison of binephrectomized and nephric patients after a decade of dialysis indicates that the total absence of any renal function is not inconsistent with rehabilitation. In co-opted papers, Scarpa and co-workers observed surprisingly minimal cardiac abnormalities in long-term hemodialysis patients. DiPillo, in a comprehensive study of coagulation and hematologic profiling of the same patients, concluded that, "It is unlikely that deranged hematologic function will limit long-term survival...." Similarly, Ricca, Rezk, and Yatto found unexplained elevated alkaline phosphate activity in Avram's long-term patients, but felt that "... patients sustained for a decade or longer need not have debilitating GI malfunction." Pulmonary functional studies in decade-treated dialysis patients discerned moderate to severe restrictive disease in the majority. Cutler and associates noted postdialysis hypoxemia acutely and advised routine oxygen administration during dialysis for patients with compromised cardiac status or significant pulmonary disease. Decreased bone density, by contrast, was found to continue progressively in all long-term patients assessed by Gelfand, Bienenstock, and co-workers. The most serious concern that "... renal osteodystrophy may yet prove to be a life and rehabilitation limiting complication..." points out an area obviously in need of further attention. The comprehensive evaluation synthesizing all of the findings by Avram in his patients recognized that "... long survivors share behavioral and personality characteristics..." including "... alertness, curiosity, aggressiveness, leadership, and assertiveness."

Cummings describes the "unpredicted rapid escalation" in costs of the U.S. chronic uremia program to over one billion dollars annually in 1980 for the support of 53,629 patients, a per-patient expenditure of $18,647. Only an amount equal to 1% of patient care costs is spent by the National Institutes of Health on research on the kidney and urinary tract. The largest category of research funding is the 38% devoted to kidney structure and function. Goodman and associates review their extensive experience with hemodialysis, commencing in 1967 when their program was selected as one of 12 federally funded demonstration projects. Their original results are impressive. Of 17 patients who survived at least a decade, 15 are still living. While absence of coronary artery disease, good blood pressure control, and adherence to the dialysis regimen argue for protracted survival, the authors, cognizant of difficulties in patient selection, urge that: "Until more science in this area is available... public policy should not be the province of physicians alone."

Levy summarizes the evidence indicating that "psychological factors somehow predispose a person to illness..." as part of a quest for the reason that some patients withstand dialysis so much better than others. Acknowledging that "we need to encourage psychological work in this area," he nevertheless is prepared to characterize long surviving patients as "givers of ulcers, rather than getters of ulcers," a view consistent with Avram's "aggressiveness and assertiveness."

M.M.A.

REFERENCE

1. Scribner BH, Buri R, Caner JEZ, et al: The treatment of chronic uremia by means of intermittent hemodialysis: Preliminary report. *Trans Am Soc Artif Intern Organs* 6:114, 1960.

13

Treatment of Chronic Renal Failure in Seattle
The First Twenty Years

BELDING H. SCRIBNER

It is my purpose here to describe for the first time some details of the early history of our maintenance dialysis program in Seattle, which began in 1960. In the second part of this chapter I deal briefly with the question of accelerated atherosclerosis, which emerged out of that early experience.[1] Finally, I present an analysis of the long-term dialysis and transplant survivors, pointing out how this analysis, as well as that of others,[2,3] may dramatically alter the prognosis of patients with chronic renal failure.

HISTORY OF THE EARLY YEARS

What made maintenance dialysis possible was the creation of the arteriovenous (A-V) shunt, which eventually turned out to be a relatively poor solution to the circulatory access problem. Nevertheless, all we had in 1960 was the original all-Teflon A-V shunt shown in Figure 1.[4] That this first experiment with long-term circulatory access worked is shown in Figure 2. Patient C.S., who was dying of uremia from chronic renal failure, had the first shunt put in place by surgeon David Dillard on March 9, 1960. Medical engineer Wayne Quinton was at the bedside, Bunsen burner in hand, bending Teflon tubing to fit the patient's anatomy. Although the first shunt lasted only 3 months, it portended a revolution in the management of end-stage renal disease, as evidenced by the fact that C.S. survived for 11 years.

During the early part of this remarkable record of survival, C.S. overcame innumerable life-threatening complications, including malig-

BELDING H. SCRIBNER ● Division of Nephrology, Department of Medicine, University of Washington School of Medicine, Seattle, Washington.

145

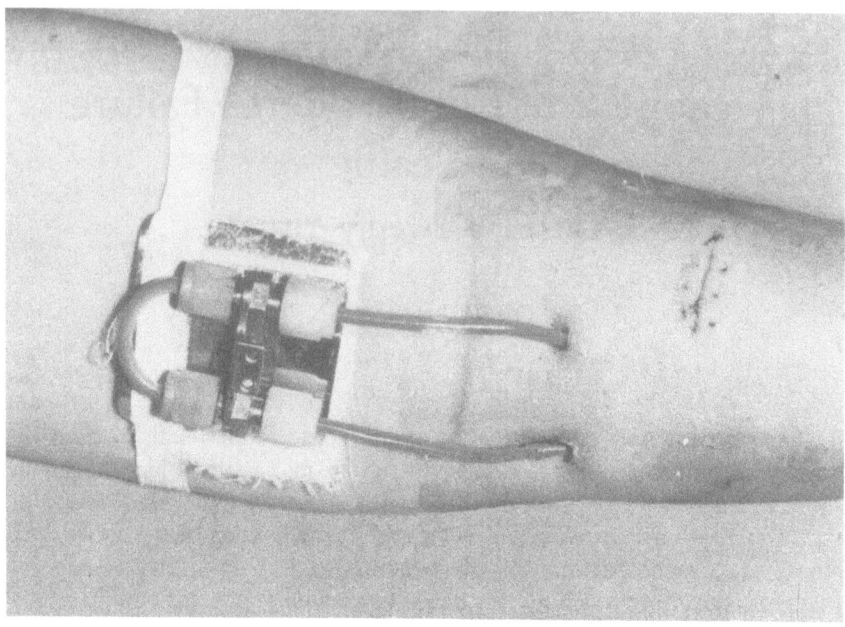

Figure 1. The all-Teflon arteriovenous shunt. Stainless steel plumbing fixtures were mounted on a small steel plate. The fixtures were used to couple the shunt to the cannula ends. They were soon replaced by a direct Teflon–Teflon joint.

nant hypertension, gout, peripheral neuropathy, massive metastatic calcification, and iron overload. As C.S. developed these complications one by one, we managed somehow to find an answer. We cured malignant hypertension by the use of aggressive ultrafiltration to control extracellular volume.[5] Gout-like attacks were recognized, proved to be due to uric acid accumulation,[6] and were prevented by hemodialyzing twice a week instead of once a week. Progression of severe peripheral neuropathy was halted and reversed by prolonging each dialysis treatment. This complication virtually disappeared from the dialysis scene when we increased hemodialysis treatments to three times a week. In the summer of 1960 our three patients literally were turning to stone (Figure 3) because of huge metastatic calcifications caused by serum phosphate levels in the 10–14 mg/dl range. Someone pointed out that an undesirable complication of antacid therapy for peptic ulcer was phosphate depletion. All patients immediately were put on antacids, and as if by magic the metastatic calcifications melted away in a matter of weeks, in what turned out to be a most dramatic therapeutic response. The use of phosphate binders by

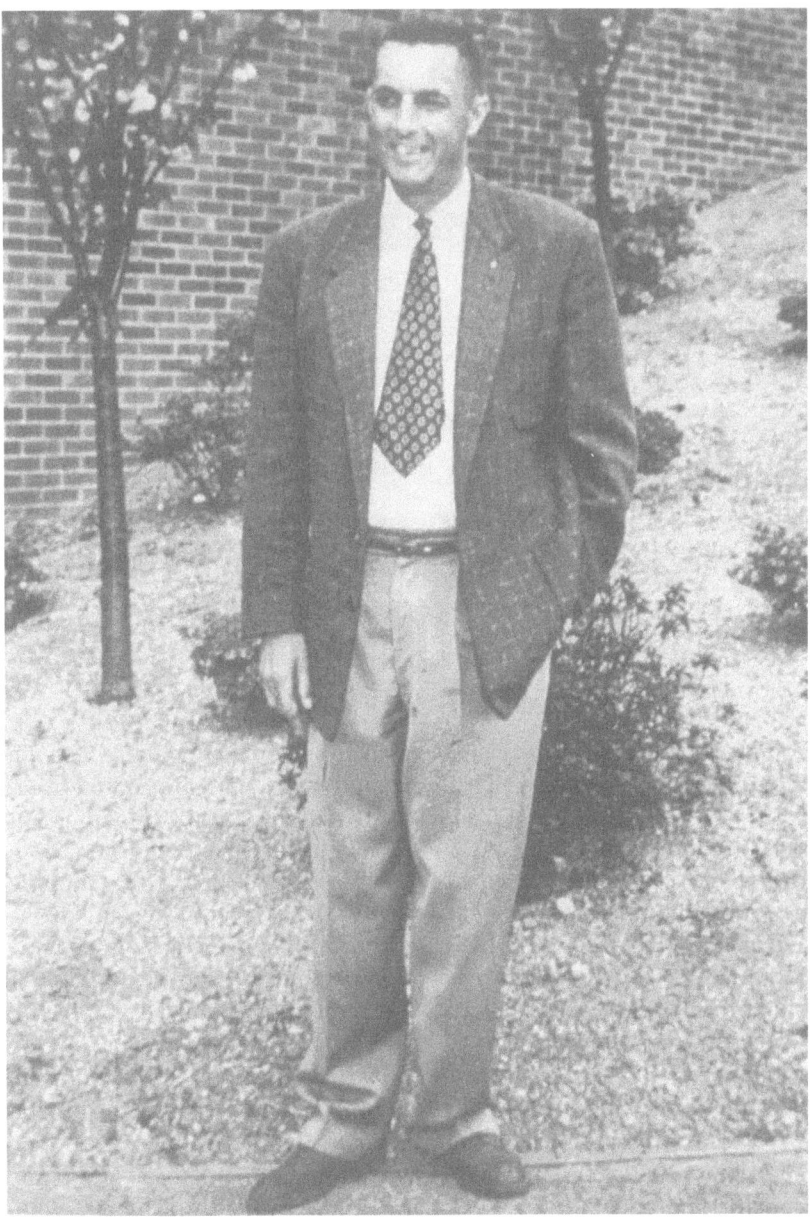

Figure 2. Patient C.S. in 1962.

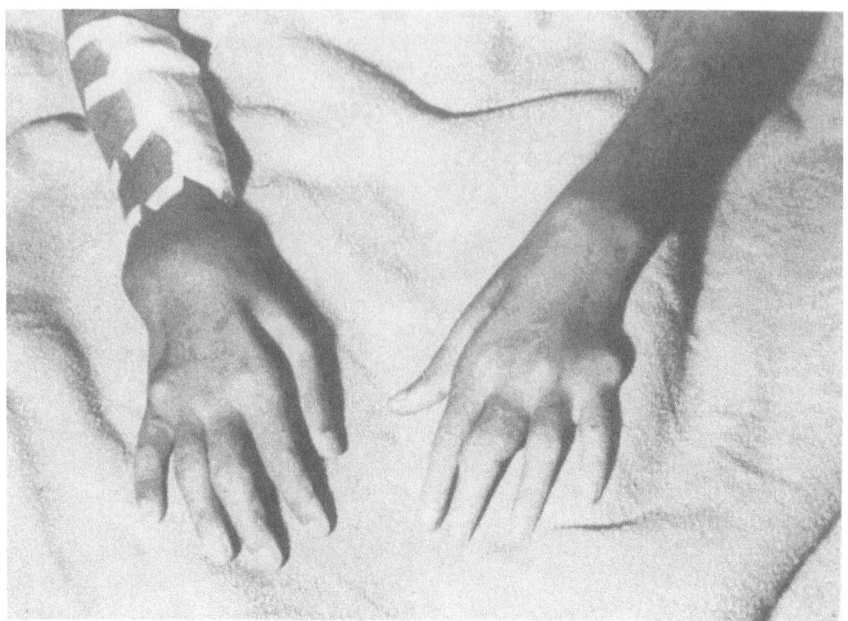

Figure 3. Metastatic calcifications in the wrists of patient R.H.

hemodialysis patients has been with us ever since. Finally, there was the problem of iron overload, which threatened to become a fatal complication. At first we tried to inject iron chelates into the dialyzer blood circuit to trap iron and remove it by dialysis.[7] Then, in careful studies of marrow iron kinetics by Eschbach et al.,[8] it was shown that, by stopping transfusions, the totally suppressed marrow slowly would become active enough to provide acceptable hematocrit levels. This increase in activity, coupled with loss of blood with each dialysis, gradually reversed the iron overload. Today, of course, all patients tend to become iron depleted unless given supplemental iron.

Patient no. 2, H.G., was cannulated on March 22, 1960. Mysteriously, he remained free of many of the above complications, including peripheral neuropathy. In contrast, patient no. 3, R.H., arrived for teatment in uremic coma in May 1960. He soon developed the fulminant form of uremic neuropathy and ended up in a Drinker respirator for several weeks while remaining on dialysis. Figure 4 shows R.H. in a wheelchair several months later, much improved, but still badly crippled by the severe muscle and nerve damage of the original neuropathic episode. He continued to improve very slowly, and at the time of the tenth anniversary of the

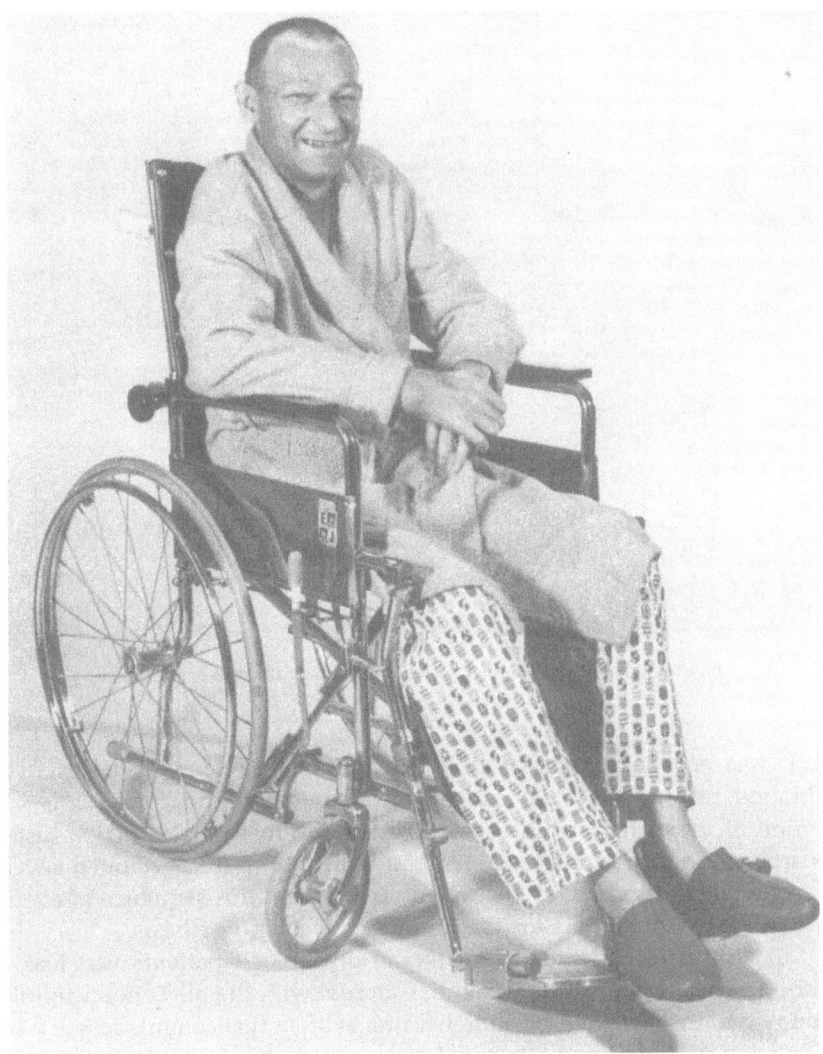

Figure 4. Patient R.H. in late 1960.

beginning of maintenance dialysis in Seattle in March 1970, he was walking with the help of a cane (Figure 5).

Not until we recognized the importance of residual renal function to dialysis patients[9] did we solve the mystery of why patient R.H. did so poorly and patient H.G. so well, with C.S. in between. Note in Table I that

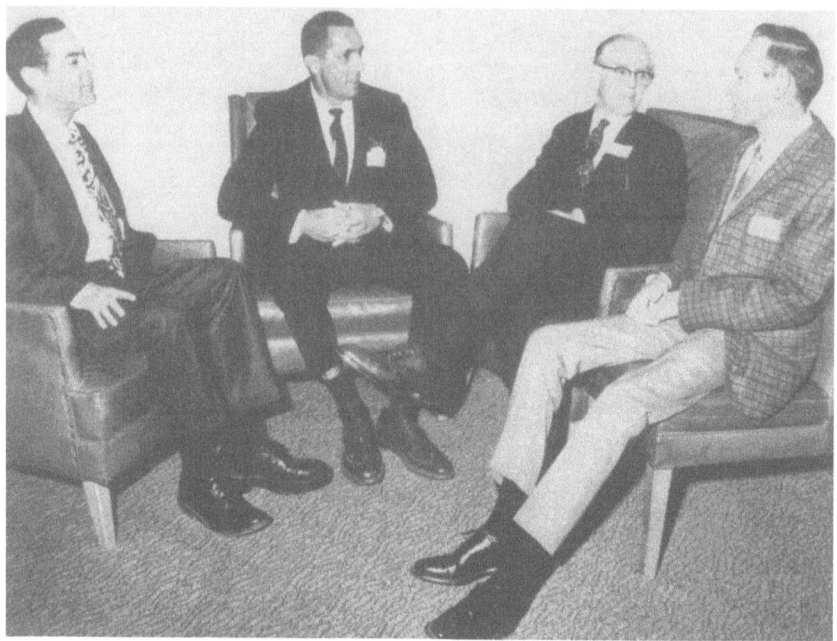

Figure 5. The three original patients with the author in March 1970.

R.H. was anuric from the outset, whereas H.G. retained a glomerular filtration rate greater than 1.0 ml/min throughout the critical 1960–61 period of underdialysis. In contrast, C.S.'s residual renal function disappeared during the summer of 1960, at which point he developed severe peripheral neuropathy. As discussed elsewhere,[10] this sequence of events provides strong support for the middle molecule hypothesis.

The greatest threat to the survival of our first patients was loss of circulatory access. Despite the initial success with the all-Teflon cannulas coupled to the armplate,[4] it soon became evident that cannula losses were occurring at an alarming rate and that the access sites in our patients would be exhausted rapidly. It was in recognition of this problem that W. E. Quinton made the tremendous advance in 1961 of introducing into the system a segment of silicone tubing that acted as a shock absorber, so that the cannula tip would remain immobile and not gouge the intima.[11] This single change in design trebled or quadrupled the life of the bypass cannula. Quinton was able to find a way to extrude silicone tubing with an inner surface of sufficient quality so that it would not promote clotting, an accomplishment that was said to be impossible by engineers at Dow-

Table I. Change in Creatinine Clearance With Time

Date	Patient R.H. UV	Patient R.H. $C_{cr}{}^a$	Patient C.S. UV	Patient C.S. C_{cr}	Patient H.G. UV	Patient H.G. C_{cr}
3/7/60			1624	3.7		
3/16/60			1510	3.3		
3/28/60			885	2.3		2.1
5/10/60	nil	nil	452	1.2	1,536	2.6
8/4/60	nil	nil	163	0.3	655	1.5
9/5/60	nil	nil	135	0.2	1,068	1.8
10/16/60	nil	nil	nil	nil	1,063	1.3
5/8/61	nil	nil	nil	nil	890	1.1

^{a} UV: urine volume (ml/day); C_{cr}: creatinine clearance (ml/min).

Corning. This change in design served us well until Brescia and Cimino made their vital contribution in 1966.[12]

After starting the first three patients on long-term hemodialysis in early 1960, the program was completely shut down because the hospital administration decreed that due to lack of funding no additional patients could be accepted until one of the first three died. Since that did not occur until 11 years later, it would have been a long wait. Later the administrators relented—mainly on the strength of a small research grant from Dr. George Aagaard, then dean of the School of Medicine, which permitted us to add two more patients. The second of these, J.R., proved to be the first failure on chronic hemodialysis, and he would have died had not Dr. Fred Boen arrived in Seattle about that time. J.R. was dying simply because he immediately clotted the same A-V shunt that was working so well in the other four patients. (Imagine what might have happened if J.R. had been patient no. 1 instead of no. 5.) The cause for this accelerated clotting never was identified. However, a small subgroup of dialysis patients with an accelerated tendency to clot recently was described[13] and J.R. may have belonged to that goup. In any event, Dr. Boen determined to try to save J.R. by means of long-term peritoneal dialysis. Figure 6 shows this patient on the cycler cleverly fashioned out of equipment that had been developed five years earlier by Dr. Thomas Marr for use in gastrodialysis.[14]

When Dr. Boen started looking after J.R. in 1962, long-term peritoneal dialysis had been abandoned because of the high incidence of peritonitis. Boen decided to eliminate the bottle change as one source of infection and developed a closed sterile system using first 20-liter and later 40-liter carboys of dialysis fluid. This remarkable system required that a "fluid factory" be built that could manufacture and sterilize fluid in 40-liter

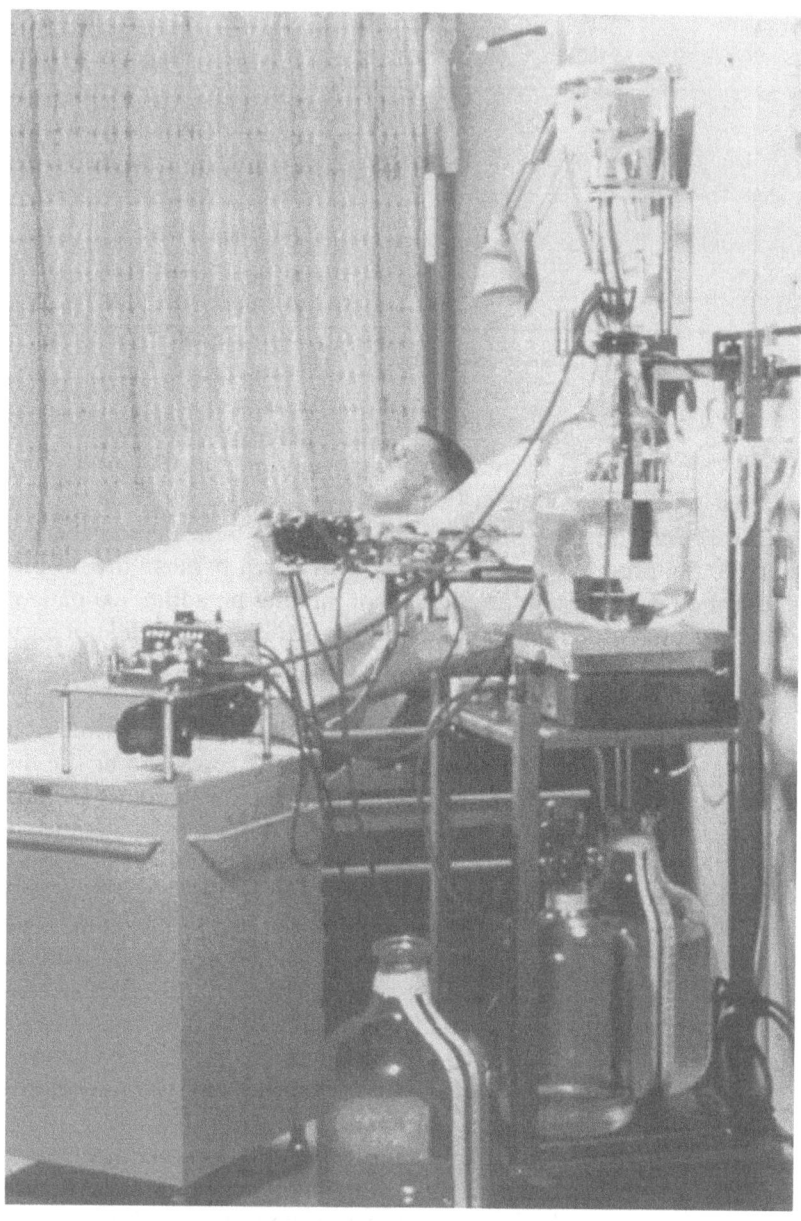

Figure 6. Patient J.R. on a 20-liter carboy dialysis system in 1962.

bottles. A remote corner in the sub-basement of the University of Washington Hospital was donated to the project, and this factory operated successfully until 1979, when it was finally refurbished and moved upstairs to more respectable quarters.

To this day all of our in-hospital peritoneal dialysis still is done with 40-liter carboys. Being completely closed and sterile, it is the safest system so far devised. It permitted Dr. Boen to keep J.R. on dialysis for many months, until J.R. finally became infected repeatedly through the access device and died. As a result, Boen decided to abandon attempts to develop a peritoneal access device, and in January 1963 he started a second patient, J.D., on peritoneal dialysis using a repeated puncture technique that involved inserting a catheter for each dialysis. J.D. did very well on peritoneal dialysis and remained virtually free of peritonitis for three years, until she was switched to hemodialysis. Eventually she received a transplant from her sister and is alive and well today, 17 years after starting peritoneal dialysis; she is one of the survivors discussed below. Dr. Boen regards his experience with J.D. as the crucial first step in proving finally the potential feasibility of long-term peritoneal dialysis in the management of end-stage kidney disease. Details of the subsequent successful development of maintenance peritoneal dialysis by Boen and Tenckhoff are presented elsewhere.[15]

It was indeed fortunate that in 1959 we were already experimenting with the technique of continuous hemodialysis for the intensive treatment of acute renal failure.[16] Experience with this technique made it possible to develop a relatively low-cost hemodialysis system without which our three original patients probably would not have survived. Figure 7 shows C.S. being dialyzed on an early version of this sytem using a large freezer as a tank for dialysis fluid. Orginally the system was designed to operate at $4°C$ to retard bacterial growth in this large dialysate reservoir. Bubble formation in the blood after rewarming was a constant problem at $4°C$. Therefore we moved the temperature up to 20°C without difficulty. The next step was to try running at 37°C. About four hours into the first run at 37°C someone noticed an unpleasant odor. Before we could discover its cause, the patient had a grand mal seizure. As we were taking him off dialysis, it became apparent that the bad smell came from the dialysate tank.

We sent a sample of the fluid, which still looked clear, to the bacteriology laboratory for culture. The next morning I received a call from Dr. John Sherris, the head of the laboratory, who said: "My God, man, I can't grow them that well down here!" The bacterial count was $>10^9$. That episode alerted us at an early stage to the extreme potential danger of bacterial contamination of dialysis fluid. The recently reported negative pyrogen studies of Bernick et al.[17] simply mean that their assay does not

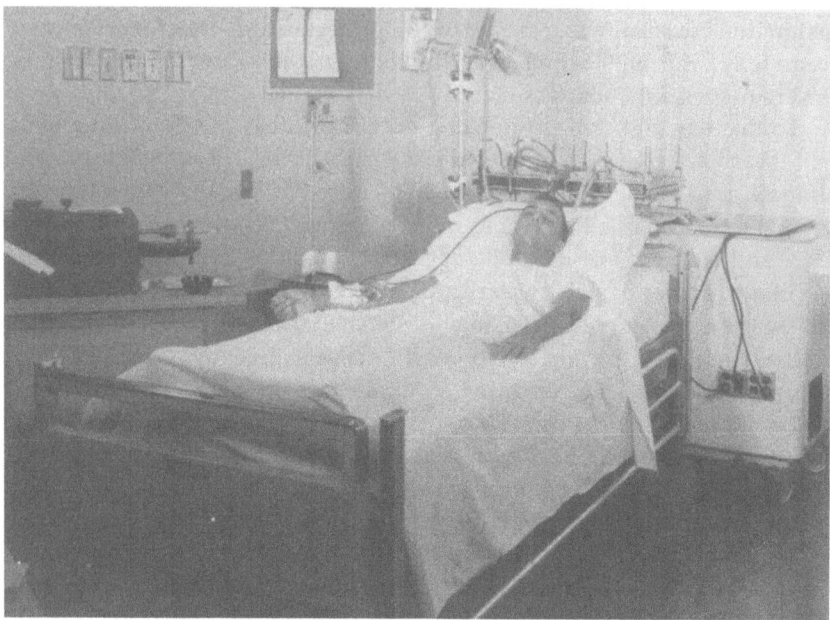

Figure 7. C.S. being hemodialyzed with a modification of the continuous-flow hemodialysis system. Note the deep-freeze that has been converted into a dialysate tank. The dialyzers were locally manufactured twin Skeggs-Leonards four-layer units selected for their low resistance to blood flow, which permitted the patient's arterial pressure to push the blood through the circuit without a blood pump.

detect the dialyzable pyrogens to which patients react. Whenever we began having adverse reactions to dialysis, one place in which we always looked for an answer was the colony count in the dialysis fluid. More often than not, a high count was found and its correction usually eliminated the problem.

Another huge problem in the first two years was the enormous difficulty in assembling and sterilizing the Skeggs-Leonards dialyzer. From the earliest moment we siliconed the little steel blood plates to reduce clotting, only to find that the steam sterilization technique advised by Dr. Jack Leonards removed the coating. We then changed to a cold sterilization technique using Zephiran®, which worked well for several months until febrile reactions recurred and it was found that spore formers that were not killed by Zephiran had contaminated the system. We changed to 2% acetic acid. Again there was no trouble for several months, until fever again recurred due to contamination with more spore formers. At that point we decided to switch to formalin, which has kept us out of trouble permanently because this agent does kill spores.

However, a great difficulty in dialyzer assembly remained in the form of a laborious assembly procedure and high leak rate. While I was visiting Dr. Claus Brun in Copenhagen in the summer of 1961, during our conversation regarding assembly problems with the Skeggs-Leonards dialyzer he said: "I have something in the closet here that you might be interested in." Whereupon he produced a four-layer Kiil dialyzer.[18] It did not take me long to realize that this unit was just what we needed to solve our dialyzer assembly problem. Claus got on the phone to Oslo, and Dr. Fred Kiil agreed to replace the Kiil dialyzer for $500—which meant that I could write out a check for that amount and take Dr. Brun's Kiil home with me. I persuaded SAS to let me stand the unit, which weighed over 100 pounds, in the coat closet of the DC-8 to New York. At New York Customs, the inspector was sure I was a diamond smuggler and proceeded to prove his point by taking out a pocket knife and digging out the gaskets on the Kiil boards, looking for precious stones. Despite this setback we soon had the Kiil in operation, and it became evident that this unit was a tremendous improvement on the Skeggs-Leonards dialyzer, and in a two-layer configuration it was just what we needed.

The difficulty was that there was no production version of the Kiil dialyzer. The few dialyzers in existence had been hand-made in Dr. Kiil's laboratory in Oslo, and there were no plans to produce it commercially. For many months thereafter Quinton labored unsuccessfully to produce the dialyzer by molding it from epoxy resin. When I discussed this problem with a colleague from Los Angeles, Dr. Jack Meihaus, he told me he had an engineering friend, Martin Headman, in charge of research at Western Gear Corporation, who probably could figure out a way to manufacture Kiil boards to an acceptable tolerance. Despite the fact that Western Gear was a manufacturer of heavy industrial equipment and not in the medical field at all, Dr. Meihaus was so persuasive that I took one of the original Kiil boards to Los Angeles and showed it to Headman. It was he who developed a technique of machining the boards out of poly-propylene slabs. As soon as the first Western Gear Kiil arrived in Seattle we knew we had a winner—and the demand for these units was instantaneous and enormous. It is a real credit to Headman and the management at Western Gear that they turned out Kiil dialyzers at an amazing pace while keeping the price just a bit above their cost. The Western Gear Kiil dialyzer became the most sought after dialyzer for many months, until production finally caught up with the demand.

Modifications on the dialysis system continued. In late 1961 the

Sweden Freezer Company, a local manufacturer of soft ice cream machines, built a commercial stainless steel version of the deep-freeze dialysate tank. Three of these units were installed in the first outpatient dialysis center, the Seattle Artificial Kidney Center (Figure 8). This Center was located in the basement of a nurses' residence adjacent to the Swedish Hospital in downtown Seattle and was made possible by a grant from the John A. Hartford Foundation.[19] The patient in the bed on the right in Figure 8 is Dr. James Albers, who began dialysis in the summer of 1961, having received the first set of Quinton silicone cannulas. It is noteworthy that after 19 years Dr. Albers still uses cannulas. Indeed, he has had cannulas in one arm only; he says he is holding the other arm in reserve! A more detailed account of Albers's history is given elsewhere.[20]

Admission to this new three-bed outpatient facility was controlled by a committee of laypersons, a selection device created by our local King County Medical Society. Figure 9 shows a picture of this committee that appeared in the November 9, 1962, issue of *Life* magazine as part of an article by Shana Alexander. The pros and cons of using such a selection device have been debated ever since, and the history and ethics of

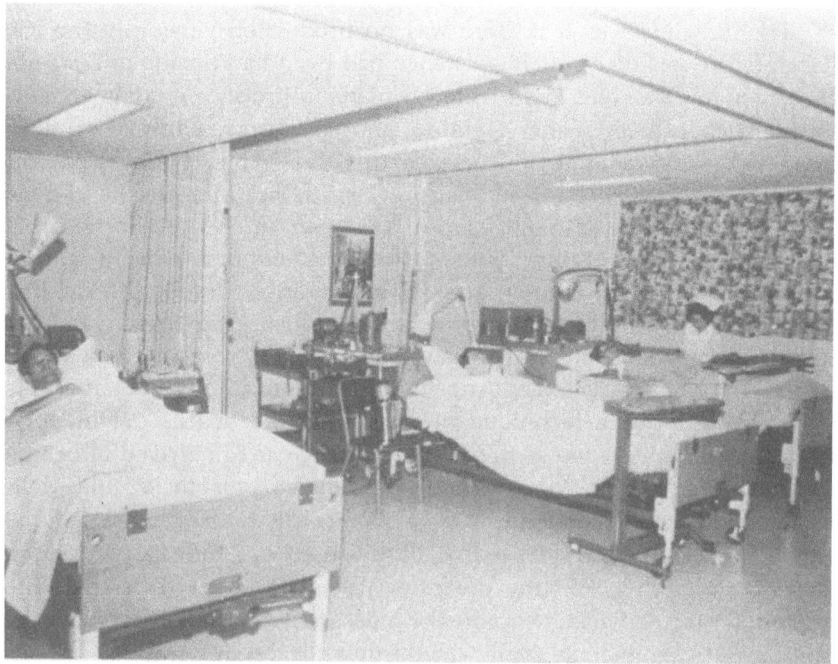

Figure 8. The first outpatient dialysis facility shortly after it opened in January 1962.

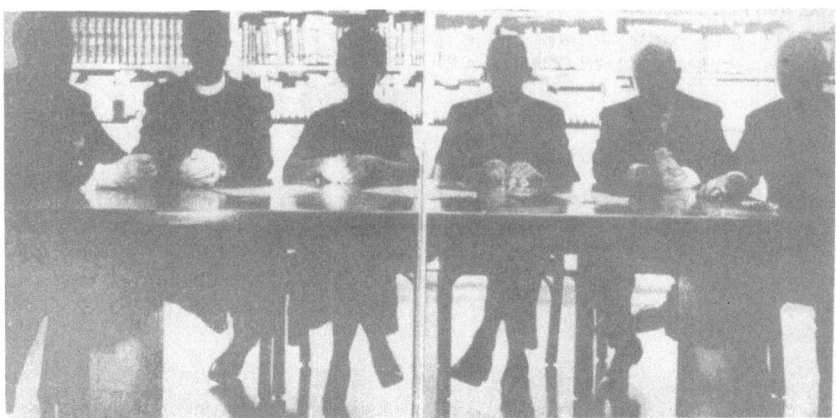

Figure 9. The committee.

the committee's activities have been described in detail by Fox and Swazey.[21]

Only one patient ever "beat the system" and was able to start long-term dialysis in Seattle despite this rigid and cruel committee selection system. That patient was Dr. Robin Eady who, in the winter of 1963, was a medical student at Guy's Hospital in London. In early January of 1963 we received a call from the British Embassy in Washington informing us that Robin Eady was dying of uremia and asking if we could help. The basic rule under which the selection committee operated was that they would consider only residents of the state of Washington. Here is how we were able to accept Dr. Eady as a patient.

Dr. Lionel McLeod was visiting us from Edmonton, Alberta, Canada, and was planning to set up a dialysis unit there. We agreed to start Robin on dialysis, to train him as a dialysis technician, and, as soon as he was well enough, to send him to Edmonton to become both patient and technician. Robin arrived in February 1963 on one of the early Pan-American transpolar flights directly from London. Had it been otherwise, I do not know whether he would have made it. He was so sick on arrival that we had to carry him off the airplane to a waiting ambulance. However, he responded very well to dialysis (Figure 10) and soon was on his way to Edmonton. From there he eventually renturned to London to become one of the first patients of Dr. Stanley Shaldon. He resumed his medical studies, and today he is engaged in research and practice of dermatology in London. Dr. Eady has described his experiences as the second longest survivor on maintenance hemodialysis.[22,23]

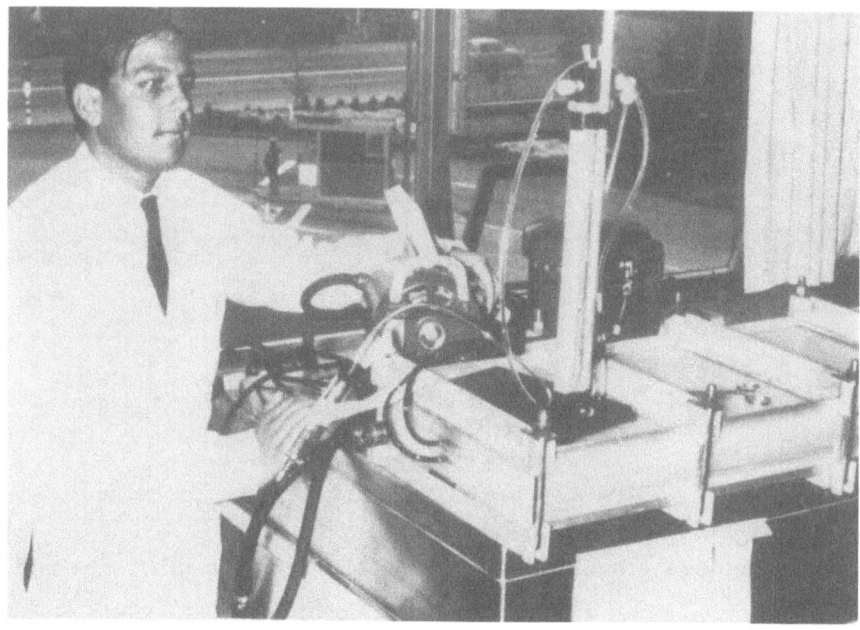

Figure 10. Robin Eady learning his trade as a hemodialysis technician in the spring of 1963. An early Western Gear Kiil dialyzer is in the foreground.

As time passed, long-term survival on maintenance hemodialysis became a real possibility. At the tenth anniversary celebration, held in Seattle in March 1970, all three original patients were doing better than ever (Figure 5). Then, in the early 1970s, it became apparent that many of these patients were developing the complications of accelerated atherosclerosis. Indeed, patient C.S. died of a myocardial infarction while on home dialysis in his basement in March 1971, 11 years after starting maintenance hemodialysis.

THE CONTROVERSIAL QUESTION OF
ACCELERATED ATHEROSCLEROSIS

In 1974 we published a retrospective analysis of survival of the 39 patients who began dialysis during those early years just described. The data supported the gloomy projection that most patients on maintenance hemodialysis were at great risk of developing accelerated atherosclerosis, which would preclude long-term survival.[1] These data were all the more convincing because the 39 patients were all under 40 years of age and carefully selected to rule out preexisting atherosclerotic complications. This report obviously was very discouraging to all who were involved in the treatment of chronic uremia, including the patients themselves. This initial report was confirmed by other investigators.[24,25] Happily, these gloomy predictions did not go unchallenged.[26]

Among the first to cast doubt on the validity of these conclusions were Rostand et al.[27] In a much larger study population, these investigators concluded that among 320 patients at risk, the incidence of myocardial infarction among men on dialysis was no greater than that in the population at large. Furthermore, most deaths from myocardial infarction that did occur in this series happened during the first year of dialysis. In women, however, the rate of myocardial infarction was twice that of the normal control population.

The Seattle group recently updated its data and reconfirmed the original conviction that accelerated atherosclerosis was indeed prevalent in the maintenance dialysis population.[28] The conclusions of Rostand and colleagues were dismissed because of the high percentage of blacks in their study population. Despite a greater occurrence of hypertension, blacks seem more resistant than whites to the development of ischemic heart disease.[29]

ANALYSIS OF LONG-TERM SURVIVORS

Although controversial, the question of accelerated atherosclerosis remained a nagging and very real concern through the late 1970s. This concern obviously prodded Dr. Peter Lundin, himself a long-term maintenance hemodialysis patient, to reexamine the question through an analysis of the long-term survival data from Downstate Medical Center.[2] This careful analysis revealed that those patients who had remained normotensive on maintenance hemodialysis did not develop accelerated atherosclerosis. Lundin et al.also concluded that smoking may have been an additional risk factor for accelerated atherosclerosis, a risk factor previously identified by Haire et al.[30] The latter study showed that smoking alone adversely affected survival, but that the combination of smoking and uncontrolled hypertension was very bad indeed.

About the time that Lundin's report appeared I was preparing a similar analysis of Seattle's long-term survivors. The results are as follows: Eleven of 36 patients who began dialysis in Seattle prior to 1966 have survived 15 years or longer. The longest survivor, patient H.G., one of the three original patients, now is beginning his 22nd year. To date none of these patients has died, and so the survival curve is flat from 15 to 21 years. Since 36 patients began dialysis in Seattle prior to 1966, the survival rate of this group of patients is 30% at 15 years.

Table II gives the essential data on these 11 patients. There are eight males and three females. Six of the 11 have had a renal transplant, of which five resulted in long-term success. Patient no. 10 had cadaveric transplants in 1965 and 1979; both were rejected within three months. All 11 patients were under 40 years of age when they began dialysis.

Table III contains a compilation of the cardiovascular complications. Note first of all the complete absence of myocardial infarction. Hypertension is virtually absent in these 11 patients. Indeed, all six dialysis patients are normotensive without antihypertensive medications. The only clinical evidence of a major cardiovascular event has been a mild cerebrovascular accident in patient no. 3. Patient no. 6 had mild peripheral vascular disease involving the small vessels of both hands. She has circulatory insufficiency in both thumbs and forefingers. Prior cannulation is not the cause, since only one arm had cannulas. Patient no. 9 has severe peripheral vascular disease involving the small vessels of the hands and feet. Two toes have been amputated. None of these 11 patients smoke.

The 36 patients used for this survival study are approximately the same as the 39 patients used to construct our earlier study.[1] However, we have not reanalyzed the data on the nonsurvivors to determine the incidence of smoking and hypertension in those patients who did develop accelerated atherosclerosis. Lundin et al.[2] did such an analysis on their

Table II. Data on 11 Patients

Patient	Sex	Age Start	Age Now	First dialysis	Transplant	Current therapy[a]	Total duration (years)
#1	M	22	42	2/60	'68—mother	Tx	21
2	M	27	46	7/61	none	Dialysis	19
3	M	37	56	11/61	'77—cadaver	Tx	19
4	F	14	31	10/62	'65—father	Tx	18
5	M	22	39	2/63	none	Dialysis	18
6	F	27	44	5/63	'71—sister	Tx	17
7	M	30	47	6/63	none	Dialysis	17
8	F	34	49	6/65	none	Dialysis	15
9	M	32	47	8/65	none	Dialysis	15
10	M	28	43	10/65	see text	Dialysis	15
11	M	34	49	10/65	'70—cadaver	Tx	15

[a]Tx: transplant.

Table III. Cardiovascular Complications

	Patient no.										
	1	2	3	4	5	6	7	8	9	10	11
Present age	42	46	56	31	39	44	47	49	47	43	49
Transplant year	1968	no	1977	1965	no	1971	no	no	no	S	1970
Complications											
MI	0	0	0	0	0	0	0	0	0	0	0
Angina	0	0	0	0	0	0	0	0	0	0	0
CVA	0	0	+	0	0	0	0	0	0	0	0
Peripheral vascular disease	0	0	0	0	0	S	0	0	S	0	0
Hypertension	+	0	0	++	0	+	0	0	0	0	+

Key: 0 = non, + = mild, ++ = moderate, S = see text

series of patients and demonstrated a very high correlation coefficient. Both of these retrospective analyses make it clear that the most striking common characteristic of long-term survivors is absence of hypertension. What is not clear is whether more vigorous treatment of those patients who remained hypertensive would have reduced the high incidence of atherosclerotic disease among the nonsurvivors in both series. An affirmative answer may be forthcoming from a study about to be reported by Charra et al.[3] from their dialysis unit in Tassin, France.

THE TASSIN EXPERIENCE

It is of great interest to me that Dr. Bernard Charra, who was second author of the original paper from Seattle by Lindner, Charra, Sherrard, et al.,[1] now is about to provide evidence, along with Dr. Guy Laurent and others, that control of hypertension can prevent accelerated athero-sclerosis among dialysis patients.

It is noteworthy that the dialysis technique used in Tassin employs old-fashioned, relatively inefficient Kiil dialyzers. Patients are dialyzed from 24 to 30 hours per week. This long dialysis facilitates excellent control of extracellular volume. Presumably as a result of this control, the incidence of hypertension in the Tassin dialysis population is extremely low, and antihypertensive medications are never used.

Charra and colleagues[3] have analyzed the long-term survival of 44 patients who began dialysis prior to 1971. Two very important conclusions emerge from this analysis. First, the ten-year survival is 84%. Compare this figure with a 50% survival at ten years of the first 36 Seattle patients, who, despite being younger and more highly selected than those from Tassin, still had a large incidence of cardiovascular deaths.[1] Second, not a single death in the Tassin series was caused by the complications of accelerated atherosclerosis and there has been no morbidity from this problem.

These encouraging conclusions from the Tassin experience receive support from a unique study by the San Francisco transplant unit. Vincenti et al.,[31] using an entirely different approach, have reached a similar conclusion, that is, that control of hypertension prevents accelerated atherosclerosis in patients on maintenance hemodialysis. These investigators looked for evidence of atherosclerosis during renal transplant surgery on 50 patients. They found that 62% had atherosclerosis, of which 31% had severe involvement. However, when patients between the ages of 25 and 40 were studied, only those who were hypertensive had significant atherosclerosis.

CONCLUSIONS

Fortunately, it seems that our 1974 paper[1] was wrong in its implication that accelerated atherosclerosis was an inevitable complication of maintenance dialysis. It may indeed be true that the maintenance dialysis patient, like the diabetic patient, has a metabolic problem that accelerates the development of atherosclerosis. However, it now appears that hypertension is a necessary catalyst. In the absence of this factor, patients on maintenance dialysis do not develop accelerated atherosclerosis. Smoking may be an additional risk factor, and when both smoking and hypertension are present, the results are devastating.[30]

Finally, it is worth pointing out that hypertension, often severe, can develop long before the patient begins maintenance dialysis. Since more than 80% of patients with chronic renal failure eventually develop hypertension, this risk factor, if neglected, can operate with severe consequences in the predialysis/transplant phase of management. Therefore careful monitoring of blood pressure of all patients with chronic renal disease becomes a vital part of long-term management, so that hypertension can be detected early and treated appropriately.

REFERENCES

1. Lindner A, Charra B, Sherrard DJ, Scribner: Accelerated atherosclerosis in prolonged maintenance hemodialysis. N Engl J Med 290:697–701, 1974.
2. Lundin AP, Adler AJ, Feinroth MV, et al: Maintenance hemodialysis. Survival beyond the first decade. JAMA 244:38–40, 1980.

3. Charra B, et al. Long term survival and improved control of blood pressure with "long" hemodialysis. *Nephron,* in press.

4. Quinton W, Dillard D, Scribner BH: Cannulation of blood vessels for prolonged hemodialysis. *Trans Am Soc Artif Int Organs* 6:104–109, 1960.

5. Hegstrom RM, Quinton WE, Dillard DH, et al: One year's experience with the use of indwelling teflon cannulas and bypass. *Trans Am Soc Artif Int Organs* 7:47–56, 1961.

6. Caner JEZ, Hegstrom RM, Decker JD: Recurrent acute (gouty?) arthritis in chronic renal failure treated with periodic hemodialysis. *Am J Med* 36:571–582, 1964.

7. Tisher CC, Barnett BMS, Finch CA, et al: DTPA in the treatment of haemosiderosis in patients on chronic haemodialysis. *Proc Europ Dialysis Transpl Assoc* 3:43–47, 1966.

8. Eschbach JW, Funk D, Adamson J, et al: Erythropoiesis in patients with renal failure undergoing chronic dialysis. *N Engl J Med* 276:653–658, 1967.

9. Ahmad S, Babb AL, Milutinovic J, et al: Effect of residual renal function on minimum dialysis requirements. *Proc Europ Dialysis Transpl Assoc* 16:107–114, 1979.

10. Babb AL, Ahmad S, Scribner BH, et al: The middle molecule hypothesis in perspective. *Am J Kidney Dis* 1:46–50, 1981.

11. Quinton WE, Dillard DH, Cole JJ, et al: Eight months' experience with silastic-teflon bypass cannulas. *Trans Am Soc Artif Int Organs* 8:236–243, 1962.

12. Brescia MJ, Cimino JE, Appel K, et al: Chronic hemodialysis using venipuncture and a surgically created arteriovenous fistula. *N Engl J Med* 275:1089–1092, 1966.

13. Kauffman HM, Edbom GA, Adams MB, et al: Hypercoagulability: A cause of vascular access failure. *Proc Dialysis Transpl Forum* 9:28–30, 1979.

14. Marr TA, Burnell JM, Scribner BH: Gastrodialysis in the treatment of acute renal failure. *J Clin Invest* 39:653–661, 1960.

15. Scribner BH: Foreword, in Nolph KD (ed): *Peritoneal Dialysis.* The Hague, Martinus Nijhoff Publishers, 1982.

16. Scribner BH, Caner JEZ, Buri R, et al: The technique of continuous hemodialysis. *Tans Am Soc Artif Int Organs* 6:88–103, 1960.

17. Bernick JJ, Port FK, Favero MS, et al: Bacterial and endotoxin permeability of hemodialysis membranes. *Kidney Int* 16:491–496, 1979.

18. Kiil F: Development of a parallel flow artificial kidney in plastics. *Acta Chir Scand Suppl* 253:142, 1960.

19. Murray JS, Tu WH, Albers JB, et al: A community hemodialysis center for the treatment of chronic uremia. *Trans Am Soc Artif Int Organs* 8:315–319, 1962.

20. Scribner BH: Preface, in Friedman EA (ed): *Strategy in Chronic Renal Failure.* New York, John Wiley & Sons, 1978, 557 pp.

21. Fox RC, Swazey JP: *The Courage to Fail,* Chicago, University of Chicago Press, 1974, 395 pp.

22. Eady RAJ: A patient's experience of over one thousand haemodialyses. *Proc Europ Dialysis Transpl Assoc* 8:50–58, 1971.

23. Eady RAJ: What seventeen-and-half years of treatment are really like: A patient's experience of dialysis. *Kidney Int* (in press).

24. Lazarus JM, Lowrie EG, Hampers CL, et al: Cardiovascular disease in uremic patients on hemodialysis. *Kidney Int* 7:S167–S175, 1975.

25. Ibels IS, Steward JH, Mahony JF, et al: Occlusive arterial disease in uraemic and haemodialysis patients and renal transplant recipients. *Q J Med* 46:197–214, 1977.

26. Burke JF Jr, Francos GC, Moore LL, et al: Accelerated atherosclerosis in chronic dialysis patients—Another look. *Nephron* 21:181–185, 1978.

27. Rostand SG, Gretes JC, Kirk KA, et al: Ischemic heart disease in patients with uremia undergoing maintenance hemodialysis. *Kidney Int* 16:600–611, 1979.

28. Haas LB, Brunzell JD, Sherrard DJ. Atherosclerotic risk factors in a chronic dialysis population. *Am Soc Nephrol* 12:118A, 1979 (abs).

29. McDonough JR, Hames CG, Stulb SC, et al: Coronary heart disease among negroes and whites in Evans County, Georgia. *J Chron Dis* 18:443–468, 1965.
30. Haire HM, Sherrard DJ, Scardapane D, et al: Smoking, hypertension, and mortality in a maintenance dialysis population. *Cardiovasc Med* 3:1163–1168, 1978.
31. Vincenti F. Amend WJ, Abele J, et al: The role of hypertension in hemodialysis-associated atherosclerosis. *Am J Med* 68:363–369, 1980.

14

The Long Island College Hospital Experience with the Decade or Longer Hemodialysis Patient

MORRELL M. AVRAM

When hemodialysis was a new therapy for chronic uremia, survival of patients for a month was regarded as miraculous by clinicians accustomed to the inevitability of failure of all regimens. As the exciting exploratory decade of the 1960s passed, rational protocols to manage hyperphosphatemia, motor neuropathy, and fluid retention were devised to cope with these complications of what was later appreciated to be underdialysis. Once it was realized that patients might live for years with artificial kidneys providing partial substitution for missing native renal function, the question of "just how long can these patients live?" became important for medical planners, and mostly for patients and their families.

At The Long Island College Hospital and other institutions committed to programs in uremia therapy, it became apparent in the mid-1960s that protracted survival on dialysis for some patients was an achievable objective. But which patients and what conditions were necessary for long life on dialysis were unclear. We were encouraged by the fact that we had been the first to successfully treat uremic diabetics by maintenance hemodialysis.

To explore the pathobiology of treated uremia in order to extract usable information that might prove translatable to new uremic patients, we utilized a unique population of patients who had "made it" for a decade or longer. Specialty divisions of the Department of Medicine each applied its own research methods, each fully aware that those patients who did not survive beyond the decade were, in most instances, nonparticipatory in the

MORRELL M. AVRAM ● The Avram Center for Kidney Diseases, Division of Nephrology, The Long Island College Hospital; and Department of Medicine, The Long Island College Hospital, and Brooklyn Kidney Center and Nephrology Foundation of Brooklyn, New York.

final conclusions. However, the final subspecialty composite provides an in-depth view of the long surviving patients, which, to our knowledge, has never been attempted before on such a large scale, or in as great detail. Dr. Joseph Schluger, chairman of the Department of Medicine, spent much energy and countless hours in helping coordinate this effort.

The papers that follow indicate that:

1. Hypertension is the most important threat to long survival on dialysis.
2. Binephrectomized patients can be fully rehabilitated for a decade or longer, even though their mean hematocrit is lower than their nephric dialysis counterparts.
3. Hematologic complications other than persistent anemia are minimal. Blood transfusion requirements do not increase with time on dialysis.
4. Gastrointestinal complications are not a major life threat, although the origin of elevated alkaline phosphatase activity must be determined.
5. Renal osteodystrophy has not been corrected by contemporary regimens and its inexorable progression could emerge as the life-limiting factor on dialysis.
6. Pulmonary disease is no threat to longevity, but restrictive lung disease is common.
7. Accelerated atherosclerosis did not occur in the absence of hypertension.

Overall, the 1980s may very well be the decade in which remaining impediments to unlimited life prolongation by hemodialysis are removed. The future is indeed brighter for this decade than it was when we began some 20 years ago at The Long Island College Hospital.

15

Pathophysiology of Anephric Patients Over a Decade

Significance of Relative Hypotension

MORRELL M. AVRAM, ABE N. PAHILAN, AMADO GAN,
PAUL A. FEIN, PAUL A. SLATER, AND MICHAEL IANCU

Although maintenance hemodialysis (MH) was introduced as a treatment for chronic uremia in 1960,[1] there have been few reports of patients surviving for more than ten years. Earlier fears that death from complications of accelerated atherosclerosis would limit dialysis longevity[2] have not been substantiated.[3] As the population of hemodialysis patients rises above 100,000 worldwide, it is of increasing importance to define the natural history of life sustained by an artificial kidney. To explore the pathobiology present in those who survived for long periods, we studied a subset of patients kept alive by repeated hemodialyses for at least a decade, and compared their clinical findings with a control maintenance hemodialysis population. From this investigation we infer that our earlier identification of parathyroid hormone as an important uremic toxin[4,5] may now be extended to this group of ten-year survivors.

METHODS

Records of all patients who were begun on MH from January 1, 1968, through December 31, 1970, in the dialysis unit of Long Island College

MORRELL M. AVRAM • The Avram Center for Kidney Diseases, Division of Nephrology, The Long Island College Hospital; Department of Medicine, The Long Island College Hospital; and Brooklyn Kidney Center and Nephrology Foundation of Brooklyn, New York.   ABE N. PAHILAN • Division of Nephrology, The Long Island College Hospital, Brooklyn, New York.   AMADO GAN, PAUL A. FEIN, PAUL A. SLATER, AND MICHAEL IANCU • Division of Nephrology, The Long Island College Hospital; and Department of Medicine, The Long Island College Hospital, Brooklyn, New York.

Hospital were analyzed. During this interval a total of 158 patients received dialytic therapy for at least three months. Of these 158 patients, 32 (20.3%) had their lives prolonged by MH for at least ten years. Currently, 16 of the 32 (50%) who survived a decade or longer are alive, representing 10.1% of the original group. Separate reports elsewhere in this volume detail the subprotocols employed to investigate gastorintestinal, cardiovascular, hematologic, pulmonary, and rheumatologic components of the composite investigation. Of the 16 currently living long survivors, 11 offered informed consent for the multidisciplinary study described herein.

In addition to the prospective study of decade or longer dialysis patients, we reviewed the course of the subset of patients who had lived for at least ten years after binephrectomy. Of the 16 long survivors, 6 (38%) had underdone binephrectomy, representing 3.8% of the total group started on dialysis. Indications for binephrectomy included malignant uncontrollable hypertension in 3 patients, and previously required pretransplant nephrectomy in 3 patients.

Uremia in the six anephric long survivors was caused by diverse etiologies. In three, lupus nephritis and hypertension were responsible, while one patient had diffuse renal cortical necrosis, one had renal tuberculosis, and one had undiagnosed renal failure. Thus three of six developed uremia as part of a systemic disease. The age, sex, race, renal diagnosis, and duration of MH for the binephrectomized patients are given in Table I. Listed in Table II for the same six patients are the mean hematocrit, current parathyroid hormone level (PTH), serum calcium and phosphorus concentrations, and motor nerve conduction velocity in an extremity (MNCV). To assess usual values to be expected as a result of MH *per se*, we collected laboratory values in a group of 50 randomly selected patients now on maintenance dialysis at Long Island College Hospital, and used these as a reference group with which the anephric ten-year-long survivors (LS) were compared (Table III). All grouped values are expressed as mean ± standard deviation. Statistical significances of the results were evaluated by the Student t test using independent data or paired samples where appropriate. Cochrane's adjustment was applied when variances were unequal. All tests of statistical significance were done at $p < 0.05$.

Blood pressure was measured at each hemodialysis in an upper extremity by sphygmomanometer. The mean of three consecutive blood pressures was taken and used as the patient's blood pressure for this study.

Hemodialysis for all patients was performed with disposable coil dialyzers and a batch-type central dialysate supply system through 1974.

Table I. Clinical Details of Patients with Bilateral Surgical Removal
of Kidneys Surviving Over Ten Years

Patient	Age	Race	Year started dialysis	Renal diagnosis	Remarks
1	35	B	1970	Systemic lupus erythematosus	HAA+ cadaveric transplant × 2
2	39	B	1969	Malignant hypertension	Related live donor 1969
3	34	B	1968	Idiopathic	HAA+ cadaveric transplant × 2
4	34	B	1970	Malignant hypertension	Cadaveric transplant 1972 Subtotal parathyroidectomy 1975
5	41	B	1969	Bilateral cortical necrosis	
6	38	B	1969	Renal tuberculosis	Cadaveric transplant 1969 Subtotal parathyroidectomy 1969

Thereafter, a central proportioning dialysate supply system was utilized. The dialysis prescription for each patient consisted of thrice-weekly five to six hour treatments, using Travenol or extracorporeal coils. Angioaccess for hemodialysis was provided via an internal arteriovenous fistula, bovine carotid heterograft, Goretex graft, or an autologous saphenous vein graft. Laboratory monitoring of patients throughout the course of dialysis consisted of a venous hematocrit done once a week, using the capillary method, and predialysis serum calcium and phosphate, measured by

Table II. Clinical Data for the Same Six Anephric Long-Term Survivors[a]

Patient	Hct	PTH	MNCV	Ca	PO$_4$	BP S	BP D
1	22	225	47	8.9	4.9	110	73.3
2	19	1036	21	10.4	4.3	96.7	60
3	19	9377	22	9.8	4.1	126.7	80
4	22	339	35	9.4	5.0	120	76.7
5	20	475	38	7.1	3.8	93.3	63.3
6	25	400	34	9.3	3.6	90	63.3
Mean	21.2	568.7	33	9.2	4.3	106.1	69.4
± SD	±2.3	±335.3	±9.9	±1.1	±0.6	±15.1	±8.3

[a] Hct: hematocrit (volume %); PTH: parathyroid hormone (pg/ml); MNCV: peroneal motor nerve conduction velocity (m/sec); Ca: serum calcium (mg/dl); PO$_4$: serum phosphates (mg/dl); S: systolic blood pressure (mm Hg); D: diastolic blood pressure (mm Hg).

Table III. Grouped Findings in 50 Control Maintenance Hemodialysis Patients
(Mean ± SD)[a]

			Hct	PTH	Ca	PO$_4$	MNCV	Blood pressure mm Hg	
Age	Sex	Race	vol. 5	pg/ml	mg/dl	mg/dl	m/sec	Systolic	Diastolic
53.7	27 M	28 B	25.8	931.3	8.5	4.9	39.0	167.4	92.2
±11.5	23 F	22 W	±3.4	±803.5	±1.1	±1.4	±11.0	±20.6	±13.7

[a] See footnote, Table II.

autoanalyzer at least monthly as part of a routine chemical screening procedure.

Parathyroid hormone levels were measured by Upjohn Laboratories (Kalamazoo, Michigan) according to the technique of Hawker.[6] The mean normal parathyroid hormone value in the Upjohn Laboratory for 20 healthy adult volunteers ranging in age from 20 to 62 years was 255 pEq/ml. The range of normal values included within two standard deviations of the mean was 163–347 pEq/ml.

Motor nerve conduction velocity was determined using a TECA TE4 electromyograph (TECA Corporation, White Plains, New York), according to the method of Johnson and Melvin as described by Nielsen.[7]

RESULTS

Key findings in the group of anephric long survivors and in the MH controls are listed in Table IV. Comparision of the two groups showed that the former were younger, a mean of 36.5 ± 3.3 years (range 33–41 years) and had begun MH at an earlier age, a mean of 25.2 ± 3.2 years (range 21–30 years) ($p < 0.05$). All of the binephric patients were black and five of six (83%) were female.

Blood pressure control in the anephric group was significantly superior to that of MH controls. Systolic blood pressure of living long-term patients, mean of 106.1 ± 5.1 mm Hg, was normal, while the MH controls, with a mean of 167.4 ± 20.6 mm Hg, were hypertensive. By contrast, diastolic pressure in the living decade patients, which was a mean of 69.4 ± 8.3 mm Hg, was also normal, while the MH controls, who had a mean of 92.2 ± 13.7 mm Hg, were hypertensive ($p < 0.05$).

Table IV. Comparison of Mean Values Between Anephric Long Survivors and Control MH Patients[a]

| | Age | Hct | PTH | Ca | PO$_4$ | BP | |
						S	D
Anephric long survivors	36.5 ± 3.3	21.2 ± 2.3	568.7 ± 335.3	9.2 ± 1.1	4.3 ± 0.6	106.1 ± 15.1	69.4 ± 8.3
Maintenance hemodialysis control	53.7 ± 11.5	25.8 ± 3.4	931.3 ± 803.5	8.5 ± 1.1	4.9 ± 1.4	167.4 ± 20.6	92.2 ± 13.7
Statistical significance	$p < 0.05$	$p < 0.05$	$p < 0.10$	NS	NS	$p < 0.05$	$p < 0.05$

[a] See footnote, Table II.

CAUSE OF DEATH OF LONG-TERM MH PATIENTS

We reviewed the cause of death of the 14 patients (anephric and controls) who had lived for at least ten years on MH. Of these, seven (50%) had developed uremia secondary to a systemic disorder. Massive gastrointestinal hemorrhage accounted for 5 of 14 (36%) deaths, although one patient also had metastastic cancer and a cerebrovascular accident. Cerebrovascular disease also caused the death of 5 patients (36%). Hepatic failure and myocardial infarction accounted for two deaths each. It is noteworthy that the number of deaths attributable to atherosclerosis was no greater than that reported by Ibels et al.[8] for shorter-term MH patients.

DEMOGRAPHICS

The MH controls had a relative predominance of men (27 of 50, 54%) and blacks (28 of 50, 56%), while the living long-term anephric patients were predominantly women and black (83.3% and 100%).

There was no significant difference between MH controls and living

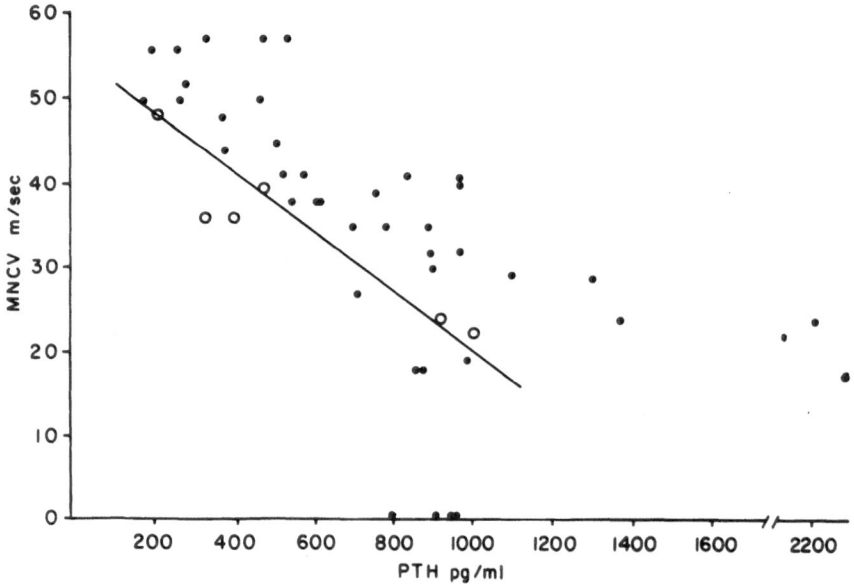

Figure 1. Relationship of nerve conduction velocity to PTH in maintenance hemodialysis control patients (O) and anephric long survivors (●).

long survivors when mean values for serum calcium phosphate or motor nerve conduction velocity were compared. The mean hematocrit in long survivors (21.2 ± 2.3%), however, was significantly lower than that of MH controls (25.8 ± 3.4%) ($p < 0.05$).

PTH AND MOTOR NERVE CONDUCTION VELOCITY

Anephric long surviving patients had a mean PTH level of 568.7 ± 335.3 pg/ml compared with the MH controls' mean level of 931.3 ± 803.5 ml. Because of the small sample ($n = 6$) size of the anephric group, their lower PTH levels did not reach statistical significances ($p < 0.10$). There was a wide range of PTH values in the MH controls whereas the anephric patients had a lower, more restrictive variation.

There was a clear inverse correlation between the height of PTH and motor nerve conduction velocity in both anephric patients and MH controls (Figure 1). An inverse relationship was present in long-term patients between hematocrit and PTH but the correlation was not present in MH controls (Figure 2).

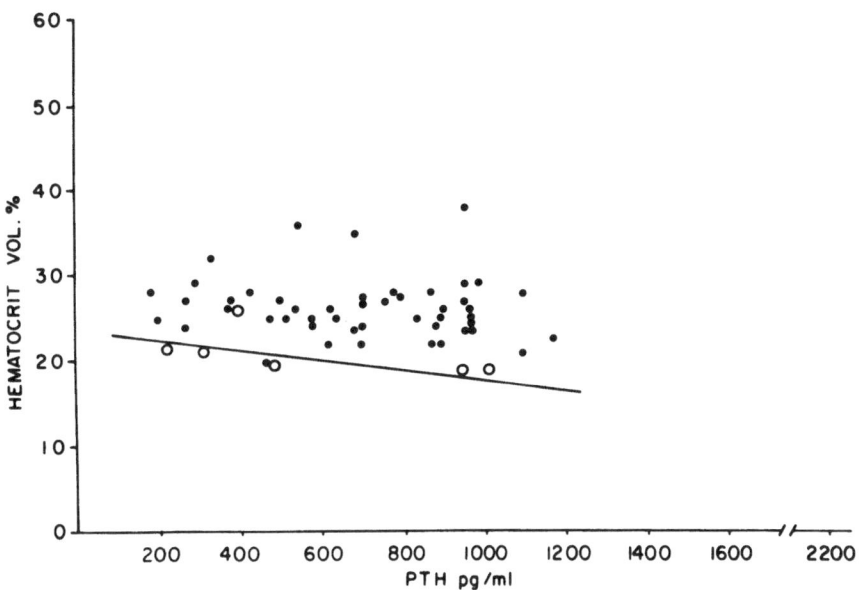

Figure 2. Relationship of hematocrit to PTH level in control (○) and anephric long survivors (●).

REHABILITATION

Most of the living decade or longer surviving MH patients were active, employed at least part-time, or maintaining their households. As a group they were suprisingly vigorous, and included a social worker, a teacher, three business persons, and a writer. The patients were gregarious human beings, as evidenced by their officerships in the Dialysis and Transplant Association (DATA), patient organization at Long Island College Hospital and services as an elected dialysis patient respresentative to the Department of Health, Education and Welfare's Network of Southern New York State. By contrast, only 29 of 50 (58%) control MH were either gainfully employed or maintaining their own homes. It has become evident that the long survivors share several behavioral and personality characteristics that have probably contributed to their longevity. These include alertness, curiosity, aggressiveness, leadership, and assertiveness.

HEPATITIS

Of the six long-term living patients, three patients have been persistently positive for hepatitis-associated antigen, though none of the three have chemical evidence of abnormal liver function or any signs of clinical hepatic disease.

ANGIOACCESS

A total of five patients who underwent at least a decade of MH, including three who are alive, have had a single functioning internal arteriovenous fistula for more than ten years. None of the other grafts lasted a decade, but one Goretex graft has been functioning for five years.

DISCUSSION

The present series details an early experience in the delivery of maintenance hemodialysis (MH) in which about one in five (20.3%) patients survived for at least a decade. Examination of this unusual group of patients who have had life prolonged by repetitive artificial kidney treatments indicates that the quality of life for those in their second decade of dialysis is consistent with social activity and fulfillment of employment and home responsibilities. We believe that personality traits of assertiveness, alertness, curiosity, and leadership are common in these long-term survivors and may have contributed to their favorable outcome.

It is noteworthy that so many of the long survivors were free of hypertension. The absence of hypertension, especially in the binephrectomized group, who had to cope with a lower hematocrit, may be the major factor promoting protracted endurance of the dialysis regimen.

Normotension in MH patients may retard development of coronary artery disease, a conclusion in agreement with the findings in non-nephrectomized, non-decade-surviving dialysis patients examined and reported by Haire et al.[9] We concur with Vincenti et al.[10] that vigorous control of hypertension in the incipient stage of renal failure might significantly reduce the frequency of ischemic heart disease developing after the onset of hemodialysis. This premise requires experimental confirmation. The importance of hypertension in development of dialysis-related atherosclerosis in our study may be questioned, however, since no age adjustments for expected rates of atherosclerosis were made and the most severe atherosclerotic disease was found in patients who were a decade older than those with either minimal or moderate disease.[11]

It is also of import to appreciate that one third of our decade or longer surviving MH patients were cigarette smokers, a risk factor of uncertain significance.

One sobering implication of our data is the realization that many of the factors shown to be strongly associated with coronary risk are beyond the control of the nephrologist seeking to extend life on MH. Of these factors—age, sex, race, predisposing systemic disease, and hypertension—only hypertension existing prior to onset of MH, and also thereafter, is amenable to correction. It may also be that duration of renal disease and the degree of control of hypertension prior to dialysis determine subsequent vascular disease.

Our surprising finding that binephrectomized patients can endure more than a decade of MH with reasonable rehabilitation provokes the speculation that the episodic hypotension usual to the course of anephric MH patients may provide protection against cardiac and vascular uremic complications. It is remarkable to observe that the consistently lower red cell mass of anephric MH patients is tolerable for more than ten years. Whatever yet to be identified secretions of the kidney are lacking in anephric MH patients clearly are not essential to life. Based on the present study, we continue to advocate a no-transfusion regimen for MH, except as an immunologic conditioning factor pretransplantation or for amelioration of angina. Far more important, these findings that anephric anemic patients survive for a decade with relative hypotension suggest the need to stress early control of hypertension in all patients, to prevent renal and cardiovascular damage before uremia, and once uremia occurs, to prolong survival.

REFERENCES

1. Scribner BH, Buri R, Caner JEZ, et al: The treatment of chronic uremia by means of intermittent hemodialysis: preliminary report. *Trans Am Soc Artif Intern Organs* 6:114, 1960.
2. Lindner A, Charra B, Sherrard DJ, et al: Accelerated atherosclerosis in prolonged maintenance hemodialysis. *N Engl J Med* 290:697, 1974.
3. Lundin AP, Adler AJ, Feinroth MV, et al: Maintenance hemodialysis: Survival beyond the first decade. *JAMA* 244:38, 1980.
4. Avram MM, Alexis H, Rahman M, et al: Decreased transfusional requirements following parathyroidectomy in long-term hemodialysis. *Proc Am Soc Nephrol* 5:5, 1971.
5. Avram MM, Feinfeld D, Huatuco AH: Search for the uremic toxin; decreased motor nerve conduction velocity and elevated parathyroid hormone in uremia. *N Engl J Med* 298:1000, 1978.
6. Hawker CD: Parathyroid hormone: Radioimmunoassay and clinical interpretation. *Ann Clin Lab Sci* 5:383, 1975.
7. Nielsen VK: The peripheral nerve function in chronic renal failure. X. Decremental nerve conduction in uremia? *Acta Med Scand* 196:83, 1974.
8. Ibels LS, Alfrey AC, Huffer WE, et al: Arterial calcification and pathology in uremic patients undergoing dialysis. *Am J Med* 66:790, 1979.
9. Haire HM, Sherrard DJ, Scardopane D, et al: Smoking, hypertension, and mortality in a maintenance dialysis population. *Cardiovasc Med* 3:1163, 1978.
10. Vincenti F, Amend WJ, Abele J, et al: The role of hypertension in hemodialysis-related atherosclerosis. *Am J Med* 68:363, 1980.
11. Bonomini V, Felletti C, Scolari MP, et al: Atherosclerosis in uremia: A longitudinal study. *Am J Clin Nutr* 33:1493, 1980.

16

Cardiovascular Effects of a Decade or Longer of Maintenance Hemodialysis
A Noninvasive Study

EDWARD M. ABRAMOWITZ, RAO S. K. MUSUNURU,
WILLIAM J. SCARPA, AND GERI MANDEL

Cardiovascular disease is the leading cause of death in patients on chronic dialysis for renal failure.[1,2] Hyperlipidemia, vascular calcification, systemic hypertension, and left ventricular hypertrophy have a high incidence in this population and have been cited as contributory to the increased cardiovascular mortality. Fernando et al.,[3] however, dispute the high incidence of ischemic cardiovascular disease and mortality therefrom. Nevertheless, it is of obvious importance to monitor the cardiovascular status in dialysis patients who, because of their frequent exposure to invasive procedures, ought to be protected from any additional traumatic procedures. Echocardiography and phonocardiography are now universally accepted as dependable means of diagnostic and prognostic evaluation of cardiac disorders. Data gathered by these noninvasive methods have been previously recorded in unmatched patients on both relatively long- and short-term hemodialysis.[3,4] We herein report the findings using these noninvasive methods in a group of patients on hemodialysis for a minimum of 11 years. They are compared with a control group on hemodialysis for a short time. All patients are age and sex matched. We found that cardiovascular dysfunction in this group of patients on long-term hemodialysis was not worse than in the control short-term hemodialysis patients.

EDWARD M. ABRAMOWITZ, RAO S. K. MUSUNURU, AND GERI MANDEL • Division of Cardiology, The Long Island College Hospital, Brooklyn, New York. WILLIAM J. SCARPA • Division of Cardiology, The Long Island College Hospital; and Department of Medicine, The Long Island College Hospital, Brooklyn, New York.

MATERIALS AND METHODS

Patients

We studied 22 patients on maintenance hemodialysis at the hemo-dialysis unit of Long Island College Hospital. All were in chronic renal failure due to a variety of disorders (Table I). Patients were subdivided into two groups.

Group A. This group included seven males and four females. All had been on maintenance hemodialysis for 11 to 14 years. Their mean age was 38.2 with a range of 27 to 54 years. Ten patients had systemic hyperten-sion. There were no diabetics. One patient suffered from angina pectoris and two had evidence of prior myocardial infarctions.

Group B. This was an age- and sex-matched group of patients who had been on maintenance hemodialysis for a maximum of one year, with the exception of one patient, who had been on hemodialysis for four years. The age range was 24 to 55 years with a mean age of 38.9. Ten patients in this group had systemic hypertension. There were three diabetics in the group. One patient had angina pectoris and an old myocardial infarction.

Echocardiographic Data

M-mode echocardiograms were performed using an IREX system II echocardiographic apparatus. All data were recorded on a fiberoptic strip chart recorder at paper speeds of 25 and 50 mm/sec with electrocardio-graphic monitoring using lead I or II. All echocardiograms were obtained with a 2.25-MHz 13-mm transducer. Patients were studied in the recumbent 45° LAO position. The transducer was placed in the fourth and fifth intercostal spaces at the left parasternal edge. Diagnostic echocardio-grams were obtained in all patients and analyzed by two investigators independently. Any discrepancies in interpretation were resolved by consensus. Echocardiographic measurements were made according to the recommendations of the Committee on M-Mode Standardization of the American Society of Echocardiography.[5]
Normal values are according to Clark[6] and Feigenbaum.[7]

Phonocardiographic Data

Phonocardiograms were obtained using an IREX 152-103 HFT-1 heart sound pulse module and recorded on a strip chart recorder at paper speeds of 50 and 100 mm/sec. Systolic time intervals were measured according to Weissler.[8] All measurements were made by two investigators independently and any discrepancies were resolved by consensus.

Echocardiographic and phonocardiographic data were obtained from all patients in the predialysis state. On their first visit to the noninvasive cardiac laboratory, all patients underwent routine clinical examination. A chest x-ray was obtained and an electrocardiogram was recorded.

Statistical Data

The following statistical procedures were used:

1. The Student t test for independent samples—when variables were unequal Cochrane's adjustment was applied.
2. A t test for prepared samples.
3. Fisher's exact test for evaluating differences in proportions.
4. All tests of statistical significance were done at $p < 0.05$.

RESULTS

There was no statistical difference between the mean ages of patients in both groups (Table I).

Echocardiographic data (Table II, Figures 1–5):

The mean end diastolic diameter was 57.9 mm ± 8.27 mm in Group A and 55 mm ± 7.03 mm in Group B (n.s.) (Table II, Figure 5).

The mean end systolic diameter in Group A was 43.1 mm ± 12.3 mm and 41 mm ± 9.58 mm in Group B (n.s.) (Table II, Figure 5).

VCF in Group A was 0.9 ± 0.33; in Group B it was 0.95 ± 0.30 (n.s.) (Table II, Figure 5).

Although Groups A and B did not differ significantly from each other in any of the above parameters, all measurements were significantly different from normal.

The E–F slope of the anterior mitral valve leaflet in Group A was 86.80 mm/sec ± 25.92 mm/sec and in Group B it was 98.50 mm/sec ± 21.87 mm/sec (n.s.). This slope measurement was not significantly different between

Table I. Echo

Patient	Age and sex	Duration of dialysis Years	Dialysis begun	Diagnoses	Left ventricle EDD (mm)	ESD (mm)	EF (Percent)	VCF (circ/sec)	Left ventricular thickness Posterior wall (mm)	Septum (mm)	Pericardium Effusion	Thickening
Normal range									7–11	7–11		
Mean ± SD					48	31	67	1.23				
					±4	±5	±7	±0.18				
											Group A—Long-Term	
T.Y.	27 M		(1970)	CGN	59	41	57	1.09	14	14	−	+
J.D.	30 M	12	(1969)	CGN	59	47	41	0.85	13	10	−	+
E.A.	33 M	14	(1967)	ESRD	54	43	42	0.68	14	14	−	+
A.E.	33 F	11	(1970)	CGN	52	30	65	1.32	12	12	+	−
E.P.	34 M	12	(1969)	HN	61	53	28	0.62	14	12	−	+
A.M.	36 M	11	(1970)	ESRD	73	61	33	0.63	13	9	−	+
R.C.	36 M	11	(1970)	CGN	61	40	63	1.15	13	12	+	−
E.R.	40 F	12	(1969)	BCN	50	30	70	1.1	11	11	−	+
E.J.	47 F	11	(1970)	CGN	70	64	17	0.26	10	12	+	−
F.J.	50 M	11	(1970)	CGN	45	27	70	1.33	11	12	−	+
S.J.	54 F	12	(1969)	CGN	53	38	54	0.91	10	10	−	+
Mean	38.2	11.6			57.9	43.1	49	0.9	12.3	11.6	3+	8+
± SD					±8.27	±12.30	±18.05	±.33	±1.56	±1.57		
											Group B—Short-Term	
H.B.	24 M	1	(1980)	PA	60	46	46	0.80	13	13	−	+
L.C.	29 M	1	(1980)	HTN	47	30	66	0.89	12	11	−	+
W.F.	33 M	1	(1980)	FS	55	35	65	1.51	10	9	−	+
T.N.	33 M	1	(1980)	HN	54	33	69	1.30	13	13	−	+
E.J.	33 F	1	(1980)	CGN	54	44	38	0.77	11	13	+	−
K.J.	39 M	4	(1977)	HTN	54	38	56	1.02	12	12	−	+
H.H.	41 M	1	(1980)	DM	61	49	40	0.76	11	11	−	+
H.T.	44 F	1	(1980)	DM	47	32	60	1.13	14	14	−	+
H.F.	48 F	1	(1980)	DM	44	33	50	0.96	10	12	+	−
G.E.	50 M	1	(1980)	MGN	65	52	40	0.87	11	11	−	+
C.W.	55 F	1	(1980)	RTN	64	59	22	0.39	11	15	−	+
Mean	38.9				55	41	50.2	0.95	11.6	12.2	2+	9+
± SD					±7.03	±9.58	±14.57	0.30	±1.29	±1.66		

Reference for normal values: Ralph D. Clark, M. D., *Case Studies in Echocardiography*; John S. Edelsen, M. D., W. B. Saunders Company, 1977. CGN: chronic glomerulonephritis; ESRD: end-stage renal disease; HN: heroin nephropathy; BCN: bilateral cortical necrosis; PA: Primary amyloidosis; HT:

the two groups or between the two groups and normal (Table II, Figure 2).

Left ventricular posterior wall thickness in Group A was 12.3 mm ± 1.56 mm and in Group B it was 11.6 mm ± 1.29 mm. The values for Group A differed significantly from normal whereas the values for Group B did not (Table II, Figure 1).

Interventricular septal thickness in Group A was 11.6 mm ± 1.57 mm and in Group B it was 12.2 mm ± 1.66 mm. This parameter was not significantly different than normal in either group (Table II, Figure 1).

In reference to the presence of aortic root calcification, pericardial effusion, or pericardial thickening, no significant difference between the two groups was noted (Table II, Figure 4).

Aortic root diameter in Group A was 34.4 mm ± 4.01 mm and 29.9 mm ± 3.15 mm in Group B. This difference between the two groups was

Cardiogram (M-Mode)

E-F slope (mm/sec)	E-IVS (mm)	Annulus calcification	Left atrial diameter (mm)	Aortic root diameter (mm)	Aortic root calcification	Right ventricular diameter (mm)	Phonocardiogram, PEP/LVET ratio	Chest x-ray/ cardiothoracic ratio
	Mitral valve							
80–150	0–5		19–40	20–37		7–23		
							0.35	0.6
							±0.04	±0.070
101	10	–	38	37	–	14	0.43	0.6
125	12	–	35	32	–	14	0.59	0.59
77	13	–	33	27	–	26	0.46	0.50
60	5	–	40	33	–	19	0.39	0.57
120	26	–	54	40	+	22	0.66	0.58
103	15	–	37	35	–	17	0.56	0.62
90	8	–	50	37	+	12	0.33	0.63
38	9	–	43	37	–	12	0.38	0.60
86	33	–	47	36	–	20	0.76	0.72
65	13	–	52	28	–	16	0.52	0.72
90	8	–	32	36	–	15	0.27	0.51
86.8	13.8	0+	41.9	34.4	2+	17	0.49	0.6
±25.92	±8.4		±7.8	±4.01		±4.38	±0.148	±0.070
87	17	–	38	35	–	18	0.41	0.50
85	3	–	33	29	–	14	0.68	0.46
70	7	–	30	28	–	15	0.48	0.52
75	10	–	37	27	–	18	0.40	0.61
122	14	–	42	32	–	26	0.70	0.60
140	9	–	40	33	–	17	0.39	0.60
90	17	–	38	31	+	19	0.33	0.60
96	10	–	41	31	+	26	0.39	0.64
87	10	–	41	23	–	16	0.27	0.68
114	20	–	54	32	–	27	0.70	0.65
118	22	–	47	30	–	32	0.66	0.68
98.5	12.6	0+	40	29.9	2+	21.0	0.49	0.59
±21.87	±5.84		±6.45	±3.15		±6.28	±1.62	±0.073

hypertension; FS: focal sclerosis; EDD: end diastolic diameter; ESD: end systolic diameter; IVS: interventricular septum; EF: ejection fraction; VCF: velocity of circumferential fiber shortening; Circ: circumference; PEP: Preejection period; LVET: left ventricular ejection time.

statistically significant; however, the difference from the normal for the two groups was not statistically significant (Table II, Figure 3).

Left atrial diameter and right ventricular diameter values were not statistically different from normal (Table II, Figure 3).

Phonocardiographic Data (Table II and Figure 6). The PEP/LVET ratio was 0.49 ± 0.148 in Group A and 0.49 ± 0.162 in Group B (n.s.). These values compared to a PEP/LVET ratio of 0.35 ± 0.04 for the normal group, a significant difference.

Chest Roentgenographic Data (Table II and Figure 6). The cardiothoracic ratio was 0.60 ± 0.070 for Group A and 0.59 ± 0.073 for Group B (n.s.).

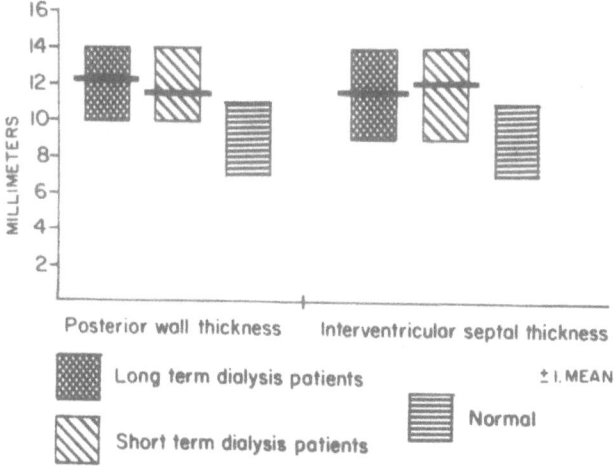

Figure 1. Measurement of the left ventricular posterior wall and intraventricular septal thicknesses by echocardiography; comparison between long- and short-term dialysis patients and normals.

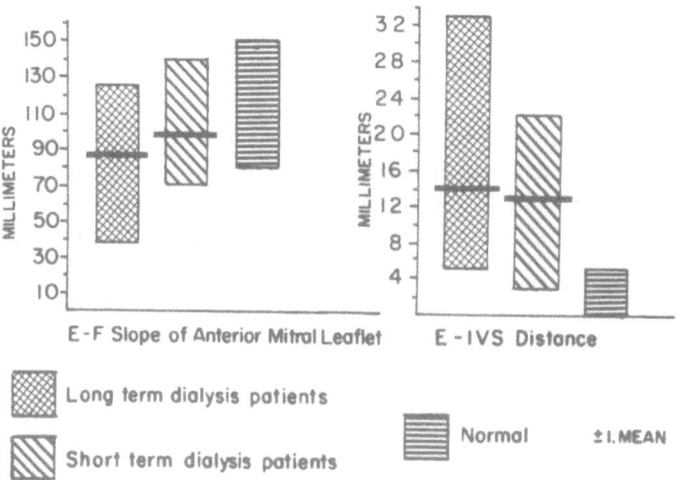

Figure 2. Measurement of the E to F slope and the E to IVS distance of the mitral valve by echocardiography.

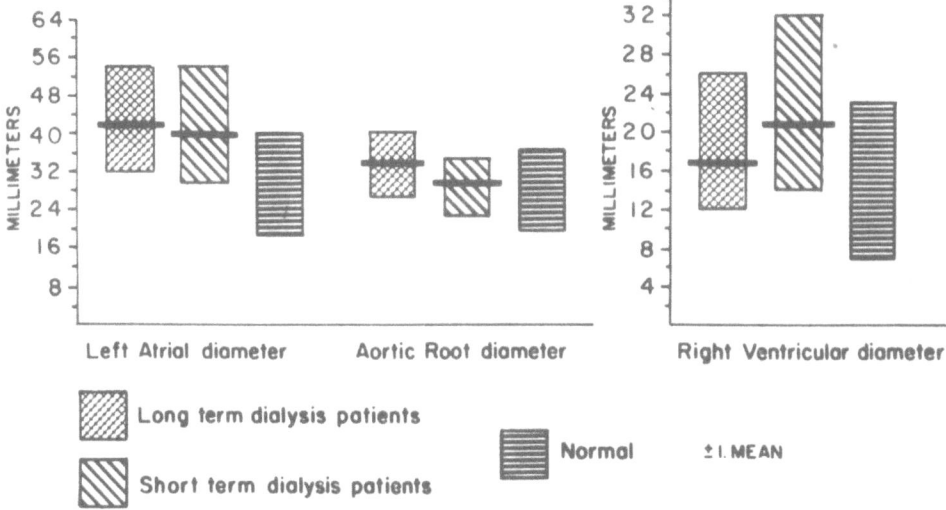

Figure 3. Measurement of the left atrial, aortic root, and right ventricular diameters by echocardiography.

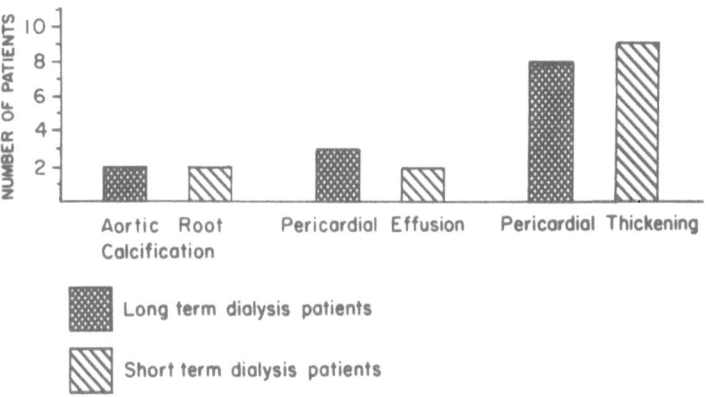

Figure 4. The presence of aortic root calcification, pericardial effusion, and pericardial thickening as noted by echocardiography in long- and short-term dialysis patients.

Table II. Comparison Between Short-Term and Long-Term Dialysis Patients

	Group A Long-term (Mean ± SD)	Group B Short-term (Mean ± SD)	Normal (Mean ± SD)
M-Mode echocardiogram			
Left ventricular end diastolic diameter	57.9 ± 8.27	55 ± 7.03	48 + 4 mm
Left ventricular end systolic diameter	43.1 ± 12.30	41 ± 9.58	31 + 5 mm
Left ventricular ejection fraction	49 ± 18.50	50.2 ± 14.57	67 + 7 %
LV velocity of circumferential fiber shortening	0.9 ± 0.33	0.95 ± 0.30	1.23 + 0.18 circ/sec[a]
LV posterior wall thickness	12.3 ± 1.56	11.6 ± 1.29	7–11 mm
Interventricular septal thickness	11.6 ± 1.57	12.2 ± 1.66	7–11 mm
Right ventricular diameter	17 ± 4.38	21.0 ± 6.28	7–23 mm
Left atrial diameter	41.9 ± 7.80	40 ± 6.45	19–40 mm
Aortic root diameter	34.4 ± 4.01	29.9 ± 3.15	20–37 mm
E-F slope of anterior mitral leaflet	86.8 ± 25.92	98.5 ± 21.87	80–150 mm
E-IVS distance	13.8 ± 8.4	12.6 ± 5.84	0–5 mm
Phonocardiogram			
PEP/LVET ratio	0.49 ± 0.148	0.49 ± 0.162	0.35 ± 0.04
Chest x-ray			
Cardiothoracic ratio	0.6 ± 0.070	0.59 ± 0.073	
Echocardiogram	Positive	Positive	
Pericardial effusion	3/11	2/11	
Pericardial thickening	8/11	9/11	
Aortic root calcification	2/11	2/11	
Mitral annulus calcification	0/11	0/11	

[a] circ: Circumference.

DISCUSSION

Cardiovascular disease is a leading cause of death among patients undergoing chronic hemodialysis.[1,2,9,10] Hypertension, lipid abnormalities, pericarditis, and left ventricular hypertrophy contribute to cardiovascular morbidity and mortality. As many as 80% of deaths in chronic renal failure have been attributed to cardiovascular causes.[11] Linder et al.[12] report that atherosclerosis is accelerated in patients with end-stage renal disease and

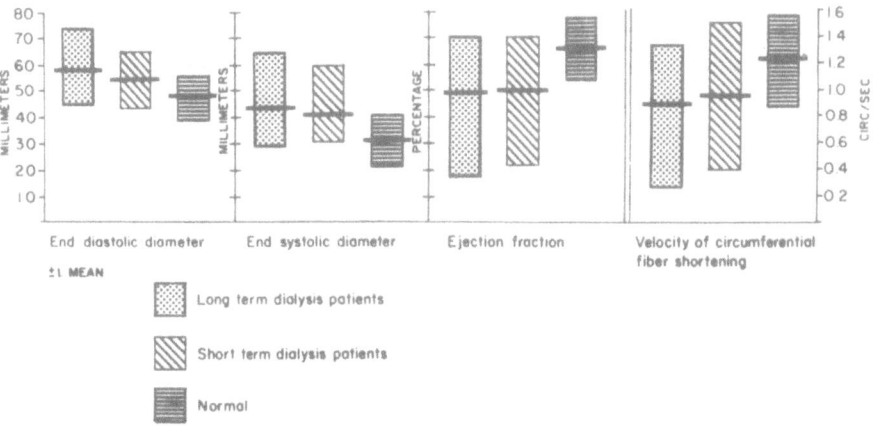

Figure 5. Left ventricular size and function as evidenced by measuring the end diastolic diameter, end systolic diameter, the ejection fraction, and the velocity of circumferential fiber shortening by echocardiography in long- and short-term dialysis patients and normals.

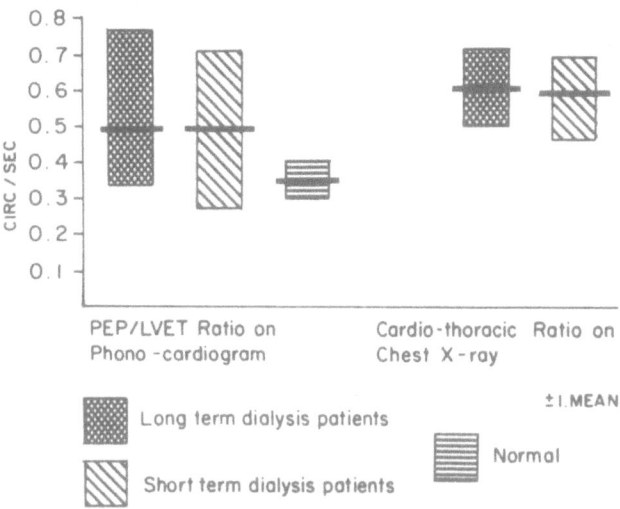

Figure 6. Comparison of the PEP/LVET ratio between long- and short-term dialysis patients and normals as noted on phonocardiogram. Comparison of the cardiothoracic ratio of long- and short-term dialysis patients as measured by chest x-ray.

that ischemic heart disease is a major mortality risk in patients undergoing maintenance hemodialysis. Moreover, they suggest that the probability of dying from this cause increases with time on dialysis. Rostand et al.[13] concluded, however, in a study of 382 dialysis patients, that the incidence of ischemic heart disease in men was not greater than that seen in a nondialysis population with similar risk factors. But they did report that the rate of ischemic heart disease in women was accelerated when compared with similar nondialysis subjects. Likewise, Roguska et al.[14] found only three deaths from myocardial infarction in 131 patients undergoing chronic dialysis.

Drueke et al.[15] and Hung et al.[16] describe a congestive cardiomyopathy in patients on long-term hemodialysis. Their reports emphasize the absence of risk factors that might precipitate such cardiomyopathic findings. Gueron et al.,[17] however, dispute the existence of a specific uremic cardiomyopathy and urge that toxic, anemic, and hypertensive causes be eliminated before this diagnosis is employed.

Other potential risk factors leading to increased cardiovascular death rate in dialysis patients include endocarditis and altered myocardial function secondary to increased cardiac output due to anemia or arteriovenous shunts.[18] Indeed, the latter has been reported as a cause of intractable pulmonary edema.[19]

Cardiovascular mortality and morbidity may also be contributed to by pericardial effusion and tamponade. Echocardiographic evidence of pericardial disease was the most common finding in our series. Previous reports have given the prevalence of pericarditis in uremia as ranging from 32% to 50%, but hemodynamically signficant effusions have been reported in only 1.3% to 5% of patients on dialysis.[20-25] The effusions in our series were, in all cases, minimal and of no hemodynamic significance. Similarly, although we detected pericardial thickening in 15 of 20 (75%) patients, none had compromised left or right ventricular function.

Myocardial calcification, including the mitral annulus, has been previously noted in patients undergoing chronic dialysis.[26,27] None of our patients showed this finding on echocardiography. Similarly, we were unable to support a reported increased incidence of asymmetric septal hypertrophy.[28]

Several workers previously recorded echo and phonocardiographic findings in patients on dialysis. D'Cruz et al.,[28] for example, in addition to detecting pericardial disease in 33 of 50 patients found cardiac dilatation, ventricular thickening, and impaired contractility in a significant number. Lewis et al.,[29] on the other hand, found systolic function of the left ventricle to be normal even in patients who were severely uremic, hypertensive, fluid overloaded, and with physical signs of heart failure. Bornstein et al.[4] reported systolic time intervals in 15 patients pre- and postdialysis. The immediate effects of hemodialysis included a reduction of stroke volume and a reduced Starling effect with or without decreased contractility.

Fernando et al.[3] assessed the echocardiographic performance in chronic renal failure following hemodialysis. They studied 12 patients pre- and postdialysis. The length of time on dialysis was not stated but all patients had impaired cardiac performance. Specifically, ejection fraction, VCF, left ventricular end diastolic volume, posterior wall velocity, and interventricular septal velocity were all found to be significantly abnormal. After hemodialysis, improvement was noted only in left ventricular end diastolic volume. They concluded that patients with chronic renal failure on maintenance hemodialysis have impaired left ventricular function. Each hemodialysis induced significant improvement of cardiac function although hemodynamic parameters remain abnormal.

Our own investigation is, we believe, the first one to address the question of the effects on ventricular function of hemodialysis for more than a decade. Although end diastolic diameter, end systolic diameter, ejection fraction, and VCF were found to be significantly abnormal, there was no significant difference between decade-long and newly started dialysis patients. Indeed, the only significant difference noted between the two groups was in aortic root diameter. The apparent aortic root dilatation on long-term hemodialysis patients is unexplained. It might be conjectured that the presence of an arteriovenous fistula over a long period of time may contribute to aortic dilatation. Although interventricular septal thickness was not abnormal in either group, left ventricular posterior wall thickness was found to be significantly increased in the long-term group only. While previously noted data may suggest a deterioration of ventricular function, it is interesting that the E-F slope, often used as a determinant of ventricular function, was normal in both groups. The PEP/LVET, on the other hand, was significantly abnormal in both groups. The significantly increased E-IVS distances are consistent with the increased systolic and diastolic diameters.

We conclude that alterations in ventricular function in decade-long hemodialysis patients can be quite slow to develop. Looked at another way, it may also indicate that the cardiovascular complication rate is related to preexisting heart disease rather than the dialysis itself and that long-term survival without cardiovascular deterioration is possible.

Overall these findings are encouraging and indicate that cardiovascular mortality may be neither inevitable nor highly prevalent in long-surviving maintenance hemodialysis patients.

REFERENCES

1. Lazarus JD, Lourie EG, Hompers CL, et al: Cardiovascular disease in uremic patients on hemodialysis. *Kidney Int* 2(suppl):167, 1975.
2. Gross JE, Alfrey AC, Vogel JHK, et al: Hemodynamic changes during hemodialysis. *Trans Am Soc Artif Organs* 13:68, 1967.
3. Fernando HA, Friedman HS, Zorman Q, et al: Echocardiographic assessment of cardiac performance in chronic renal failure and following hemodialysis. *Clin Res* 24:613A, 1967.
4. Bornstein A, Zambrano SS, Morrison R, et al: Cardiac effects of hemodialysis noninvasive monitoring by systolic time intervals. *Am J Med Sci* 269:189, 1975.
5. Sahn DJ, DeMaria A, Kisslo J, et al: The Committee on M-Mode Standardization of the American Society of Echocardiography: Recommendations regarding quantitations of echocardiographic measurements. *Circulation*, 58. 1978.
6. Clark R: *Case Studies in Echocardiography.* Philadelphia, WB Saunders Co, 1977.
7. Feigenbaum H: *Echocardiography.* Philadelphia, WB Saunders Co, 1981.
8. Weissler AM: *Noninvasive Cardiology.* New York, Grune & Stratton, 1974.
9. Lowrie EG, Lazarus JM, Hampers CL, et al: Cardiovascular disease in dialysis patients. *N Engl J Med* 290:737, 1974.
10. Burton TC, Kruger KK, Bryon FA: National Registry of long term dialysis patients. *JAMA* 218:718, 1971.
11. Samuels S, Charra B, Olsheisen K, et al: Twelve years experience of treatment of chronic renal failure. *Trans Am Soc Artif Intern Organs* 20:62, 1974.
12. Lindner A, Charra B, Sherrard DJ, et al: Accelerated atherosclerosis in prolonged maintenance hemodialysis. *N Engl J Med* 290:697, 1974.
13. Rostand SG, Gretes JC, Kirk KA, et al: Ischemic heart disease in patients with uremia undergoing maintenance hemodialysis. *Kidney* 16:600, 1979.
14. Roguska J, Simon NM, Delgreco F, et al: Ten years' experience with maintenance hemodialysis for chronic uremia. *Trans Am Soc Artif Intern Organs* 20:579, 1974.
15. Drueke T, Le Pailleur C, Meilhoc B, et al: Congestive cardiomyopathy in uremic patients on long term hemodialysis. *Brit Med J* July 1:350, 1979.
16. Hung J, Harris P, Uren RF, et al: Uremic cardiomyopathy. Effect of hemodialysis on left ventricular function in end-stage renal failure. *N Engl J Med* 302:547, 1977.
17. Gueron M, Berlyne GM, Nord E, et al: The case against the existence of a specific uremic myocardiopathy. *Nephron* 15:2, 1975.
18. Riley SM, Blackstone EH, Sterling WA, et al: Echocardiographic assessment of cardiac performance in patients with arteriovenous fistulas. *Surg Gyn Obstet* 146(2):203, 1978.
19. Ahern DJ, Maher JF: Heart failure as a complication of hemodialysis arteriovenous fistula. *Ann Int Med* 77:201, 1972.
20. Luft FC, Qilman JK, Weyman AE: Pericarditis in the patient with uremia. Clinical and echocardiographic evaluation. *Nephron* 25:160, 1980.
21. Bailey GL, Hampers CL, Hager EB, et al: Uremic pericarditis: Clinical features and management. *Circulation* 38:582, 1968.
22. Goldberg M, Lazarus JM, Gottlieb MN, et al: Treatment of uremic pericardial effusion. *Proc Clin Dial Trans Forum* 5:20, 1975.
23. Gilman JK et al: Echocardiography in the diagnosis of pericarditis in patients with uremia. *Proc Clin Dial Trans Forum* 8:121, 1978.
24. Horton JD, Gelfand MC, Shinbar HS: Natural history of asymptomatic pericardial effusions in patients on maintenance hemodialysis. *Proc Dial Trans Forum* 76:81, 1977.

25. Wray T, Stone WJ: Uremic pericarditis. A prospective echocardiographic and clinical study. *Clin* 6:295, 1976.
26. Arora KK, Lacy JP, Schackt TA, et al: Calcific cardiomyopathy in advanced renal failure. *Arch Intern Med* 135:603, 1975.
27. Sehott CR, Kotler MN, Parry WR, et al: Mitral annular calcification. Clinical and echocardiographic correlations. *Arch Intern Med* 137:1143, 1977.
28. D'Cruz IA, Bhatt GR, Cohen HC, et al: Echocardiographic detection of cardiac involvement in patients with chronic renal failure. *Arch Intern Med* 138:720, 1978.
29. Lewis BS, Milne FJ, Goldberg B: Left ventricular function in chronic renal failure. *Br Heart* July 38:1229, 1976.

17

Over-Decade Maintenance Hemodialysis
Its Effect on Uremic Anemia and Coagulation

FRANK W. DIPILLO AND HARSH GANDHI

Anemia is an almost invariable component of the uremic syndrome. The pathogenesis of uremic anemia has been related to: (1) failure of renal excretory function resulting in a metabolic and/or mechanical environment unfavorable to red cells; (2) subnormal red cell iron utilization; (3) decreased marrow responsiveness to erythropoietin; (4) the effect of impaired renal secretion of erythropoietin; (5) increased blood loss from ecchymoses, gastrointestinal, or gynecologic bleeding[1,2]; and (6) the erythropotoxic effect of excess parathyroid hormone, a common concomitant abnormality in uremia. The major factor in the genesis of uremic anemia appears to be a lack of renal erythropoietin stimulation of erythroid marrow.[3-5] The Long Island College Hospital group has, for more than a decade, implicated the possible role of parathyroid hormone (PTH) as a uremic toxin.[6,7]

It is now accepted that the most important coagulation defect in uremic patients is an acquired, reversible, platelet dysfunction[8-11] produced by at least two dialyzable compounds—guanidinosuccinic acid[12] and phenols.[13] An exact mechanism for thrombocytopathy in uremia is not understood, but it is recognized that several known platelet functions are affected, with considerable improvement induced by dialysis. While abnormalities in plasma coagulation factors may be present in some uremic patients, by themselves these are usually not responsible for bleeding. The present study aims to evaluate the degree of anemia and integrity of the coagulation in a group of patients treated by maintenance hemodialysis for uremia for a decade or longer.

FRANK W. DIPILLO AND HARSH GANDHI • Division of Hematology/Oncology, The Long Island College Hospital, Brooklyn, New York.

METHODS AND MATERIALS

Two groups of patients were investigated. A group of 12 patients (Group A) with chronic renal failure on thrice-weekly hemodialysis for ten years or longer was studied from January 1981 to March 1981. All patients were treated with disposable dialyzers and received intravenous heparin during each four- to six-hour hemodialysis. The following factors were noted:

1. Frequency of prior blood transfusions.
2. Blood transfusion records for the past three years for each patient.
3. Red blood count, hemoglobin, hematocrit, corrected reticulocyte index (RI), serum ferritin level, serum B12 level, and serum folic acid level.
4. Coagulation screening included platelet count, Ivy bleeding-time (BT), one-stage prothrombin time (PT), activated partial thromboplastin time (PTT), and thrombin time (TT). For fibrin degradation products (FDP), the Thrombo Wellco test kit was used.
5. Prothrombin consumption.
6. Platelet factor-3 availability (PF3a) by the method of Spaet and Cintron. A shortening of Stypen time by 20 seconds or greater with kaolin at 30 minutes' incubation was considered evidence of normal PF3 availability.
7. Platelet aggregation with collagen, ADP, and epinephrine measured in a lumi aggregometer. All blood samples were drawn from a peripheral vein immediately prior to a hemodialysis treatment. All were fasting specimens.

RESULTS

Anemia

All but two patients in Group A (Table I) (E.P. and E.J.) were anemic and had a low reticulocyte index, reflecting a hypoproliferative marrow function. Five of 11 patients (Table II) were receiving blood transfusions of more than three to four units per year to maintain their hematocrits above 20%. Only one of these five (J.D.) had an increasing frequency of blood transfusions over the past three years coincident with the onset of chronic myelogenous leukemia. One patient (C.B.) was not transfused routinely, even though her hematocrit was below 20. She is 61 years old, sedentary, and usually tolerates her hematocrit well.

Table I. Study Group

Patient	Age (years)	Sex	Race	Renal disease[b]	On dialysis since
T.Y.	27	M	Oriental	CGN	1970
J.D.[a]	30	M	White	CGN	1969
A.E.	33	F	Black	CGN	1970
E.P.	34	M	Black	Heroin nephropathy	1969
R.C.	36	M	Hispanic	CGN	1970
E.R.	40	F	Black	Acute cortical necrosis	1969
E.J.	47	F	Black	CGN	1970
F.J.	50	M	Black	CGN	1970
F.M.	59	F	Black	CGN	1970
C.B.	61	F	Black	Hypertensive/nephropathy	1971
S.J.	64	F	Black	CGN	1969
D.W.	34	M	Black		

[a]Patient has chronic myelogenous leukemia. [b]CGN: chronic glomerulonephritis.

Six of 11 Group A patients received occasional transfusions, mainly necessitated by episodes of bleeding from the GI tract, or an arteriovenous fistula. None of these patients had had a recent increase in the frequency of transfusion. There were no statistical differences between Groups A and B in mean hematocrit, reticulocyte indices, serum ferritin, serum B12, or serum folate level. In Group B (Table II), however, fewer patients (2/11) required routine transfusions than did Group A.

Coagulation

Table III summarizes the results of testing of coagulation in Group A patients (on hemodialysis for ten years or more). The PT, PTT, and thrombin time were within normal limits in all patients except one (J.D.), who has prolonged PTT secondary to circulating anticoagulant (not to factor 8). FDP was normal in nine of 11 patients, mildly elevated in one, and moderately elevated in one (J.D.). J.D. had chronic myelogenous leukemia. None of the patients were bleeding at the time of the study. However, most (eight of ten) interviewed reported easy bruisability and/or gum bleeding on brushing their teeth. Platelet counts were normal in eight of ten patients and two had mild thrombocytopenia (102,000 and 118,000/mm^3). Ivy bleeding time was prolonged in six of eight Group A patients (75%). Eight of the nine patients had normal prothrombin consumption times and all of seven patients studied had normal platelet factor-3

Table II. Comparison of Study Group (A) with Short-Term Hemodialyzed Patients[a]

Patient group		Hematocrit		Reticulocyte index		Transfusion requirements		Transfusion changes in past 3 years in group	Serum ferritin (nl 12–230 ng per ml)		Serum B12 (nl 220–940 ng per ml)		Serum folate (nl 2–14 ng per pl)	
A	B	A	B	A	B	A	B	A	A	B	A	B	A	B
T.Y.	1	30	20[c]	0.7	0.8	Occ.[d]	qm.	No	1818	2670	683	1015	14.3	16
J.D.	2[b]	21[c]	22	1.3	0.16	q 2–4 wk	Occ.	Yes	111	212	1053	270	16	4
A.E.	3	16	33	1.0	1.9	q 1–2 wk	None	No	5000	81	1099	734	16	15.1
E.P.	4	38	28[c]	3.0	—	Occ.	Occ.	No	600	5000	858	690	4.8	16
R.C.	5	27	20	1.3	0.65	Occ.	None	No	443	1966	438	809	15.7	16
E.R.	6	22	21	1.2	0.36	q 2–4 wk	None	No	117	28.3	461	666	4.7	10.8
E.J.	7	39	28[c]	2.5	2.5	Occ.	Occ.	No	6.6	—	314	784	8.2	8.7
F.J.	8	25[c]	32	1.8	0.9	q 2–4 mo	Occ.	No	1853	55	386	659	5	16
F.M.	9	21	30	—	2.1	q 3–4 mo	Occ.	No	37	170	697	738	14.6	16
C.B.	10	17	28	0.8	0.5	Occ.	None	No	2791	18.2	517	693	11.1	11.4
S.J.	12	27	20	0.9	—	Occ.	q 4–8 wk	No	62.3	931	—	428	—	1.6
Mean		25.7	25.5	1.45%	1.09%				1167.1	1113.1	650.6	680.5	11	11.9
± S.D.		±7.6	±5.1	±0.8%	±0.8%				±1583.3	±1651.3	±227.2	±204.1	±4.9	±5.3

[a] Group A: Study group on hemodialysis for more than ten years. Group B: Patients on hemodialysis for less than one year; age and sex matched with Group A. [b] Patient has chronic myelogenous leukemia. [c] Transfused within past six weeks (two–six weeks). [d] Patients requiring transfusion once a year or less are categorized as having occasional transfusion requirement (Occ.).

Table III. Coagulation Profile of Long-Term (Ten Years) Hemodialysis[a,b]

Patients	One-stage PT (Control 11–13 sec)	Activated PTT (Control 30–40 sec)	TT (within 4 sec of control)	FDP (Normal <10 μg/ml)	BT (Normal <9 min)	Platelet count 150–450 × 10³/CMM	Prothrombin consumption (>35 sec)	PF–3	Platelet aggregation	History—easy bruising and/or bleeding
T.Y.	11.2	36.2	12.8	<10	>20	138	39.2	—	Normal	Yes
J.D.[c]	12.8	48[d]	11.6	>20<40	8.5	227	—	Normal	Normal	Yes
A.E.	9.6	30.6	11.2	10	18	153	33.4	Normal	Abnormal w/collagen and epinepherine	Yes
E.P.	12.4	40.2	14.7	<10	19	102	—	Normal	Abnormal w/ADP, collagen, and epinepherine	Yes
R.C.	10.6	30.8	11.4	<10	13	219	57	Normal	Normal	Yes
E.R.	10.4	31.8	12.2	<10	12.5	253	>60	Normal	Normal	No
F.J.	10.4	24	13	<10	7.5	152	55.4	Normal	Normal	Yes
F.M.	11.3	30.2	11.7	<10	—	—	60	—	Normal	No
C.B.	11.9	29	16	<10	>20	148	53.4	Normal	Abnormal w/epinepherine	Yes
S.J.	11.3	31.4	12.6	<10	—	186	35.8	—	Abnormal w/epinepherine	Yes
D.W.	13	39.8	11.3	>10<20	—	118	>60	—	Abnormal w/epinepherine	—

[a] None of the patients was bleeding at the time of the study. [b] PT: prothrombin time; PTT: partial prothrombin time; TT: thrombin time; FDP: fibrin degradation products; BT: bleeding time; PF—3: platelet factor —3. [c] Patient has chronic myelogenous leukemia. [d] Prolonged PTT is 2° to circulating anticoagulant.

availability. Five of ten patients (50%) have normal platelet aggregation studies and the other 50% (five of ten) had varying degrees of impairment in aggregation in response to one or more of the following: epinephrine, collagen, and ADP.

Anemia in CRF has been attributed to:

1. Failure of renal excretory function, resulting in a metabolic environment that is responsible for shortened red cell survival,[1-3,14] diminished iron utilization,[14] and suboptimal marrow responsiveness to erythropoietin.[15,16]
2. Failure of renal endocrine function.[3-5]
3. Increased blood loss,[1,2] etc.

With regard to the second item, loss of renal erythropoietin appears to be the major factor in the chronic anemia of the uremic syndrome. The combined effect of shortened RBC survival, decreased iron utilization, and increased blood loss exerts a moderate stress on the marrow's synthetic ability, which could be met easily by a normal marrow. In uremia the bone marrow is not capable of this compensatory response because of concomitant failure of renal endocrine function. Though improvements in RBC survival,[17] iron utilization,[18] and presumably increased marrow responsiveness to erythropoietin[1] have been reported with dialysis, the anemia of chronic renal failure understandably persists despite intensive maintenance hemodialysis precisely because of loss of renal erythropoietin. Barring development of any deficiency state (e.g., iron or folate) and bleeding, one would expect the uremic anemia to be stable since erythropoietin is undetectable by the time the patient requires dialysis[1,5] and further deterioration is unmeasurable. Our results confirm this presumption since no significant difference was found between the mean hemocrit of patients on hemodialysis for ten years or more and of patients on dialysis for less than a year. The fact that there was no progressive increase in transfusion requirements was noted in the study group with duration of dialysis also consistent with this view.

The difference in numbers of patients requiring routine transfusions between the two groups (five of 11 decade or longer dialysis patients versus two out of 11 in the one-year or less dialysis group) is not significant if one considers that two short-term patients who had had occasional transfusions had been on the dialysis program for only three months.

Two patients in study Group A (E.P. and E.J.) not only had near-normal hematocrits, but high reticulocyte indices as well. This is unusual in uremic patients. It is possible that these patients have significant extrarenal sources of erythropoietin. It is now accepted that the most important coagulation defect in uremic patients is an acquired platelet dysfunction produced by the least two dialyzable substances, guanidino-succinic acid and phenols. Considerable improvement in platelet functions follows within 48 hours after dialysis.[9,10] The present study shows that it is possible to maintain good hemostasis in uremic patients during protracted maintenance hemodialysis even after a decade or longer. Our observations also confirm the minor role plasma coagulation factors play in bleeding disorders of uremia, as PT, PTT, TT, and platelet counts were within normal limits in most patients.[19]

We found that Ivy bleeding time was prolonged in six of eight decade or longer dialysis patients (75%). It has been shown that Ivy bleeding time shortens to normal with peritoneal dialysis, but normalizes incompletely with hemodialysis,[20] possibly because the hemodialysis membrane is less physiologic than the peritoneal membrane and incompletely removes some middle molecular weight substances or conversely removes some small molecular weight plasma consitutents necessary for normal platelet function.

SUMMARY

In this investigation of anemia and the coagulation system in decade or longer hemodialysis patients, we found that there was no deterioration with time in either the severity of anemia or the tendency to hemorrhage sufficiently to require transfusions. Deficient coagulation factors play a minor role at most in uremic bleeding disorders. It is unlikely that deranged hematologic function will limit long-time survival in treated uremic patients.

ACKNOWLEDGMENTS

The authors greatly appreciate the technical assistance of Marcia K. Albano, B.S., M.T. (ASCP), Elena B. Goddy, B.S., M.T., and J. Michael Rivera, B.S., M.T. (ASCP).

REFERENCES

1. Allan JE: Anemia of chronic renal disease. Arch Int Med 126, Nov. 1970.
2. Desforges JF: Anemia in uremia. Arch Int Med 126, Nov 1970.
3. Adamson JW, Eischback J, French CA: The kidney and erythropoiesis. Am J Med 44:725, 1968.

4. Naets JP, Heuse AF: Measurement of erythroid stimulating factor in anemic patients with or without disease. *J Lab Clin Med* 60:365, 1962.
5. Brown R: Plasma erythropoietin in chronic uremia. *Br Med J* 2:1036, 1965.
6. Avram, MM, Alexis H, Rahman M, et al: Decreased transfusional requirement following parathyroidectomy in long term hemodialysis. *Proc Am Soc Nephro* 5:5, 1971.
7. Avram MM, Feinfeld DA, Huatuco AH: Search for the uremic toxin:Decreased motor-nerve conduction velocity and elevated parathyroid hormone in uremia. *N Engl J Med* 298:1000–1003 (May 4), 1978.
8. Lewis JH, Zucker MB, Fregusen JH: Bleeding tendency in uremia. *Blood* 11:1073, 1956.
9. Castaldi PA, Rosenberg MC, Steward JH: The bleeding disorder of uremia. *Lancet* 2:66, 1966.
10. Stewart JH, Castaldi PA: Uremic bleeding: A reversible platelet defect corrected by dialysis. *Q J Med* 36:143, 1967.
11. Rabiner SF, Hrodek O: Platelet factor 3 in normal subjects and patients with renal failure. *J Clin Invest* 47:901, 1968.
12. Horowitz HI, Stein IM, Cohen BD: Further studies on platelet inhibiting effect of guanidinosuccinic acid and its role in uremic bleeding. *Am J Med* 49:336, 1970.
13. Rabiner SF, Molinas F: The role of phenol and phenolic acids on thrombocytopathy and defective platelet aggregation of patients with renal failure. *Am J Med* 49:346, 1970.
14. Magid E, Hilden M: Ferrokinetics in patients suffering from chronic renal disease and anemia. *Scand J Hemat* 4:33, 1967.
15. VanDyke DC, Pollycove M, Lawrence JH: Erythropoietin therapy in renoprival patients, in the semiannual *Report on Biology and Medicine*. Berkley, Calif, Donner Laboratory, Lawrence Radiation Laboratory, 1967, p 127.
16. Essers U, Müller W: Decreased sensitivity to erythropoietin in chronic uremic man. *Int Soc Nephrol* 950:1972 (abs).
17. Berry ER, Rambach WA, Alt HA, et al: Effect of peritoneal dialysis on erythrokinetics and ferrokinetic of azotemic anemia. *Trans Am Soc Artif Int Organs* 10:415, 1964.
18. Eschback JW, Funk D, Adamson J: Erythropoiesis in patients with renal failure undergoing chronic dialysis. *N Eng J Med* 276:653, 1967.
19. Stewart JH: Platelet numbers and life span in acute and chronic renal failure. *Thromb Diath Macmersch* 17:532, 1967.
20. Eschback JW, Harker LA, Dale DC: The hematological consequences of renal failure in Brenner BM, Rector FC (eds): *The Kidney*. Philadelphia, WB Saunders, 1976, p 1522.

18

The Effects of Long-Term Hemodialysis on Gastrointestinal Function

JOSEPH J. RICCA, GEORGE J. REZK, AND ROBERT P. YATTO

Numerous studies indicate the prominence of gastrointestinal disturbance in uremia; however, to our knowledge there are no reports comparing the effects of a decade or longer of hemodialysis versus short-term hemodialysis on gastrointestinal function. Previous reports have shown that patients on maintenance hemodialysis have an increased incidence of hiatus hernia and diverticulosis coli,[1] as well as gastrointestinal hemorrhage from a variety of lesions, including gastritis, duodenitis, and peptic ulcer disease.[2-4] Ascites is occasionally seen and is often of uncertain origin.[5,6] An increased incidence of pancreatitis has been found postmortem.[7] Enzymatic evidence of hepatic malfunction,[8-10] as well as alterations in serum gastrin[11,12] and serum amylase,[13] have also been described.

Because of our institution's unusual resource of maintenance hemodialysis patients treated for more than a decade, we undertook a study to compare the effects of long- versus short-term hemodialysis in certain clinical and biochemical aspects of gastrointestinal function.

METHODS AND MATERIALS

Two study groups matched for age and sex were established. Group I consisted of 13 patients treated by maintenance hemodialysis for at least ten years. Two patients (C.G. and F.M.), however, were included, although they have completed only eight years of dialysis, in order to match both groups for age and sex. Group II contained 13 patients on dialysis for a

JOSEPH J. RICCA ● Division of Gastroenterology, The Long Island Hospital; and Department of Medicine, The Long Island College Hospital, Brooklyn, New York.   GEORGE J. REZK AND ROBERT P. YATTO ● Division of Gastroenterology, The Long Island College Hospital, Brooklyn, New York.

period of about one year. Two patients (T.R. and J.O.) were included for age and sex match, although they have been on dialysis for four years with only the last year spent at our institution. Groups I and II were compared with established values for nonuremic patients where applicable.

The following statistical tests were used to compare Groups I and II:

1. Student's t test for independent samples. When variables were unequal Cochrane's adjustment was applied.
2. The t test for paired samples.
3. Fisher's exact test for including differences in proportions. All tests of statistical significance were done at a $p < 0.05$.

HISTORY

Gastrointestinal symptoms were elicited by careful history and chart review and tabulated (Table I).

Specimens of peripheral venous blood were obtained in the fasting state from each patient on three separate occasions prior to hemodialysis over a three- to five-month period from October 1980 through February 1981 for SGOT, alkaline phosphatase, and total bilirubin. The SMA method (Technicon Autoanalyzer) was used. Hepatitis B surface antigen was routinely tested for in all patients by radioimmune assay (RIA). Prehemodialysis fasting venous blood specimens were drawn for analysis of total serum gastrin by radioimmune assay (Becton-Dickinson RIA kit). Serum amylase was determined by the Perkin-Elmer colorimetric method and gamma glutamyl transpeptidase (GGTP) was determined by the

Table I. Gastrointestinal Symptoms in Long-Term and Short-Term Hemodialysis Patients[a]

	Group I ($n = 13$)	Group II ($n = 13$)
Weight loss	6 (46)	7 (54)
Nausea/vomiting	4 (31)	6 (46)
Abdominal pain	4 (31)	5 (38)
Ascites	4 (31)	3 (23)
Hemorrhoids	6 (46)	2 (15)
Constipation	4 (31)	6 (46)
Gastrointestinal bleeding	2 (15)	1 (8)

[a] There was no statistically significant difference ($p < 0.05$) in the incidence of symptoms between Groups I and II.

Biodynamics (BMC) colorimetric method. Determinations of gastrin, amylase, and GGTP were made once for 13 Group I patients and 12 Group II patients.

RESULTS

Twelve of 13 long-duration dialysis patients (Group I) and 12 of 13 short-term dialysis patients (Group II) reported the subjective experience of one or more manifestations of gastrointestinal disturbance (Table I). Most patients maintained a good appetite, but 6 of 13 (46%) in Group I reported weight loss since beginning hemodialysis, as did 7 of 13 patients (54%) in Group II. Nausea and vomiting were commonly reported in both groups, as was abdominal pain. Constipation and symptomatic hemorrhoids were noted frequently, especially in Group I. Ascites was seen in 31% of Group I and 23% of Group II patients. Manifestations of serious life-threatening gastrointestinal disease were uncommon in both groups. There was no statistically significant difference in the incidence of symptoms in Group I and Group II.

In Group I, 37 of 39 determinations of SGOT (95%) were within normal ranges (7–45 IU) (Table II). The values ranged from 5 to 53 IU (mean 25.8 IU). In Group II 29 of 39 SGOT determinations (76%) were in the normal range with values ranging from 4 to 147 IU (mean 34.3 IU). There were no significant abnormalities in bilirubin levels in either Group I or II patients.

Twenty-one percent of serum alkaline phosphatase determinations in Group I were within the normal range (normal—25–115 U/dl). Values ranged from 105 to 1,086 U/dl (mean 331.6 U/dl). Fifty-one percent of Group II had normal alkaline phosphatase values ranging from 49 to 210 U/dl (mean 115.4 U/dl). [The mean alkaline phosphatase of both groups had statistically significant ($p < 0.05$) elevations when compared with a normal midrange value of 70 ($n = 25$–115.) In addition, there was a significant difference ($p < 0.05$) between the elevated alkaline phosphatase of Groups I and II.]

Twenty-three percent of serum amylase determinations in Group I fell within the normal range (normal, 40–180 U). (Range was 155 to 655 U, mean 308 U.) In Group II only one was normal (range 88–490 U, mean 288 U). [The mean serum amylase levels of both Groups I and II were significantly elevated ($p < 0.05$) above a normal midrange value of 110 U ($n = 4$–180 U). There was no statistically significant difference between Groups I and II.]

Total serum gastrin levels in 7 of 13 (54%) patients in Group I were normal ($n = 0$–184 U, range 117–1,000 U, mean 294 U). In Group II only 2 of 12 (17%) were normal (range 131–1,000 U, mean 436.1 U). [The mean gastrin levels of both Groups I and II were significantly elevated ($p < 0.05$) above a normal midrange value of 92 U ($n = 1$–184 U). There was no statistically significant difference between Groups I and II.]

Gamma glutamyl transpeptidase levels in Group I were normal in 4 of 13 patients (31%) ($n = 6$–28 U, range 6–604 U, mean 95.2 U). In Group II 4 of 12 (33%) had values in the normal range (range 9–165 U, mean 72.8 U). [The mean GGTP levels of both groups were significantly elevated ($p < 0.05$) above a normal midrange value of 17 U ($n = 6$–28 U).] There was no statistically significant difference between both groups.

Mean alkaline phosphatase values for each patient in Group I and II were compared with corresponding GGTP levels in both groups (Figures 1 and 2). No patients in Group I and three (25%) in Group II had both alkaline phosphatase and GGTP normal. Two patients in Group I (15%) and four patients in Group II (33%) had normal alkaline phosphatase levels but elevated GGTP levels. Six patients in Group I (46%) but only one patient in Group II (8%) had elevated mean alkaline phosphatase levels with a normal GGTP activity. Five patients in Group I (38%) and four patients in Group II (33%) had both GGTP and alkaline phosphatase activity elevated. Table II summarizes the comparison of Group I and Group II versus normal midrange values and between each other.

DISCUSSION

Gastrointestinal complaints have a high prevalence in both long- and short-term hemodialysis patients but are most often benign with life-threatening manifestations uncommon. We found that both long- (46%) and short- (54%) duration hemodialysis patients reported weight loss since beginning dialysis, though the extent to which this represented extraction of excess extracellular fluid was not determined. Nausea, vomiting, and abdominal pain afflicted a third (Group I) to a half of patients (Table I). Margolis et al.[4] attributed similar findings to endoscopically proven gastric and duodenal mucosal changes. Dorph[14] found mucosal edema as the cause of these symptoms. Avram[7] suggests that pancreatitis, as seen postmortem, may explain some gastrointestinal symptoms during life on hemodialysis. We are unable to distinguish between these etiologies, all of which may have been present, though in different patients.

The high incidence of constipation in our patients (31% to 46%) may be explicable by the universal ingestion of constipating medications such

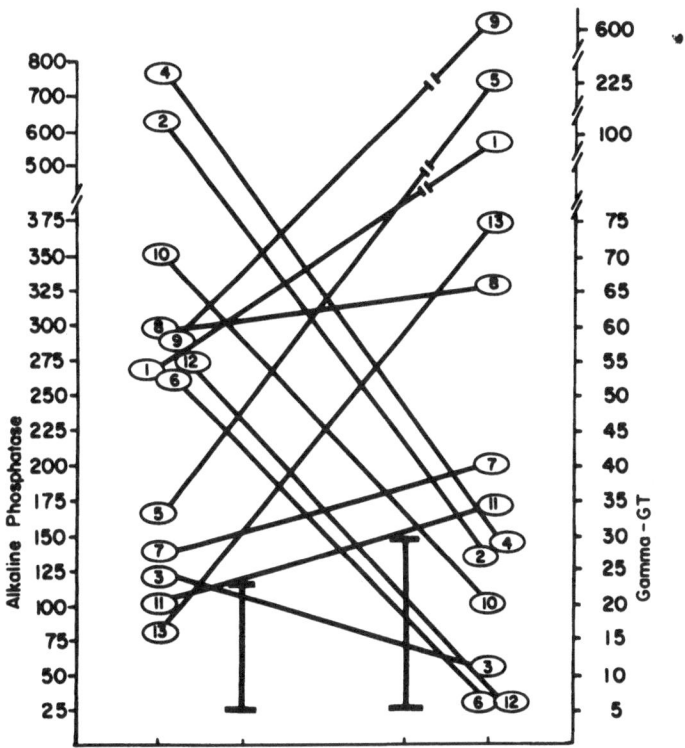

Figure 1. Relationship of alkaline phosphatase to GGT in long-term hemodialysis patients. The numbered ovals correspond to individual patients. The GGT represents a single value and the alkaline phosphatase represents the average of three separate values for each patient.

as aluminum hydroxide and calcium gluconate as part of the dialysis regimen. The incidence was similar in both groups.

Since Jaffe and Laing[15] reported diffuse gastrointestinal hemorrhagic lesions in the majority of 136 autopsied uremics, attempts have been made to define the occurrence of ulcer disease in dialysis patients. Incidence ranged from 0% by Margolies[4] to 60% by Shepherd.[3] Hampers et al.[16] suggested that their 11% incidence of ulcer was no greater than the general population. Most of these studies are not comparable and it has been suggested that a true determination depends on survey techniques, ulcer criteria, and duration of the investigation. None of our long-term group gave a history of ulcer disease, but 15% did have gastrointestinal bleeding. Erosive gastritis was determined to be the cause in one case.

The mean SGOT was normal in both of our groups. Crawford[9] and

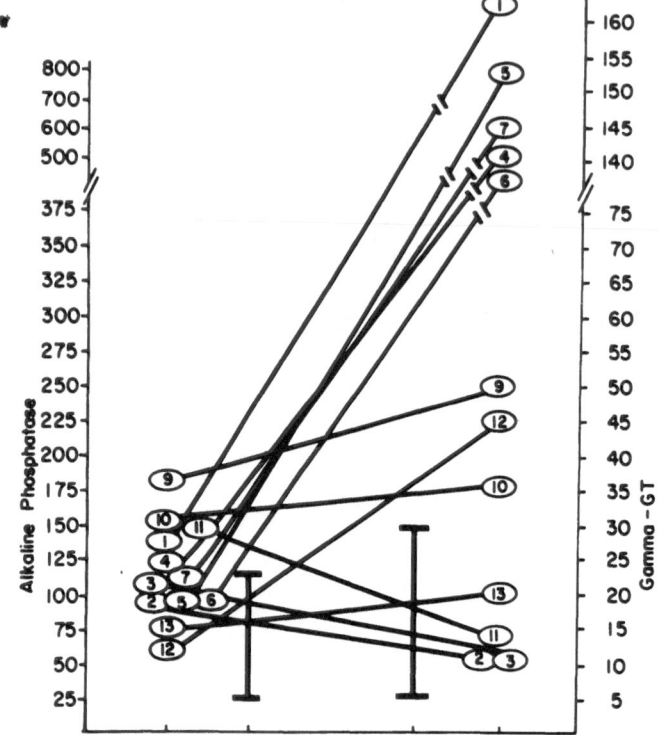

Figure 2. Relationship of alkaline phosphatase to GGT in short-term hemodialysis patients. The numbered ovals correspond to individual patients. The GGT represents a single value and the alkaline phosphatase represents the average of three separate values for each patient.

Table II. Comparison of Laboratory Values—Long-Term versus
Short-Term Dialysis Patients

	Group I	Group II	
Bilirubin (mg/dl)	0.39	0.46	n.s.
SGOT (U/dl)	25.8	34.3	n.s.
Alkaline phosphatase (U/dl)	331.6	115.4	$p < 0.05$
Amylase (U/dl)	307.8	288	n.s.
GGTP (U/dl)	95.2	72.8	n.s.
Gastrin (U/dl)	294.2	436.1	n.s.

Cohen[10] found predialysis SGOT to be decreased or absent as compared with postdialysis specimens, which were normal. They postulated that there may be some unidentified inhibitor substance present in the serum of chronic uremics that interferes with the SGOT determination and is removed by dialysis. Bailey[8] also found the SGOT to be normal in 73% of 76 chronic uremics. The fact that the increased incidence of viral hepatitis in chronic dialysis patients[17,18] can still be assessed by SGOT elevations would seem to minimize any artifact induced by the testing methods.

We know of no study determining the incidence of biliary tract disease in long-term hemodialysis patients. Although we found no elevation of the total bilirubin in either group, this does not imply the absence of biliary tract disease or defects of bilirubin metabolism or excretion, nor does it preclude the possibility of developing pathology at some future date. Other biochemical and diagnostic parameters would be needed to adequately investigate the hepatobiliary system.

A significant finding in this study was the marked elevation of AP in those patients on long-term hemodialysis as compared with those on short-term dialysis, which showed no elevation. The mean elevation of Group I was 331.6. Serum AP is derived mainly from bone, intestine, placenta, and the hepatobiliary system.[19] Thus elevations of AP are seen in Paget's disease,[20] primary hyperparathyroidism,[21] pregnancy,[22] the aged,[23] and growing children.[24] Increased AP of liver origin is due to impairment of intra- or extrahepatic bile flow, which, in turn, causes increased synthesis of hepatic AP. This is eventually leaked into the serum.[25,26] Thus elevations in this instance are noted in cholestatic and obstructive liver disease, hepatitis, and such infiltrative diseases as lymphoma, sarcoid, TB, metastases, and cirrhoses.[27,28] To identify that which was elevated hepatic AP in our study, GGTP was measured in both our groups. Although GGTP is found in greatest concentration in kidney tissue,[29] its greatest value lies in its extreme sensitivity to liver cell dysfunction. In fact, elevations of GGTP of renal origin were found by Orlowski[30] only in the nephrotic syndrome and certain renal neoplasms. On the other hand, Zein[31] found GGTP elevated in obstructive jaundice, chronic hepatitis, hepatic metastases, hepatoma, and chronic alcoholic liver disease. Levinson[32] showed that GGTP helps differentiate liver AP from other tissue sites by pointing out that elevations in GGTP parallel rises in liver AP. Other refinements in comparing AP and GGTP have been noted. Orlowski[30] and Dragosics[33] demonstrated in chronic hepatitis that the GGTP may be elevated when the AP and SGOT are normal. Zein[31] demonstrated a similar finding in chronic alcoholics. In this study, the GGTP was found elevated in both groups: Group I, mean 95.2; Group II,

mean 72.8. The comparison of the individual GGTP with the corresponding AP in each group (Figures 1 and 2) demonstrates four basic enzymatic
patterns (Table III). These patterns may be explained in this manner:

1. Those patients with both a normal GGTP and AP presumably have no
   detectable bone or liver dysfunction. No patients in Group I and only
   three (25%) in Group II fit this category.
2. Those patients with an increased GGTP and a normal AP might have an
   as-yet-undetected liver disease. Two patients in Group I (15%) and four
   in Group II (33%) fit this pattern. Five of these particular patients (nos.
   11, 13, 5, 6, and 12) also had a normal SGOT and a negative HbsAg.
   These patients might warrant a closer follow-up for the presence, or the
   future development, of chronic active hepatitis as noted by Orlowski.[30]
   The one patient (no. 7) in Group II with an elevated GGTP and a
   normal AP also had an increased SCOT with a positive HbsAg and
   would require a liver biopsy for a pathologic tissue diagnosis.[31]
3. The six patients in Group I (46%) and the one patient in Group II (8%)
   with an elevated AP and a normal GGTP might have the rise, not from
   hepatic origin, but from bone origin, presumably due to renal osteodystrophy. The much higher incidence in the long-term dialysis group
   might truly reflect the combined effects of long-term dialysis and
   uremia.
4. The five patients in Group I (38%) and four patients in Group II (33%)
   with both GGTP and AP elevations may have either hepatobiliary
   disease alone or possibly a combination of bone and hepatobiliary

Table III. The Four Basic Enzymatic Patterns Found Comparing
Mean Alkaline Phosphatase Levels with Corresponding
GGTP Levels[a]

Pattern of enzymes	Group I no. patients (percent)	Group II no. patients (percent)	Clinical correlation
GGTP =	0(0)	3(25)	Liver −
AP =			Bone −
GGTP ↑	2(15)	4(33)	Liver +
AP =			Bone −
GGTP =	6(46)	1(8)	Liver −
AP ↑			Bone +
GGTP ↑	5(38)	4(33)	Liver +
AP ↑			Bone +

[a] The percent refers to the total number of patients in each group. Clinical correlation refers to the possible
presence or absence of bone and liver diseases (see text for details). ↑, increase; =, normal.

disease. Further investigations would be needed to explain the elevations and separate those possibilities.

Since the initial report of normal serum gastrin in five uremics on hemodialysis by Reeder and Thompson,[11] other reports by Korman,[12] Christensen,[34] and Owyang[35] have demonstrated elevations in serum gastrin in chronic renal failure patients. Recently Gokal[36] found no elevation of gastrin in patients with chronic renal failure who were not on dialysis but a group of patients who were on maintenance hemodialysis showed significant elevations. Both our groups showed marked elevations of mean gastrin levels. However, it should be noted that 54% of patients in Group I had normal gastrin. Two patients in Group I and three in Group II with gastrin levels over 500 gave no history of peptic ulcer disease or evidence of gastrointestinal bleeding. One might expect some significant ulcer disease, but this lack of correlation between gastrin and peptic ulcer disease in uremics has been previously cited by Gokal.[36]

Since the kidney is the major site of gastrin degradation, these elevated levels in patients with chronic renal failure are not surprising and, in fact, they return to normal following renal transplantation. Gastrin elevation is also partly due to the hypochlorhydria from atrophic gastritis that is present in some uremics. This is due to the loss of acid feedback inhibition, which leads to uncontrolled gastrin release. The large increase in gastrin in our cases may be a reflection of atrophic gastritis.

Total serum amylase was elevated in 32% of patients with uremia studied by Bailey[8] with the greatest elevations seen in patients on dialysis. Berk[13] found elevated amylases in 50% of patients but did not report those patients on hemodialysis separately. In our study 77% of Group I and 92% of Group II had elevated amylase with the mean values not differing significantly (Group I, 308; Group II, 228). The high percentage of elevations may be due to the fact that we measured only chronic uremic patients who were also on maintenance hemodialysis. Our data also tend to substantiate the observation of Berk[13] that total serum amylase in uremics, when elevated, tends to be less than three times normal. The elevations are a reflection of impaired renal clearance.

SUMMARY

Figure 3 summarizes the mean values of Group I and Group II as they compared with established normal values. Our data correlate with data of others regarding the incidence of hyperamylasemia, hypergastrinemia, and normal SGOT levels. The relationships between total bilirubin,

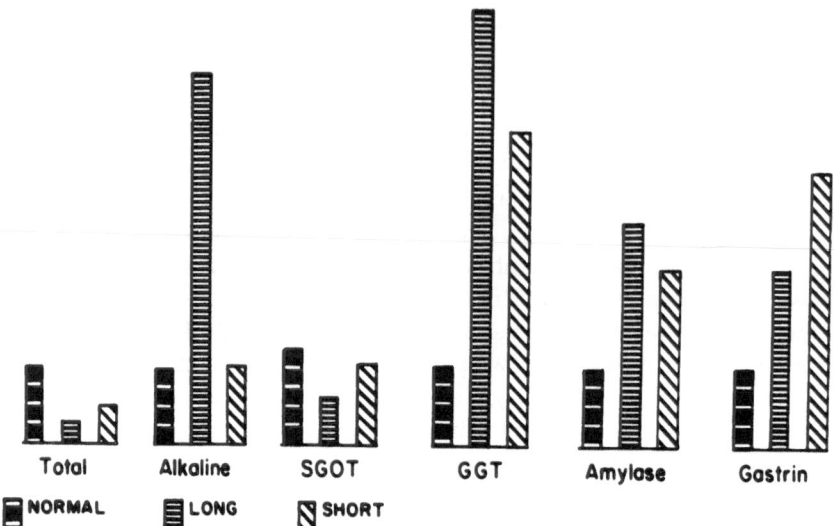

Figure 3. Comparison of all mean values for Group I (long-term) and Group II (short-term) patients with established normal values.

alkaline phosphatase, and GGTP, and the further delineation of the enzymatic patterns of the latter two, would require more detailed and individualized investigations to determine the true incidence of hepato-biliary disease in long-term hemodialysis patients. It is of great importance to appreciate that patients sustained by an artificial kidney for a decade or longer need not have debilitating GI malfunction.

ACKNOWLEDGMENTS. We wish to thank Mrs. Alice Rezk for her invaluable assistance in interviewing patients and coordinating all of the blood collections. We would also like to thank Ms. Frances Celentano for her help in collecting data.

REFERENCES

1. Bailey GL, Griffiths H, Locke JP, et al: Gastrointestinal abnormalities in uremia. *Am Soc Nephrol* 5:5, 1971.
2. Boner G, Berry EM: Gastrointestinal hemorrhage complicating chronic hemodialysis. *Isr J Sci* 4:66, 1968.
3. Shepherd AMM, Stewart WK, Wormsely KG: Peptic ulceration in chronic renal failure. *Lancet* 1:1357, 1973.
4. Margolus DM, Saylor JL, Geisse G, et al: Upper gastrointestinal disease in chronic renal failure: A prospective evaluation. *Arch Intern Med* 138:1214, 1978.

5. Eknoyan G, Dichoso C, Hyde S, et al: "Overflow ascites"—The safety valve of the volume expanded patient on dialysis. *Proc Clin Dial Transpl Forum* 3:156, 1973.
6. Gotloib L, Servadio C: Ascites in patients undergoing maintenance dialysis. *Am J Med* 61:465, 1976.
7. Avram MM: High prevalence of pancreatic disease in chronic renal failure. *Nephron* 18:68, 1977.
8. Bailey GL, Katz AI, Hampers CL, et al: Alterations in serum enzymes in chronic renal failure. *JAMA* 213:2263, 1970.
9. Crawford DR, Reyna RS, Weiner MW: Effects of *in vivo* and *in vitro* dialysis on plasma transaminase activity. *Nephron* 22:418, 1978.
10. Cohen GA, Goffinet JA, Donabedian RK, et al: Observations on decreased serum glutamic oxalacetic transaminase (SGOT) activity in azotemic patients. *Ann Int Med* 84:275, 1976.
11. Reeder DD, Thompson JC: Effect of hemodialysis on serum gastrin levels in uremic patients. *Gastroenterology* 60:795, 1971.
12. Korman MG, Laver MC, Hansky J: Hypergastrinemia in chronic renal failure. *Brit Med J* 1:209, 1972.
13. Berk JE, Fridhandler L, Ness RL: Amylase and isoamylase activities in renal insufficiency. *Ann Int Med* 90:351, 1979.
14. Dorph S, Oigaard A, Pederson G: Gastroduodenal mucosal changes in chronic uremia. *Scand J Gastroent* 7:589, 1972.
15. Jaffe RH, Laing DR: Changes of the digestive tract in uremia: A pathologic anatomic study. *Arch Intern Med* 53:851, 1934.
16. Hampers CL, Schupak E, Lowrie EF: The gastrointestinal system, in Hampers CL, Schupak E, Lowriie EF, et al (eds): *Long Term Hemodialysis*. New York, Grune & Stratton, 1974, p 136.
17. Sengar DPS, Rashid A, McLeish WA, et al: Hepatitis B surface antigen infection in a hemodialysis unit. *CMA J* 113:945, 1975.
18. Snydman DR: Hemodialysis associated hepatitis in the United States—1972. *CDS News* 109.
19. Posen S: Alkaline phosphatase. *Ann Intern Med* 67:183, 1967.
20. Nagant de Deuxchaisnes C, Krane SM: Paget's disease of bone: Clinical and metabolic observations. *Medicine* 43:233, 1964.
21. Dent CE, Harper CM: Plasma alkaline phosphatase in normal adults and in patients with primary hyperparathyroidism. *Lancet* 1:599, 1962.
22. Robinson JC, Pierce JE, Blumberg BS: The serum alkaline phosphatase of pregnancy. *Am J Obstet Gynec* 94:559, 1966.
23. Heino AE, Jokipii SG: Serum alkaline phosphatase levels in the aged. *Ann Med Intern Tenn* 51:105, 1962.
24. Clark LC, Beck E: Plasma alkaline phosphatase activity. *J Pediat* 36:335, 1950.
25. Kaplan MM, Righetti A: Induction of rat liver alkaline phosphatase: The mechanism of the serum elevation in bile duct obstruction. *J Clin Invest* 49:508, 1970.
26. Kaplan MM: Alkaline phosphatase. *Gastroenterology* 62:452, 1972.
27. Breeensilver HL, Kaplan MM: Significance of elevated liver alkaline phosphatase in serum. *Gastroenterology* 68:1556, 1975.
28. Kaplan MM: in Davidson CS (ed): *Problems in Liver Disease*. New York, Stratton Intercontinental Medical Book Corp, 1979, p 79.
29. Goldberg JA, Pineda EP, et al: A method for the colorimetric determination of gamma glutamyl transpeptidase in human serum; enzymatic activity in health and disease. *Gastroenterology* 44:127, 1963.

30. Orlowski M: Role of gamma glutamyl transpeptidase in the internal diseases. *Clin Arch Immunol Ther Exp* 1:11, 1963.
31. Zein M, Discombe G: Serum gamma glutamyl transpeptidase as a diagnostic aid. *Lancet* 2:748, 1970.
32. Levinson M, Holbert J, Blackwell C, et al: Serum gamma glutamyl transpeptidase: Its specificity and clinical value. *S Med J* 72:837, 1979.
33. Dragosics B, Ferenci P, Pesendorfer F, et al: Gamma glutamyl transpeptidase: Its relationship to other enzymes for diagnosis of liver disease, in Popper CF (ed): *Progress in Liver Diseases*. New York, Grune & Stratton, Vol. 5, 1976, p 436.
34. Christensen CK, Nielsen HE, Kamstrup KJ, et al: Serum gastrin and serum calcitonin in patients with chronic renal failure. *ACTA Endocrin* 91:564, 1971.
35. Owyang C, Miller LJ, DiMagno EP, et al: Gastrointestinal hormone profile in renal insufficiency. *Mayo Clin Proc* 54:769, 1979.
36. Gokal R, Kefflewell M, Drexler E, et al: Gastrin levels in chronic renal failure, hemodialysis and renal transplant patients. *Clin Nephrol* 14:96, 1980.

19

Pulmonary Function and Arterial Blood Gas in the Long-Term Hemodialysis Patient

SANTOSH B. SUREKA, MOHAMED H. SHAHJAHAN,
MORRELL M. AVRAM, AND SEYMOUR S. CUTLER

Very little is known about pulmonary mechanical function and blood gas exchange in uremic patients undergoing maintenance hemodialysis over a prolonged period. Because of the presence at our institution of a unique group of maintenance hemodialysis patients who had survived for a decade or longer, we initiated a study to assess their pulmonary function. We also investigated pulmonary function before and after dialysis in patients who had been treated by dialysis for a shorter period.[1-4] The purpose of our study was to determine whether or not pulmonary abnormalities develop in hemodialysis patients after 8 to 11 years, as compared with the normal population. We attempted to ascertain whether these abnormalities, if present, improve acutely after each dialysis.

The study population's clinical diagnoses, the year begun on dialysis, smoking habits, and chest x-ray findings are given in Table I. Forced vital capacity, forced expiratory volume in one second, ratio of forced expiratory volume in one second to forced vital capacity, maximum midexpiratory flow rate, inspiratory capacity, functional residual capacity, expiratory reserve volume, residual volume, and total lung capacity are

SANTOSH B. SUREKA • Division of Pulmonary Medicine, The Long Island College Hospital, Brooklyn, New York.   MOHAMED H. SHAHJAHAN • Division of Respiratory Services, The Long Island College Hospital, Brooklyn, New York.   MORRELL M. AVRAM • The Avram Center for Kidney Diseases, Division of Nephrology, The Long Island College Hospital; Department of Medicine, The Long Island College Hospital; and Brooklyn Kidney Center and Nephrology Foundation of Brooklyn, Brooklyn, New York.   SEYMOUR S. CUTLER • Division of Pulmonary Medicine, The Long Island College Hospital; and Department of Medicine, The Long Island College Hospital, Brooklyn, New York.

Table I. Clinical and Radiological Data

Patient	Age	Sex	Year dialysis began	Clinical diagnoses	Smoker	Chest x-ray findings
A.E.	33	F	1970	Chronic glomerulonephritis	Yes	Slight bilateral interstitial fibrosis
E.M.	36	M	1972	End-stage renal disease	Yes	Minimal bilateral interstitial fibrosis
E.R.	40	F	1969	Cortical necrosis	Yes	Minimal bilateral interstitial fibrosis
E.A.	33	M	1969	End-stage renal disease	No	Slight bilateral interstitial fibrosis
C.B.	61	F	1972	Hypertension	No	Slight bilateral interstitial fibrosis
R.C.	36	M	1970	Chronic glomerulonephritis	No	Minimal bilateral interstitial fibrosis
T.Y.	27	M	1970	Chronic glomerulonephritis	No	Moderate bilateral interstitial fibrosis with left-sided pleural reaction
E.J.	47	F	1970	Chronic glomerulonephritis	No	Moderate bilateral interstitial fibrosis
E.P.	34	M	1969	Heroin nephropathy	Yes	Minimal bilateral interstitial fibrosis
F.M.	59	F	1970	Chronic glomerulonephritis	No	Minimal bilateral interstitial fibrosis with left-sided pleural reaction
F.J.	50	M	1970	Chronic glomerulonephritis	No	Minimal bilateral interstitial fibrosis with right-sided pleural effusion
S.J.	54	F	1969	Chronic glomerulonephritis	Occasional	Minimal bilateral interstitial fibrosis with bilateral pleural reaction

presented in Table II. Lung dynamics and lung volumes presented in Table II were measured before and after hemodialysis and were compared with normal predicted values.[5,6] In one patient, F.J., a lung volume study was not completed. Arterial blood gases and diffusion studies before and after hemodialysis are reported in Table III, and were compared with normal established standards.[7] Results could not be obtained in four patients because of their inability to cooperate. Alveolar to arterial oxygen gradients were calculated by using the alveolar gas equation.

Statistical significance of the results was evaluated by the use of the Student's t test, using independent samples or paired data, where appropriate. Cochrane's adjustment was applied when variants were unequal. All tests of statistical significance were done at $p < 0.05$.

Lung dynamics, lung volumes, and lung diffusion capacity were performed on a Warren E. Collins Computerized Modular Lung Analyzer. Lung volumes were measured by helium dilation and diffusion capacity by the single-breath method, using 0.3% carbon monoxide. Arterial blood gas analyses were performed using the Radiometer BMS-3 blood gas analyzer. Arterial blood was collected from the arterial side of the arteriovenous fistula or graft fistula used for hemodialysis. The pulmonary function equipment was calibrated and checked periodically with a 4-liter super syringe for volume and an accurate stopwatch for speed. The helium meter was calibrated and the volume calculated by adding a known volume of air to a known volume of diluted helium. The carbon monoxide meter was calibrated against a known concentration of carbon monoxide. The arterial blood gas analyzer was checked using commercially available blood gas controls.

Abbreviations

FVC: forced vital capacity
FEV_1: forced expiratory volume in one second
MMEFR: maximum midexpiratory flow rate
IC: inspiratory capacity
FRC: functional residual capacity
ERV: expiratory reserve volume
TLC: total lung capacity
RV: residual volume
DLCO: diffusion capacity by single-breath carbon monoxide
PCO_2: partial pressure of carbon dioxide
PO_2: partial pressure of oxygen
$A\text{-}aDO_2$: alveolar to arterial oxygen gradient

PROTOCOL

A smoking history was obtained from each patient. Each patient's chest roentgenogram was studied and, in particular, reviewed for pulmonary fibrosis. Weight was recorded before and after dialysis. One hour before initiating hemodialysis and immediately afterward we

Table II. Lung Dynamics and Volumes Before and After Dialysis

Patient	Pulmonary function	Weight (lbs)	FVC (liters)	FEV₁ (liters)	FEV₁/FVC	MMEFR (l/sec)	IC (liters)	FRC (liters)	ERV (liters)	RV (liters)	TLC (liters)
A.E.	Predialysis	128	3.44	2.90	84%	3.42	2.68	1.46	0.74	0.72	4.10
	Postdialysis	122	3.37	2.90	86	3.96	2.38	1.35	0.76	0.59	3.73
	Predicted		2.80	2.23	80	2.92	1.92	1.81	0.88	0.93	3.73
E.M.	Predialysis	144	3.71	3.25	87	4.30	2.26	2.67	1.29	1.38	4.93
	Postdialysis	138	4.15	3.40	82	4.61	2.20	2.91	1.65	1.26	5.10
	Predicted		4.92	3.84	78	4.09	3.10	3.68	1.82	1.86	6.78
E.R.	Predialysis	162	2.71	2.14	79	1.98	2.57	1.53	0.29	1.24	4.10
	Postdialysis	156	2.98	2.44	82	2.66	2.44	1.44	0.46	0.98	3.88
	Predicted		3.64	2.83	78	3.22	2.49	2.89	1.15	1.74	5.37
E.A.	Predialysis	136	2.65	2.23	84	2.76	1.89	1.42	0.78	0.64	3.31
	Postdialysis	133	2.87	2.41	84	2.91	2.14	1.55	0.87	0.68	3.68
	Predicted		4.41	3.57	81	4.04	2.78	3.16	1.63	1.53	5.94
C.B.	Predialysis	139	1.92	1.82	95	3.05	1.56	1.60	0.41	1.19	3.16
	Postdialysis	136	2.05	1.88	92	3.01	1.63	1.64	0.37	1.27	3.27
	Predicted		2.93	2.15	73	2.50	2.03	2.60	0.90	1.70	4.68
R.C.	Predialysis	180	2.81	2.33	83	2.74	2.47	1.70	0.68	1.02	4.16
	Postdialysis	174	3.34	2.74	82	3.01	2.64	1.74	0.64	1.10	4.38
	Predicted		4.60	3.63	79	4.46	2.84	3.29	1.64	1.65	6.13

T.Y.	Predialysis	120	2.45	1.80	74	1.36	1.47	1.82	1.15	0.67	3.29
	Postdialysis	114	2.56	2.12	83	2.37	1.53	2.01	0.98	1.03	3.53
	Predicted		4.26	3.58	84	4.21	2.65	2.90	1.61	1.29	5.55
E.J.	Predialysis	137	1.59	1.23	77	1.15	1.53	1.22	0.11	1.11	2.75
	Postdialysis	136	1.70	1.38	81	1.54	1.43	1.11	0.17	0.94	2.54
	Predicted		3.15	2.41	77	2.86	2.77	2.53	0.98	1.55	4.70
E.P.	Predialysis	148	1.56	1.14	73	0.80	1.29	1.24	0.17	1.07	2.52
	Postdialysis	143	1.44	1.01	70	0.61	1.39	1.27	0.28	0.99	2.66
	Predicted		3.79	3.17	84	3.80	2.43	2.64	1.37	1.27	5.06
F.M.	Predialysis	140	1.41	1.31	93	1.75	1.23	1.54	0.16	1.38	2.77
	Postdialysis	138	1.49	1.47	99	2.17	1.39	1.64	0.27	1.37	3.04
	Predicted		2.98	2.22	74	2.56	2.06	2.65	0.91	1.74	4.71
F.J.	Predialysis	145	1.13	0.99	88	1.48					
	Postdialysis	138	1.55	1.20	78	1.04					
	Predicted		4.13	3.12	76	3.32					
Mean	Predialysis	144	2.30	1.92	84	2.25	1.89	1.62	0.58	1.04	3.51
	Postdialysis	139	2.50	2.08	84	2.53	1.92	1.67	0.65	1.02	3.58
	Predicted		3.78	2.95	79	3.45	2.51	2.81	1.29	1.53	5.25
SD	Predialysis	±2.01	±0.85	±0.73	±7.05	±1.08	±0.56	±0.41	±0.42	±0.28	±0.78
	Predicted		±0.74	±0.64	±3.66	±0.70	±0.38	±0.51	±0.37	±0.28	±0.09

Table III. Gas Exchange and Diffusion Studies

Patient	ABG and DLCO	pH	PCO_2 mm Hg	PO_2 mm Hg	A-a DO_2	DLCO ml/min/mm Hg
A.E.	Predialysis	7.27	42	103	0	7.7
	Postdialysis	7.34	41	79	20	10.5
	Predicted					19.6
E.M.	Predialysis	7.36	42	80	17	12.0
	Postdialysis	7.39	34	66	42	11.7
	Predicted					30.9
E.R.	Predialysis	7.33	33	94	15	5.2
	Postdialysis	7.43	35	96	10	5.3
	Predicted					21.3
E.A.	Predialysis	7.33	37	104	0	12.6
	Postdialysis	7.42	40	80	20	10.9
	Predicted					30.0
C.B.	Predialysis	7.31	43	82	14	11.4
	Postdialysis	7.38	34	69	38	11.9
	Predicted					18.8
R.C.	Predialysis	7.41	34	81	26	18.8
	Postdialysis	7.36	29	77	37	19.6
	Predicted					30.2
T.Y.	Predialysis	7.33	39	74	27	16.4
	Postdialysis	7.37	41	40	29	Denied
	Predicted					31.0
E.J.	Predialysis	7.31	31	70	41	
	Postdialysis	7.45	31	64	47	
	Predicted					
E.P.	Predialysis	7.25	35	76	30	
	Postdialysis	7.28	32	68	42	
	Predicted					
F.M.	Predialysis	7.40	30	98	14	
	Postdialysis	7.39	30	76	36	
	Predicted					
F.J.	Predialysis	7.36	34	75	32	
	Postdialysis	7.35	39	77	24	
	Predicted					
S.J.	Predialysis	7.32	38	89	13	
	Postdialysis	7.39	34	72	35	
	Predicted					
Mean	Predialysis	7.33	37	86	19	12.1
	Postdialysis	7.38	35	75	32	11.65
	Predicted					25.97

Table IV. Mean Values of Pulmonary Function

Parameters	Predicted	Predialysis	Postdialysis
FVC	3.78	2.30	2.50
FEV_1	2.95	1.95	2.08
FEV_1/FVC	79	84	84
MMEFR	3.45	2.25	2.53
IC	2.51	1.89	1.92
FRC	2.81	1.62	1.67
ERV	1.29	0.58	0.65
RV	1.53	1.04	1.02
TLC	5.25	3.51	3.58
pH	7.40	7.33	7.38
PCO_2	40	37.0	35.0
PO_2		86.0	75.0
$A\text{-}aDO_2$	10	19	32
DLCO	25.97	12.01	11.65

determined lung dynamics, lung volumes, lung diffusing capacity, and arterial blood gases.

Predicted normal values were obtained from the following sources:

FVC; FEV_1; MMEFR—from Morris, Koski, and Johnsen[6]
FRC; RV; TLC; ERV; and IC—from Protti, Craven, Haimark, et al.[8]
DLCO single breath—from Cadigan, Marks, Ellicott, et al.[7]
Arterial blood gases:
  pH—7.35–7.45
  PCO_2—35–45 mm Hg
  PO_2—For 60 years of age or less, 80 mm Hg or higher.
    After 60 years of age the predicted PO_2 was calculated by subtracting 1 mm Hg from 80 mm Hg for each additional year of age.

RESULTS

Clinical Data (Table I)

Four out of 12 (33%) patients had a history of heavy smoking (over 20 cigarettes daily), and one was a light smoker (less than 20 cigarettes daily). One patient had a history of asthma until 15 years of age, but has been free of symptoms for the past 19 years. Chest roentgenograms of all 12 patients showed interstitial fibrosis, with a slight to moderate increase of interstitial markings. Four patients also showed evidence of pleural effusion, ranging from blunting of the costophrenic angles to a moderate amount of fluid.

As shown in Table II, 10 out of 11 patients had FVCs and FEV₁s below the predicted value and 8 of the 11 were below the commonly applied standard of normality, 75% of the predicted value. After dialysis, both the FVC and FEV₁ improved consistently, with a mean increase of 8%. The changes in FVC and FEV₁ before and after dialysis are significant ($p < 0.05$). FEV₁/FVC ratio remained normal or above normal in all patients before and after dialysis since both measurements changed proportionately. The MMEFR improved significantly ($p < 0.05$) after dialysis, with a mean increase of 12%. Lung volumes were studied in ten patients and IC was found to be reduced from a mild to moderate degree in five of ten, without improvement after dialysis. The FRC was reduced, from a mild to severe degree, in eight of ten patients, without improvement after dialysis. The ERV was reduced, from a mild to severe degree, in nine of ten patients and improved after dialysis with a mean increase of 12%, which may be physiologically, though not statistically, significant. The RV was reduced in five of ten patients, from a mild to severe degree, and did not increase after dialysis. The TLC was reduced, from mild to severe degree, in seven out of ten patients without increase after dialysis.

Gas Exchange and Diffusion Studies (Table III)

PO₂ dropped to a significant degree ($p < 0.05$) in ten of 12 patients, mean decrease of 10 mm Hg, after dialysis. The lowest PO₂ observed either before or after dialysis was 40 mm Hg. No clinically detectable complication due to postdialysis hypoxemia was observed in any patient. The DLCO was depressed significantly from a moderate to severe degree, in all seven patients where it could be measured. After dialysis, one patient showed a substantial increase in DLCO.

DISCUSSION

This study demonstrates that patients treated by hemodialysis for 8 to 11 years have lung function abnormalities, including decreased lung dynamics, lung volumes, and diffusion capacity, as well as a drop in arterial PO₂ after dialysis.

Of interest to further survival is the fact that although 36% of patients were smokers, none showed evidence suggestive of large airway obstruc-

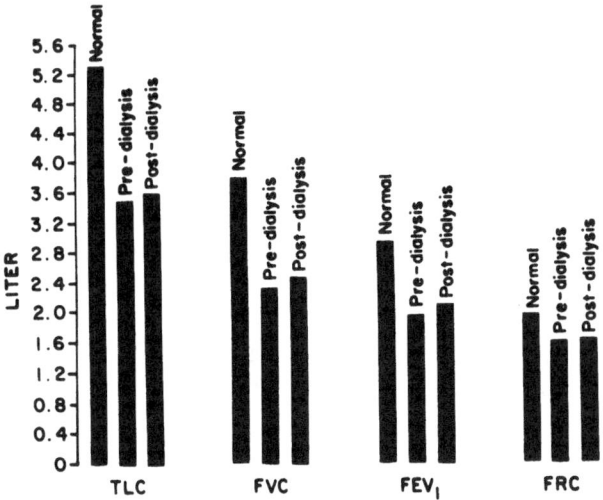

Figure 1. Mean values of TLC, FVC, FEV$_1$, and FRC before and after dialysis as compared with predicted normal values. There is restrictive lung pattern with statistically significant improvement ($p < 0.05$) after dialysis.

tion. Previous studies[1,3,4,9] of shorter duration dialysis patients also found a significant incidence of restrictive lung function. In our patient group, there was significant improvement in lung function after dialysis (Figure 1), corroborating the findings of Zidulka.[4] A reduced MMEFR that had been previously described[1,4] was noted in 75% of our patients. This abnormality may result from small airway resistance due to peribronchial edema, which improves after fluid extraction during dialysis. Fairshter[2] reported a decrease of ERV before dialysis, which worsened after dialysis. Our results show, however, no decrease of ERV after dialyisis (Figure 2), which actually improved postdialysis by 12% (p = n.s.). Since we did not measure expiratory force, we cannot comment on Fairshter's suggestion that expiratory muscle strength was lessened by dialysis. The significant decrease of IC, FRC, ERV, RV, and TLC in our patients demonstrates restrictive lung function. As reported previously,[2,10–14] we also found a significant drop in PO$_2$ after dialysis (Figure 3) in 83% of our patients. Mechanisms postulated for a fall in PO$_2$ after dialysis include hypoventilation secondary to carbon dioxide loss during dialysis, a decrease of the respiratory quotient, or hemodialysis-induced leukoaggregation. Patterson, Nissenson, Miller and associates[15] have concluded that the decline in PO$_2$ after dialysis results from a concomitant drop in partial pressure of alveolar oxygen (PAO$_2$) and a decreased respiratory quotient.

Santosh B. Sureka et al.

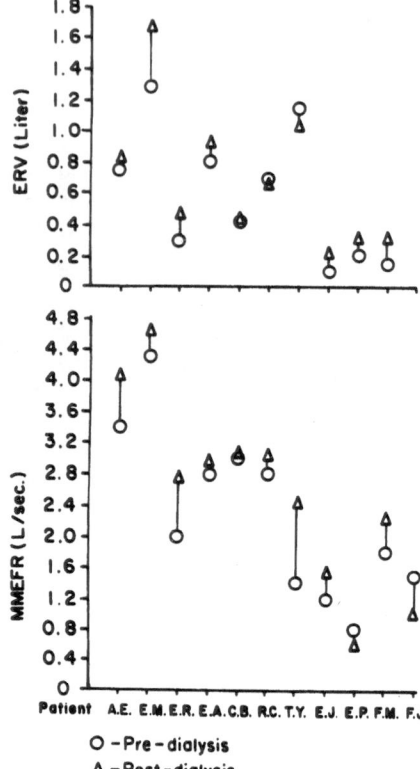

Figure 2. MMEFR and ERV for each patient before and after dialysis showing significant improvement ($p < 0.05$) after dialysis.

As is apparent from the above discussion, no definitive explanation can be given for the drop in PO_2 after dialysis. We advise that patients who have a compromised cardiac status, coronary artery disease, or significant pulmonary disease be monitored closely and treated with supplemental oxygen therapy during and after dialysis. Moderate to severely decreased diffusion capacity noted in all of our patients, when considered with the radiologic evidence of some interstitial fibrosis that was discerned, may indicate thickening of the alveolar membranes due to chronic pulmonary fibrosis, possibly resulting from chronic exposure to still undefined uremic toxins.[16,17]

SUMMARY

Pulmonary function tests and arterial blood gas measurements performed one hour before and immediately after dialysis were obtained

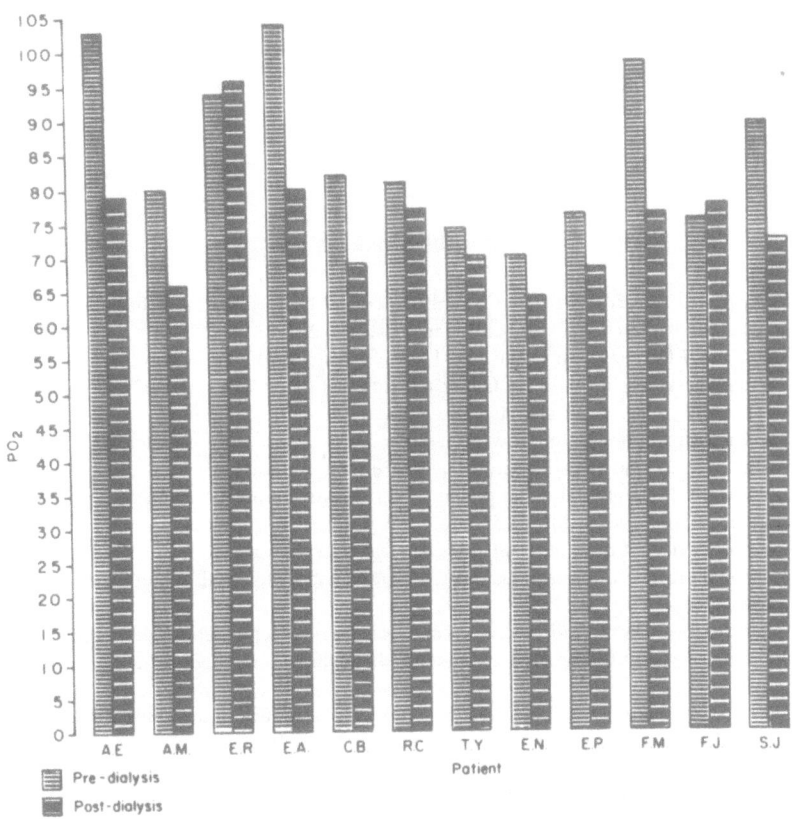

Figure 3. PO$_2$ before and after dialysis in 12 patients showing a signficant drop in PO$_2$ after dialysis in 83% of patients.

in 12 patients who had undergone maintenance hemodialysis for 8 to 11 years. Lung diffusion studies were performed in seven patients before dialysis and in six of these seven after dialysis. Eight out of 11 patients showed evidence of moderate to severe restrictive lung function as compared with predicted values. These functions improved significantly after dialysis. Although 33% of the patients were heavy smokers, we did not find any evidence suggestive of large airway obstruction. Maximum midexpiratory flow rate was significantly decreased in 8 of 11 patients before dialysis, and improved significantly after dialysis. We suggest that this improvement may be attributed to a decrease in peribronchiolar edema occurring after dialysis associated with a mean weight decrease of 9 pounds following dialysis. After dialysis, arterial oxygen tension decreased significantly by a mean value of 10 mm Hg. Though none of these patients were clinically hypoxemic, we advise that patients with compromised cardiac status, coronary artery disease, or significant pulmonary disease be monitored closely and be given routine supplemental oxygen therapy during and after dialysis.

REFERENCES

1. Meyers BD, Rubin AE, Schey G, et al: Functional characteristics of the lung in chronic uremia treated by renal dialysis therapy. *Chest* 68:2, 1975.
2. Fairshter RD, Vaziri ND, Wilson AF, et al: Respiratory physiology before and after hemodialysis in chronic renal failure patients. *Am J Med Sci* 278:1, 1979.
3. Stanescu DC, Veriter C, DePlaeu JF, et al: Lung functions in chronic uremia before and after removal of excess of fluid by hemodialysis. *Clin Sci Molecular Med* 47:143, 1974.
4. Zidulka A, Despas PJ, Milic-Emili J, et al: Pulmonary function with acute loss of excess lung water by hemodialysis in patients with chronic uremia. *Am J Med* 55:134, 1973.
5. Goldman HI, Becklake MR: Respiratory function test: Normal values at median altitudes and prediction of normal results. *Am Rev Tuberc* 79:457, 1959.
6. Morris JF, Koski A, Johnson LC: Spirometric standards for healthy non-smoking adults. *Am Rev Respir Dis* 103:57, 1971.
7. Cadigan JB, Marks A, Ellicott MF, et al: An analysis of factors affecting the measurement of pulmonary diffusing capacity by the single breath method. *J Clin Inves* 40:1495, 1961.
8. Protti DJ, Craven N, Naimark A, et al: Computer assistance in the clinical investigations of pulmonary function studies. *Meth Info Med* 12:102, 1973.
9. Zolton Z, Benjamin JJ, Koeruer SK, et al: Effects of hemodialysis and renal transplantation on pulmonary function. *Chest* 63:4, 1973.
10. Aurigemma NM, Feldman NT, Gottlieb M, et al: Arterial oxygenation during hemodialysis. *N Engl J Med* 297:16, 1977.
11. Sherlock J, Ledwith J: Reflex hypoventilation and decreased arterial oxygen tension during ultrafiltration. In *Proceedings Dialysis Transplant Forum* 1978, p 250.
12. Carlon GC, Campfield RN, Goldinger PL: Hypoxemia during hemodialysis. *Crit Care Med* 7:11, 1979.
13. Mahajan S, Gardiner H, Detar B, et al: Relationship between pulmonary functions and hemodialysis induced leukopenia. *Trans Am Soc Artif Intern Organs* 23:411, 1977.
14. Craddock PR, Fehr J, Brighan KL, et al: Leukocyte mediated pulmonary dysfunction in hemodialysis. *N Engl J Med* 296:769, 1977.
15. Patterson RW, Nissenson AR, Miller J, et al: Hypoxemia and pulmonary gas exchange during hemodialysis. *J Appl Phys* 50:2, 1981.
16. Henkin RI, Maxwell MH, Murray JF, et al: Uremic pneumonitis. *Ann Intern Med* 57:1001, 1962.
17. Borgstron KE, Ising U, Linder E, et al: Experimental pulmonary edema. *Acta Radiol* 54:97, 1960.

20

Musculoskeletal Abnormalities of the Ten-Year Hemodialysis Patient

GILBERT F. GELFAND, HARRY BIENENSTOCK,
MORRELL M. AVRAM, AND DAVID ROSENBLUM

Hemodialysis and renal transplantation have increased longevity in the chronic renal failure patient. Increased longevity, however, has been associated with many new medical problems. These problems derive from both ongoing chronic renal failure and the hemodialysis regimen.

Musculoskeletal abnormalities associated with chronic renal failure and hemodialysis have been well described.[1,2] Terms such as "renal osteosdystrophy" and "dialysis osteodystrophy" describe clinical, laboratory, and radiologic signs and symptoms that are observed more frequently in long-duration dialysis patients.

In this study we attempted to ascertain how an unusual group of hemodialysis patients treated for longer than a decade withstood the stress of uremia and its therapy in terms of the musculoskeletal system.

METHODS

Eleven patients entering the dialysis program at the Long Island College Hospital between 1968 and 1971 and now still on hemodialysis, the long-dialysis group (LDG), and 11 randomly selected age-matched

GILBERT F. GELFAND • Division of Rheumatology, The Long Island College Hospital, Brooklyn, New York. HARRY BIENENSTOCK • Division of Rheumatology, The Long Island College Hospital; and Department of Medicine, The Long Island College Hospital, Brooklyn, New York. MORRELL M. AVRAM • The Avram Center for Kidney Diseases, Division of Nephrology, The Long Island College Hospital; Department of Medicine, The Long Island College Hospital; Brooklyn Kidney Center and Nephrology Foundation of Brooklyn, Brooklyn, New York. DAVID ROSENBLUM • Department of Radiology, The Long Island College Hospital.

patients on hemodialysis one year or less, the short-dialysis group (SDG),
were studied (Table I). The LDG consisted of seven men and four women
who ranged in age from 27 to 54 years. The SDG consisted of five men and
six women aged 24 to 55 years. The primary causes leading to renal failure
in the LDG were chronic glomerulonephritis (eight), heroin nephropathy
(one), hypertension (one), and cortical necrosis (one). In the SDG the
primary diagnoses were diabetic nephropathy (three), hypertension (two),
primary amyloidosis, membraneous glomerulonephritis, chronic glomerulonephritis, focal sclerosis, polycystic kidney, and heroin nephropathy
(one each).

Hemodialysis was performed three times a week for five hours with a
batch-type central dialysate supply system until 1974 and thereafter a
proportioning central dialysate delivery system was used. Dialysate
calcium concentration was 4.1 mEq/dl.

Three patients from the LDG received a renal transplant. Acute

Table I. Patient Profile[a]

	Age	Race	Sex	Hemodialysis begun	Diagnosis
LDG					
T.Y.	27	O	M	1970	CGN
J.D.	30	C	M	1969	CGN
E.A.	33	B	M	1968	CGN
A.E.	33	B	F	1970	CGN
E.P.	34	B	M	1969	Heroin nephropathy
A.M.	36	B	M	1971	HTN
R.C.	36	B	M	1970	CGN
E.R.	40	B	F	1969	Cortical necrosis
E.J.	47	B	F	1970	CGN
F.J.	50	B	M	1970	CGN
S.J.	54	B	F	1969	CGN
SDG					
H.B.	24	C	M	1980	Amyloidosis
W.F.	33	B	M	1980	Focal sclerosis
T.N.	33	B	M	1980	Heroin nephropathy
E.J.	33	B	F	1980	CGN
H.H.	41	B	M	1980	Diabetic nephropathy
M.T.	44	B	F	1980	Diabetic nephropathy
M.F.	48	H	F	1980	Diabetic nephropathy
G.E.	50	B	M	1980	MGN
C.W.	55	B	F	1980	HTN
A.R.	53	C	F	1980	Polycystic kidney
M.C.	35	B	F	1980	HTN

[a] O: oriental; B: black; C: Caucasian; H: Hispanic; CGN: chronic glomerulonephritis; MGN: membranous
glomerulonephritis; HTN: hypertension.

rejection occurred in two patients; in a third the transplant survived for 1½ years. Four patients in the LDG had undergone partial parathyroidec- tomies during the course of dialysis treatment (Table II). One patient (M.F.) from the SDG was interviewed, examined, and underwent the required radiologic studies; however, she died before laboratory evalua- tions could be completed.

Evaluation of each patient included a review of musculoskeletal symptoms and roentgenologic and laboratory findings. Patients were evaluated for the musculoskeletal signs and symptoms listed in Table III. All available bone and joint x-rays were reveiwed. In every case recent x- rays of the chest, pelvis, spine, hands, and skull were available. These radiographs were evaluated for the specific changes listed in Table III.

All laboratory evaluations were performed immediately prior to hemodialysis. The mean values of at least five different determinations (serum calcium, phosphorous, uric acid, alkaline phosphatase, BUN, and creatinine) over the preceding one to six months were taken as represen- tative. The Technicon SMAC automated methods # 4001 PCg (Technicon, Tarrytown, New York) was used for these determinations. Other labora- tory investigations performed included: serum protein electrophoresis (Helena serum protein electrophoresis procedure: super Z and Zip Zone procedure), parathyroid hormone assay (method of Hawker[3]), rheumatoid factor (Ra-Test Reagent Kit [4]), antinuclear antibodies (immunofluorescent tumor technique[5]), C3 and C4 (RID diffusion plate[6]), and VDRL.

Statistical significances of the results were evaluated by the use of the Student t test using independent samples or paired data where appro- priate. Cochrane's adjustment was applied when variances were unequal. All tests of statistical significance were done at the $p < 0.05$ level.

RESULTS

The results of the symptom inquiry are summarized in Table III. Joint pain, the most common symptom, was present in 91% of the LDG and in 54% of the SDG. Knee joint symptoms were the most common, occurring in 54% of the LDG and 45% of the SDG.

Two patients in each group had swelling of a single joint (the knee in three patients and the elbow in another). No bone or joint infections were detected. Soft-tissue calcifications, gout, specific muscle group weakness, and fractures were seen less frequently. Two patients (one in each group) had clinical findings consistent with carpal tunnel syndrome. One patient in the LDG had symptoms consistent with Raynaud's phenomenon.

Musculoskeletal symptoms were present in a higher percentage of

Gilbert F. Gelfand et al.

Table II. Laboratory Summary,

	Ca	P	Ca × P	UA	AP	BUN	Creatinine	PTH/CA
Normal values	8.5–10.5 mg/dl	2.5–4.2 mg/dl		M—3.9–9 F—2.2–7.7 mg/dl	30–115 μ/liter	10–26 mg/dl	0.7–1.5 mg/dl	163–347 pgEq/ml
T.Y.	10.6	4.6	48.8	9.9	72	102.8	20.8	217 10.7
J.D.[b]	10.4	5.5	57.2	8.9	105.1	80.2	9.2	230 10.8
E.A.	9.3	5.5	51.2	11.1	100.3	117	22.4	238 8.5
A.E.[b]	8.8	5.4	47.5	8.8	166.8	63.5	14.8	311 8.3
E.P.[b]	7.5	4.0	30.0	9.4	237.8	75.8	18.0	240 6.5
A.M.	9.7	6.1	59.2	6.9	297.5	83.8	19.6	2100 8.9
R.C.	10.1	4.4	44.4	8.9	744[b]	102.8	18.5	645 9.6
E.R.	8.0	5.4	43.2	8.2	466.3[b]	90.9	22.3	703.5 7.35
E.J.[b]	9.4	4.6	43.2	10.5	177	67.2	16.6	337 8.7
F.J.	9.2	4.5	41.4	7.9	401.7	77.4	14.5	2447.0 9.1
S.J.	8.8	4.0	35.2	9.6	205.2	109	20.9	315 8.9
Mean	9.3	4.9	45.6	9.1	270.3	88.2	18	690 8.75
Parathyroidectomy mean	9.0	4.8	44.5	9.4	171.7	71.6	14.7	285.8 8.5
Non-Parathyroidectomy mean	9.4	4.9	46.2	8.9	326.6	97.6	19.9	279.5 8.6

[a]Ca: calcium; P: phosphorus; Ca × P: calcium–phosphorus product; UA: uric acid; AP: alkaline phosphatase; BUN: Blood urea nitrogen; PTH: parathyroid hormone; ANA: antinuclear bodies; RF rheumatoid factor; TP: total protein.

patients in the LDG than in the SDG. This was especially apparent when comparing joint, bone, and back pain in both groups. The total number of symptoms elicited in the LDG was 39 as compared with 20 in the SDG. Three patients in the LDG reported that their symptoms were transiently relieved by hemodialysis.

We also compared symptoms prevalent in 1981 with symptoms described at any time during the ten-year period (Table III). The only

Ten-Year Patients

ANA	RF	VDRL	C3	C4	TP	Alpha	Alpha 1	Alpha 2	Beta	Gamma
—	—	—	83–177	15–45	6–8	3.5–5	0.2–0.4	0.6–1.0	0.6–1.0	0.7–1.3
—	1/160	—	75	251	7.6	4.0	0.29	0.75	0.72	1.81
—	—	—	106	34.1	6.9	3.3	0.14	0.82	0.74	1.89
—	—	—	90	36.8	6.8	3.5	0.38	0.43	0.78	1.76
—	—	—	71	25.5	6.3	3.5	0.18	0.66	0.56	1.40
—	—	—	67	16.2	7.7	4.0	0.21	0.69	0.60	2.19
—		—	120	40.2	7.5	4.3	0.25	0.85	0.71	1.32
—	—	—	115	16.5	7.5	3.9	0.17	0.72	0.74	2.0
—	—	—	93	26.7	7.2	4.3	0.18	0.67	0.6	1.45
—	1/20	—	94	16.4	9.2	3.9	0.25	0.88	0.88	3.30
—	—	—	96	11.0	8.5	3.6	0.17	0.71	0.64	3.4
—	—	1:2 FTS+	112	26.2	7.9	4.6	0.19	0.71	0.72	1.70
—	—	—	95.4	25.7	7.6	3.9	0.22	0.72	0.70	2.0
—	—	—	88.8	25.2	7.52	3.7	0.19	0.76	0.70	2.19
—	—	—	100.1	26.1	7.57	4.6	0.23	0.79	0.70	1.92

[b] Parathyroidectomy.

differences observed were a decrease in bone and joint pain frequency (1981). These differences were accounted for by the four patients who underwent parathyroidectomies. All four experienced bone and joint pain prior to surgery. In two patients pain was significantly reduced following surgery; in one patient it completely disappeared. A fourth patient experienced an increase in bone and joint pain.

The location of specific joints affected is summarized in Table IV. The

Table III. Musculoskelatal Symptoms in Hemodialysis Patients

Symptoms	LDG (11 patients)				SDG (11 patients)	
	Number	(Percent)	1981	(Percent)	Number	(Percent)
Morning stiffness	5	(45)	5	(45)	1	(9)
Bone pain	7	(64)	4	(36)	3	(27)
Joint pain	10	(91)	9	(82)	6	(54)
Back pain	4	(36)	4	(36)	3	(27)
Swelling	2	(18)	1	(9)	2	(18)
Fractures	2	(18)	2	(18)	1	(9)
Infections						
Bone	0		0		0	
Joint	0		0		0	
Raynaud's syndrome	1	(9)	1	(9)	0	
Restriction of movement	2	(18)	2	(18)	1	(9)
Muscle weakness	3	(27)	3	(27)	1	(9)
Soft-tissue calcifications	1	(9)	1	(9)	0	
Gout	1	(9)	1	(9)	1	(9)
Extremity numbness	1	(9)	1	(9)	1	(9)
Total number of symptoms	39		34		20	

Table IV. Joint Pain Distribution

Joint	LDG (11 patients)		SDG (11 patients)	
	Number	(Percent)	Number	(Percent)
Shoulder	5	(45)	1	(9)
Elbow	0		1	(9)
Wrist	3	(27)	0	
Fingers	1	(9)	0	
Hips	3	(27)	2	(18)
Knees	6	(55)	5	(45)
Ankles	1	(9)	0	
Feet	2	(18)	1	(9)
Back	4	(36)	3	(27)
Great toe	1	(9)	0	
Temporomandibular	0		1	(9)
Ribs	0		1	(9)
Total number of joints	26		15	

total number of joints affected in the LDG was 26 as compared with 15 in the SDG. Joint pain was most frequently noted in the knees, shoulders, wrists, and hips. It was described less frequently in the feet, ribs, and temporomandibular joint.

The laboratory findings for both groups are summarized in Tables II, V, and VI. The mean serum calcium values for the LDG and SDG were 9.3 mg/dl and 9.1 mg/dl respectively. Values ranged from 7.5 to 10.4 mg/dl in the LDG and from 8.2 to 10.4 mg/dl in the SDG.

The mean phosphorous levels for the LDG and the SDG were 4.9 and 4.4 mg/dl. Values ranged from 3.8 to 6 mg/dl in the SDG and from 4 to 6.1 mg/dl in the LDG.

The mean serum uric acid levels for the LDG and SDG were 9.1 and 8.8 mg/dl. In the LDG values ranged from 6.9 to 11.1 mg/dl and in the SDG from 6.3 to 11.4 mg/dl. The two patients with gout had mean serum uric acid levels of 7.5 and 9.5 mg/dl.

There was no statistically significant difference between the LDG and SDG for the mean values of any of the previous laboratory determinations.

The mean alkaline phosphatase value in the LDG was 270.3 μ/liter compared with 114.3 μ/liter in the SDG (normal: 25–115 μ/liter). Two patients in the LDG had two values listed as 600 μ/liter (no dilutions were done). These values were arbitrarily averaged into their mean alkaline phosphatase score as 700 μ/liter. There was a significant difference ($p < 0.05$) between the mean values for both groups.

The mean BUN values were 88.2 mg/dl for the LDG and 76.9 mg/dl for the SDG. The creatinine mean values were 17.9 and 12.4 mg/dl for the LDG and SDG respectively. Only the difference in mean creatinine values was statistically significant at the $p = 0.05$ level.

Parathyroid hormone levels for the LDG and the SDG were 690 pgEq/ml and 344 pgEq/ml. In the SDG PTH values were obtained in only four patients. The difference between the groups was not statistically significant.

Antinuclear antibody tests were performed on ten patients in each group. All test results were reported as negative. Rheumatoid factor was found to be present (1/160 dilution) in one patient in each group.

VDRL was nonreactive in all patients tested (not done in one patient in the SDG), save one who also had a positive FTS-ABS.

The mean serum C3 and C4 levels in the LDG were 95.4 mg/dl and 25.7 mg/dl, respectively, compared with 102.1 and 30.3 mg/dl in the SDG. There was no significant difference between the two groups.

A serum protein electrophoresis was done on all patients. The mean values for LDG were (g/dl): total protein, 7.6; albumin, 3.9; alpha 1,

Table V. Laboratory Summary, One-Year Patients

	Ca	P	Ca × P	UA	AP	BUN	Creatinine	PTH/CA
Normal values	8.5–10.5 mg/dl	2.5–4.2 mg/dl		M—3.9–9 F—2.2–7.7 mg/dl	30–115 μ/liter	10–26 mg/dl	0.7–1.5 mg/dl	163–347 pgEq/ml
H.B.	10.4	3.9	40.6	7.6	149.7	97.3	16.0	287 9.7
W.F.	9.5	4.4	41.8	11.4	102	72	8.8	
E.J.	10.3	4.6	47.4	8.8	127	55.7	12.4	
T.N.	8.6	4.2	36.1	9.6	141.8	89.6	16.1	
H.H.	8.2	4.1	33.6	6.3	116.8	42.2	10.3	
M.T.	9.1	6.0	54.6	8.9	61.5	90.2	11.7	226 9.0
M.F.	8.4	3.9	32.8	6.7	128.6	43	8.2	
G.E.	8.8	4.3	37.8	8.2	85.8	77	16.0	
C.W.	9.0	3.8	34.2	9.8	156.2	85.9	11.6	625 8.8
A.R.[b]	9.1	4.8	43.7	9.5	102.4	131.4	11.4	238 9
M.C.	9.2	4.5	41.4	10.4	85.5	61.8	13.6	
Mean	9.1	4.4	40.4	8.8	114.3	76.9	12.4	344 9.1
Standard deviation	0.7	0.6	6.6	1.71	29.3	19.7	2.18	184.3 0.4

[a] See footnote, Table II.
[b] Gout.

0.22; alpha 2, 0.72; beta, 0.70; and gamma, 2.0. The normal values for all laboratory determinations are listed in Table II.

The roentgenologic findings of the LDG and SDG are summarized in Table VII. The most common radiologic finding in the LDG was decreased bone density or coarsening of bone. This was found in all 11 patients. Subperiosteal resorption was also a common finding, occurring in 91% (LDG). The "pepperpot skull" (thickening of the tables with areas of increased and decreased density seen throughout the skull) was observed in 73%, whereas thickening of the table of the skull alone was seen in only one patient.

Vascular calcifications were observed in 64% of the LDG. Soft-tissue calcifications were found in two patients and only around the arteriovenous fistula in both.

ANA	RF	VDRL	C3	C4	TP	Alpha	Alpha 1	Alpha 2	Beta	Gamma
—	—	—	83–177	15–45	6–8	3.5–5	0.2–0.4	0.6–1.0	0.6–1.0	0.7–1.3
—	—	—	77	17.7	5.9	3.4	0.25	0.65	0.56	1.03
—	1/160 1/40	—	129.5	36.5	7.75	3.4	0.36	0.93	0.89	2.10
—	—	—	101	26.9	6.9	3.8	0.33	0.55	0.83	1.37
—	—	—	99	30.4	7.7	2.9	36	81	42	3.13
—	—	—	120	36.4	7.6	3.4	0.32	1.21	0.81	1.90
—	—	—	117.5	28	6.0	3.0	0.43	0.80	0.86	0.92
—	—	—	88	50.5	7.2	3.7	0.27	0.80	0.79	1.61
—	—	—	88	18.9	6.8	3.5	0.38	0.43	0.78	1.76
—	—	—	112	27.2	7.3	3.4	0.29	1.16	1.07	1.34
—	—	—	89	30.5	8.3	3.8	0.30	0.36	0.91	2.13
			102.1	30.3	7.13	3.43	0.33	0.77	0.79	1.73
									0.18	0.64
			17.1	9.42	0.76	0.32	0.05	0.28		0.64

Pseudo-enlargement (osteolysis of the joint surface and replacement by a poorly mineralized woven bone and fibrous tissues) and erosions of the sacroiliac joint were observed in 64%, while true sacroiliac joint obliteration was seen in only one patient. A widening and erosions of the symphysis pubis were seen in 55% of the LDG. The "rugger jersey" spine (coarsening at both ends of the vertebral body with a central lucency) was also observed in 55%. Acroosteolysis (resorption of bone at the outer ends of clavicle) of the clavicles was seen in six patients (55%), while periosteal elevation, cortical striations of the phalanges, decreased volume of the vertebral bodies, and joint narrowing were each seen in 27%.

Other less common radiologic signs included kyphosis, tubular bone fractures, protrusio acetabuli, periarticular erosions, and periarticular calcifications.

In the SDG there were only two patients who exhibited radiologic changes. One patient showed subperiosteal erosions, decreased bone

Table VI. Laboratory

	Ca	P	Ca × P	UA	AP	BUN	Creatinine
LDG							
Mean	9.3	4.9	45.6	9.1	270.3	88.2	17.9
Standard deviation	0.96	0.7	8.6	1.2	128.8	17.6	4
SDG							
Mean	9.1	4.4	40.4	8.8	114.3	76.9	12.4
Standard deviation	0.7	0.6	6.6	1.71	29.3	19.7	2.2
	ns	ns	ns	ns	$p < 0.05$	ns	$p > 0.05$

[a] See footnote, Table II.

density and coarsening, vascular calcifications, a tubular bone fracture, and acroosteolysis of the clavicle. A second patient had early evidence of diffuse decreased bone density.

In the LDG there were 75 total x-ray changes (Table VII) as compared with seven in the SDG. Meniscal calcifications or vertebral fractures were not seen in either group.

Table VIII presents a summary of the radiologic findings in each of the bones and joints. Decreased bone density and coarsening were seen most frequently in the dorsal and lumbar spine (100%) and in the skull (82%), and also frequently seen in the pelvis, femur, and humerus. Decreased bone density of the hands was present in 45%.

Subperiosteal erosions were most commonly observed in the hands (73%). They were especially prevalent on the radial side of the second and third middle phalanges. Erosions were also commonly seen in the ischium (64%) and clavicles (55%). They occurred somewhat less frequently in the sacroiliac joints (45%), ribs (36%), symphysis pubis (27%), and humerus (27%).

Vascular calcifications, when present, were widespread, most often involving the vessels of the hands, tibia, femur, knees, and feet.

Periosteal new bone formation was observed four times in three patients in the LDG. The femur was involved in three cases and the humerus was involved once.

Two patients from the LDG had joint narrowing. Both had protrusio acetabuli and one additionally had narrowing of both knees.

Summary Comparison[a]

PTH/CA	C3	C4	TP	Alpha	Alpha 1	Alpha 2	Beta	Gamma
630 / 8.8	95.4	25.7	7.6	3.9	0.22	0.72	0.70	2.0
764.3 / 1.21	18.0	9.6	0.73	0.4	0.07	0.12	0.09	0.71
344 / 9.1	102.1	30.3	7.1	3.4	0.33	0.77	0.79	1.73
184.3 / 0.4	17.1	9.42	0.76	0.32	0.05	0.28	0.18	0.64
ns	ns	ns	ns	$p < .05$	$p < .05$	ns	ns	ns

DISCUSSION

The incidence of musculoskeletal complaints in patients receiving hemodialysis has been variable. Katz[1] studied 195 patients who were on hemodialysis or who had received a kidney transplant, and found only three patients who complained of bone pain. Most complaints in his study were related to metastatic calcium deposits. Alvarez-Ude et al.[7] report bone pain in 44% of 85 patients on regular hemodialysis. Other authors report from 10% to 100% incidence of symptomatic dialysis osteodystrophy.[8–12] Bone pain is often associated with the onset of osteomalacia[1,7,12] but it is observed in osteitis fibrosa in only a small minority. It has also been suggested that hemodialysis may activate or worsen in clinical symptoms of bone pain.

In our ten-year dialysis group we found musculoskeletal complaints in a majority of patients to be the rule. Ninety-one percent of our patients complained of joint pain while 63% complained of bone pain at some time during the ten-year period. Three patients noted reduced bone and joint pain immediately after dialysis. Other complaints included morning stiffness, back pain, muscle weakness, restriction in shoulder motion, and joint swelling.

No patients complained of symptoms related to metastatic calcifications (a frequently reported symptom finding in previous studies). Interestingly, we had only two patients with soft-tissue calcifications; both were around the arteriovenous fistulae. We observed one patient with periarticular calcifications around the proximal and distal interphalangeal

Gilbert F. Gelfand et al.

Table VII. Radiographic Changes in Hemodialysis Patients

Radiographic changes	LDG (11 patients)		SDG (11 patients)		
	Number	Percent	Number	Percent	
Subperiosteal resorption	10	(91)	1	(9)	$p < 0.05$
Periarticular erosions	1	(9)	0		$p < 0.05$
Decreased bone density	11	(100)	2	(18)	$p < 0.05$
Calcifications					
Soft tissue	2	(18)	0		n.s.
Periarticular	1	(9)	0		n.s.
Vascular	0	(64)	0	(9)	$p < 0.05$
Meniscal	0		0		
Rugger jersey spine	6	(55)	0		$p < 0.05$
Fractures					
Vertebral	0				
Tubular	1	(9)	1	(9)	n.s.
Skull					
Pepperpot	8	(73)	1	(9)	$p < 0.05$
Thick tables	1	(9)	0		n.s.
Acroosteolysis					
Clavicle	6	(55)	1	(9)	n.s.
Cortical striations					
Phalanges	3	(27)	0		n.s.
Pseudo-enlargement					
Sacroiliac joint	7	(64)	0		$p < 0.05$
Symphysis pubis	6	(55)	0		$p < 0.05$
Vertebral volume loss	3	(27)	0		n.s.
Kyphosis	2	(18)	0		n.s.
Periosteal elevation	3	(27)	0		n.s.
Joint narrowing	2	(27)	0		n.s.
Protrusio acetabuli	2	(18)	0		n.s.
Total number of changes	75		6		

joints. The mean calcium/phosphorous product was 45.6 (LDG), the highest individual product being 59.2. It has previously been reported that a calcium/phosphorous product of 75 is associated with metastatic calcifications.[1,12] We felt that the paucity of metastatic calcifications in our study was related to the strict dialysis regimen and phosphate control under which these patients were maintained as well as the consequent lowered calcium/phosphorous product.

Only two patients described previous fractures. One patient had a chip fracture of the elbow and the other a fracture of one of the metatarsal bones. These findings are not in agreement with other studies,[11,13–15] which suggest that vertebral and rib fractures are more common and are found in 13% to 50% of dialysis patients. This again is thought to be related to the

Table VIII. Skeletal Distribution of Radiologic Changes Number and (Percent)

	Decreased bone density Number	Erosions	Vascular calcification	Periosteal	Joint narrowing	Fractures	Periarticular calcification	Periarticular erosions
Skull	9 (82)							
C-Spine	4 (36)							
D-Spine	11 (100)							
LS-Spine	11 (100)							
Humerus	5 (45)	3 (27)		1 (9)				
Elbows	3 (27)		1 (9)			1 (9)		
Wrist	1 (9)							
Phalanges	5 (45)	8 (73)	3 (27)					
Hips	1 (9)		3 (27)		2 (18)		1 (9)	1 (9)
Knees	3 (27)		3 (27)		1 (9)			
Tarsal								
Toes	1 (9)	1 (9)	2 (18)					
Pelvis	10 (91)	7 (64)						
Sacroiliac		5 (45)						
Symphysis pubis		3 (27)						
Femur	6 (54)		4 (36)	3 (27)				
Ribs	5 (45)	4 (36)						
Tibia	2 (18)	1 (9)	4 (36)					
Clavicles		6 (55)						
Total number of changes	77	38	17	4	1	3	1	1

low calcium/phosphorous product that resulted from the strict dialysis regimen and phosphate control.

None of our patients developed bone or joint infections. Mathews et al.[16] reported six episodes of septic arthritis in 450 patient-years of dialysis. Infection is the second leading cause of death in chronic maintenance hemodialysis patients.[17,18] The organisms are thought to originate in the A-V fistula.[19,20] The high incidence of infection may be related to the compromised immune system in patients with renal insufficiency.[21] It is interesting to note that none of our ten-year group representing 126 patient-years of hemodialysis developed bone or joint infections.

Two patients in the LDG and one patient in the SDG had marked reduction in shoulder range of motion. In two cases the restriction was bilateral and in all three patients abduction was less than 90°. There was no evidence of periarticular or soft-tissue calcifications on any of the shoulder x-rays. We have not encountered any other reports of restriction in shoulder motion in patients undergoing long-term hemodialysis.

Two of the 11 patients in LDG experienced joint swelling. One patient had recent transient knee swelling, while the other had swelling of the great toe secondary to gout. We found no other evidence of crystal-induced arthritis. The mean uric acid for the LDG was 9.1 mg/dl. Secondary gout is an infrequent complication of hemodialysis.[2,22] Pseudo-gout has also been described.[2] We found no radiologic evidence of chondrocalcinosis, and only one patient had periarticular calcification. We were, therefore, not surprised that episodic pseudo-gout was not observed. Pseudo-gout has also been reported as a postparathyroidectomy complication. This did not occur in any of the four patients who underwent parathyroidectomy (LDG).

One patient in the LDG and one in the SDG had signs and symptoms consistent with carpal tunnel syndrome. Warren and Otieno[23] reported carpal tunnel syndrome in 23 of 36 patients on maintenance hemodialysis. Vijay et al.[24] reported five symptomatic and five asymptomatic patients with carpal tunnel syndrome in 62 maintenance hemodialysis patients. Most reports suggest that the extremity bearing the A-V fistula is usually affected. One of our patients had symptoms suggestive of carpal tunnel in both hands (no EMG was performed). Vijay et al. reported a tight and thickened flexor retinaculum as the principal findings in those patients who underwent surgery for this condition.

All patients complained of generalized weakness, yet only three patients in the LDG complained of weakness in a specific muscle group.

The knees and shoulders were most commonly affected by pain in both groups (Table IV). We cannot readily explain this since there was no apparent correlation between radiographic changes and clinical symptoms.

Musculoskeletal symptoms in 1981 varied little from those observed over the ten-year period in general. A significant reduction in bone and joint symptoms was noted in the four patients who underwent partial parathyroidectomy. Hemodialysis did not improve symptomatology in the remainder of our patients.

There was a significant difference in the number, but not the distribution, of musculoskeletal complaints between the LDG and SDG. The LDG had a total of 39 complaints while the SDG had 20 (Table III).

Review of the laboratory data (Tables II, and V, VI) reveals that the mean calcium and phosphorous levels were maintained at normal or near-normal levels throughout the period of dialysis. The calcium/phosphorous product was well below the level of 75, a value that has been associated with metastatic calcifications.

Serum alkaline phosphatase levels were elevated in the LDG. There was a significant difference between the mean levels in the LDG and SDG, and also a significant difference between patients who underwent parathyroidectomy and the remainder of the group (LDG). It has been reported that 30% of the circulating alkaline phosphatase found in patients on intermittent hemodialysis represents the intestinal alkaline phosphatase enzyme rather than the isoenzyme produced by the osteoblast.[25] Alvarez-Ude et al.[7] reported that 45% of 85 patients on long-term hemodialysis were found to have elevated alkaline phosphatases. He also confirmed, as have other authors, its association with osteitis fibrosa (hyperparathyroidism).[1,14] Most studies, however, have underscored the difficulty of correlating laboratory, histologic, and clinical parameters in a meaningful way with any consistency.[26] In the long-term hemodialysis patient, the mean level of serum alkaline phosphatase was higher and the numbers of radiographic changes (75 in the LDG and 6 in SDG) and symptoms (39 in the LDG and 20 in SDG) were greater than those observed in patients in the short-term group. There was, however, no correlation of any of these two parameters in individual patients. In fact, quite often, the highest alkaline phosphatase levels were found in those patients who had the fewest complaints. It has been reported that bone pain in patients undergoing regular hemodialysis results from osteomalacia and is not related to hyperparathyroidism.[7] This may explain the nonrelationship between alkaline phosphatase and clinical symptomatology that was found in this study.

Although increased levels of PTH have clearly been correlated with the bone changes associated with hyperparathyroidism, the extent of this relationship is still controversial. O'Riordan et al.[11] reported that dialyzed patients may have lower levels of circulating PTH than nondialyzed uremics. Furthermore, they report that dialyzed patients with bone disease may have less immunoreactive PTH than their counterparts without osteodystrophy. They concluded that while hyperparathyroidism contributes to osteodystrophy, it is unlikely to be its prime cause. It has also been stated that the bone disease of dialyzed patients may heal in the presence of persistently elevated PTH.[27] PTH levels were elevated in both groups in our study, and there was no significant difference between the values in the LDG and SDG, although there was a difference in the mean PTH levels between those patients who underwent parathyroidectomies and those who did not. Again, we could find no relationship between bone pain and elevated PTH levels, perhaps for reasons similar to those proposed for the lack of alkaline phosphatase correlation; that is, that bone pain is associated with osteomalacia and not osteitis fibrosa (hyperparathyroidism).

Nolph et al.[28] report that 25% of 77 long-term hemodialysis patients had either antibodies to native DNA or ENA. They previously had shown that free nuclei of damaged leukocytes adhere to hemodialysis membranes and postulated that the nuclear debris could be flushed back into the patient during dialysis. This then might result in the formation of antibodies to nuclear components. Das Gupta et al.[29] report no significant increase in anti-DNA antibodies in long-term hemodialysis patients. FANA assays were negative in every case in both studies. The ENA, FARR, and hemoagglutinin assays are thought to be much more sensitive than the FANA. FANA in ten of ten patients in the LDG and in ten of ten patients in the SDG was negative.

Ten patients in each group were tested for rheumatoid factor. It was found to be positive at a low titer (1–160) in one patient from each group. Neither of these patients had any stigmata of synovial disease.

VDRL was nonreactive in ten of ten patients in the LDG and was reactive in one of 11 patients in the SDG. This patient also had a positive FTS-ABS.

Craddock[30] has demonstrated that both alternate and classical complement pathways may be activated by the cellophane membrane hemodialysis apparatus. Mean C3, C4 values were well within normal limits in our study. Further scrutiny of the data reveals that three of our patients had C3 values below normal. One patient had a low C4 value associated with a normal C3 level. These laboratory abnormalities appear to be insignificant. Patients in the SDG had significantly higher mean C3, C4 values than patients in the LDG, although these values were still within the normal range. These findings were again of no clinical significance.

Serum protein electrophoresis was performed in all patients in the LDG. Mean values for all protein components were normal, with the exception of gamma globulins, which were significantly elevated. Preliminary immunoelectrophoresis results (in four patients) reveal IgG values ranging from 1,380 to 1,510 (normal = 639–1349). Gamma globulin values were also elevated in the SDG. We cannot explain these elevated levels. It is generally thought that both cellular and humoral immunologic defenses may be impaired in chronic renal failure[26] and that the incidence of infection is increased. We hypothesize that this increased susceptibility to infection may reflect the hypergammaglobulinemia that we have encountered in all of our patients.

In the LDG we also note that six of 11 patients had a decreased alpha 1 fraction. We again cannot explain this. HDL is an alpha 1 component and, given the increased atherogenic incidence in chronic renal failure, we speculate that HDL levels might be lower and thereby contributory to this increased incidence of atherosclerosis. In the SDG the alpha 1 levels were normal, except in one patient, where it was elevated. There was a significant difference between the mean alpha 1 values of both groups. Preliminary HDL levels on some of these patients revealed a uniformly higher level than normal. This is opposite to what we would expect. If we consider that the LDG represents a group of survivors, it may well be that they survive because they were intrinsically less prone to developing arteriosclerotic complications.

Bone disease is a well-recognized complication of chronic renal failure. Histologically, there are reports of a combination of osteitis fibrosa, osteomalacia, or osteosclerosis[31,32] present in this setting. Bone disease seems to appear and progress more rapidly after hemodialysis has started.[33,34] Some authors actually consider bone loss to be specific for hemodialysis.[35] It seems clear that there is little relationship between bone histology, the severity of bone disease, and radiologic changes.

Massry[36] found that 92% of hemodialysis patients had roentgenographic evidence of bone disease within two years. Johnson[13] reported that hypomineralization occurred in 85% of 33 patients on hemodialysis for as long as 75 months. Katz[1] found demineralization of the spine to be the most common roentgenographic sign. Resorption of the clavicles and spotty demineralization of the skull were the next most common findings. Subperiosteal bone resorption localized to the radial border of the middle phalanges of the second and third fingers was also commonly observed.

All of our patients in the LDG had radiologic evidence of renal osteodystrophy. In the SDG only two of 11 patients had evidence of bone disease.

Decreased bone density was the most common finding and was present in 100% of the LDG. The dorsal and lumbar spines were involved in all patients, the pelvis in 91%, and the skull in 82%. The long bones were involved in 55% of the cases and the hands in 50%. These findings were not unexpected, and they are consistent with what has previously been reported.

Subperiosteal erosions were observed in ten of 11 patients in the LDG. This was most commonly seen in the phalanges (73%), ischium (64%), and the distal clavicles (55%). Schwartz et al.[37] report erosions in the distal clavicle in 50% of two-year or longer dialysis patients. In our study erosions were also found in the sacroiliac joints, symphysis pubis, ribs, and humerus. These findings are consistent with previous reports.[32,38–41] It is interesting that such a high percentage of our LDG patients had superiosteal resorption (91%), especially when compared with SDG where only one patient had such findings.

Periosteal new bone formation has infrequently been described in association with renal osteodystrophy. Meema et al.[42] report that 85% of 117 patients with severe chronic renal disease had evidence of new bone formation. These changes were always accompanied by subperiosteal resorption in the phalanges. In this study new bone formation was most commonly found in the metatarsal bones, pelvis, tibia, and phalanges, in that order. There were only 11 previously reported cases before this review. It seems logical to assume that this is a change found more frequently in the long-term dialysis patient. We observed periosteal new bone formation in three patients in the LDG. These changes were seen only in the femur and humerus. No evidence of periosteal new bone formation was observed in any patient from the SDG. None of the three patients in the LDG had evidence of the bronchogenic carcinoma, cyanotic heart disease, Crohn's disease, polyarteritis nodosa, scurvy, or thyroid acropachy with which this radiologic finding has been associated.

Although 55% of patients in the LDG were found to have a "rugger jersey spine" (central radiolucency with sclerosis of the upper and lower thirds of the vertebral body), only three had loss of vertebral body volume and only two were judged to have a significant kyphosis. There were no such changes in the SDG. Thus this appears to be an uncommon change more likely to be seen in the long-term dialysis patient.

Joint disease was found in surprisingly few patients. Two were found to have protrusio acetabuli and another had minimal narrowing of the hips and knees. One of the patients had periarticular erosions of the proximal interphalangeal joints. These findings do not appear to correlate with the aforementioned incidence of joint symptoms. No radiologic abnormalities of the joints were noted in any of the SDG patients.

Vascular calcifications have previously been reported in 3% to 83% of patients on long-term hemodialysis.[1,15,43] The radiologic appearance is due to the deposition of calcium in the media and the internal elastic membrane of the artery.[2] The lumen is not involved.[2] Tatler et al.[15] suggest that at ten years 82% of patients on long-term hemodialysis should be expected to have vascular calcification. After a year of hemodialysis they report the presence of calcification of 27% of patients. Most studies have agreed that the incidence of vascular calcification is not altered by hemodialysis.[1,15,43] Vascular calcifications have not been reported to be associated with ischemic vascular lesions. In our study 64% of the patients in LDG had radiologic evidence of vascular calcifications, while only one patient (9%) had such evidence in the SDG. The areas most commonly affected included the tibia (36%) and femur (36%) and somewhat less commonly the phalanges (27%) and the knees (27%). Tatler et al. have reported a high incidence (36%) of vascular calcifications in the arteries of the foot. We had only two patients in whom x-rays of the foot were performed. Both had vascular calcifications. The difference between the LDG and SDG suggests that long-term hemodialysis does not prevent vascular calcification and that with time on dialysis vascular calcification increases.

Tatler et al. found periarticular calcifications in 9% of patients after one year of hemodialysis. They project that 42% of their patients would have been expected to develop periarticular calcifications after eight years of hemodialysis. We had only one patient in the LDG with periarticular calcifications. There were none in the SDG.

As previously mentioned, the calcium/phosphorous levels in our patients were consistently below 75, which may account for the low incidence of metastatic calcification. It is possible that this may be the result of better control of the phosphate level and other parameters in this group of hemodialysis patients under our care.

Apparent differences in the levels of PTH, alkaline phosphatase, BUN, and creatinine levels were noted when the four patients who underwent subtotal parathyroidectomies were compared with the remainder of the LDG. Patients who underwent parathyroidectomy did not exhibit an increase in symptoms or radiologic abnormalities. This, of course, is not surprising. Of note was the fact that there was a gradual healing of the skull abnormalities on roentgenographic examination, with complete healing in one patient six years after parathyroidectomy (Figures 1 and 2). In another patient, healing of the subperiosteal resorption of the phalanges was observed.

In summary, evaluation of a group of patients who have undergone hemodialysis for ten years or more has revealed to us a population that

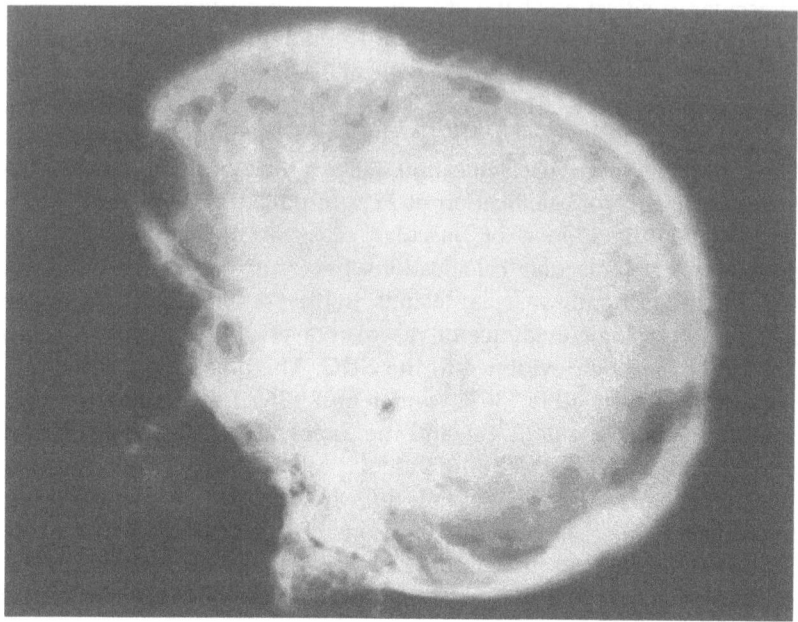

Figure 1. Preparathyroidectomy skull radiograph. Note "pepperpot" skull with thickened tables.

appears to differ from the short-term group, not so much in the type or distribution of musculoskeletal and radiographic changes, but more in the incidence of these changes. Interesting findings revealed by this study include: the universal presence of decreased bone density in the LDG group (100%); the decreased incidence of vascular calcifications and the almost complete absence of metastatic calcifications in the LDG group; the decreased range of shoulder mobility in some of our LDG patients; the hypergammaglobulinemia and decreased alpha 2 levels found in most of the LDG patients; and the high incidence of musculoskeletal complaints in almost all of our patients in the LDG group. We can further add that the excellent phosphate and PTH control under which these patients were maintained seems to have actually diminished the incidence of findings such as metastatic calcifications, which were amply and frequently reported in the literature. We agree with the previous studies cited that there appears to be little correlation between laboratory abnormalities, radiologic changes, and musculoskeletal symptoms. Musculoskeletal symptoms seemed to worsen with time, suggesting that they were either independent of or negatively correlated with the hemodialysis process.

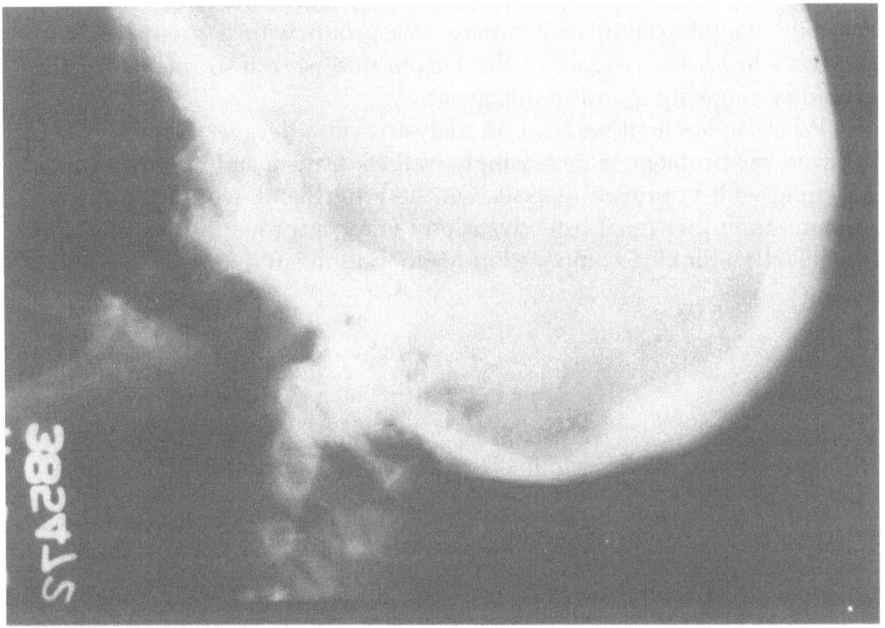

Figure 2. Skull radiographs of the same patient (Figure 1) taken six years after para-thyroidectomy. Note healing of the original bony lesions.

Parathyroidectomy, on the other hand, clearly ameliorated musculo-skeletal symptoms in the majority of those patients who underwent the procedure. This is interesting considering that bone pain has been more frequently associated with osteomalacia than with osteitis fibrosa (which is thought to be pathognomonic for hyperparathyroidism).

Few radiologic joint changes were noted. Restricted shoulder move-ment in some of the long-term dialysis patients suggests that a greater awareness of this potential complication and the more aggressive use of such therapeutic modalities as physical therapy and exercise programs may ameliorate this problem before it becomes irreparable.

No bone or joint infections were observed in any of our patients, underscoring the high-quality clinical care our patients received.

Some parameters that may deserve further investigation are the abnormal alpha 1 and gamma globulin fractions of the serum protein electrophoresis found in some of our patients—a new finding we speculatively attribute to altered immunity with resultant repeated subclinical infections and increased gammaglobulinemia.

It should be stressed that our long-term hemodialysis group represents a group of survivors, perhaps inherently less prone to complication. It would be interesting to compare this group with a group of non-survivors to ascertain some of the factors that were instrumental in the extended longevity found in this group.

What factors limit survival on dialysis over a decade? Hypertension, an awesome problem, is increasingly well controlled, and nephropathy is lessening with improved dialysis. On the other hand, we infer from the present study that renal osteodystrophy may yet prove to be a life- and rehabilitation-limiting complication for long-term survivors.

REFERENCES

1. Katz AI, Hampers CL, Merrill JP: Secondary hyperparathyroidism and renal osteo-dystrophy in chronic renal failure. *Medicine* 48:333, 1969.
2. Massry S, Bluestone R, Klinenberg J, et al.: Abnormalities of the musculoskeletal system in hemodialysis patients, in *Seminars in Arthritis and Rheumatism*, vol. 4, no. 4, May 1975, pp 321–349.
3. Hawker CD: Parathyroid hormone: Radioimmunoassay and clinical interpretation. *Ann Clin Sci* 5:383–398, 1975.
4. Singer JM, Plotz CM: The latex fixation test. 1. Application to the serological diagnosis of rheumatoid arthritis. *Am J Med* 21:888, 1956.
5. Bunnham TK, Fine G, Neblett TR: The immunofluorescent tumor imprint technique. 11. The frequency of anti-nuclear factors in connective tissue diseases and dermatoses. *Ann Int Med* 65:9, 1966.
6. Mancini G: Immunochemical quantitation of antigen by simple radialdiffusion. *Immunochemistry* 2:235–254, 1965.
7. Alvarez-Ude F, Feest TG, Ward MK, et al.: Hemodialysis bone disease: Correlation between clinical, histologic and other findings. *Kidney Int* 14:68–73, 1978.
8. Massry SG, Coburn JW, Popovtzer MM, et al.: Secondary hyperparathyroidism in chronic renal failure: The clinical spectrum in uremia during hemodialysis and after renal transplantation. *Arch Int Med* 124:431–441, 1969.
9. Simpson W, Kerr DNS, Hill AVL, et al.: Skeletal changes in patients on regular hemodialysis. *Radiology* 107:313–320, 1973.
10. Siddiqui J, Kerr DNS: Complications of renal failure and their response to dialysis. *Br Med Bull* 27:153–159, 1971.
11. O'Riordan JLH, Page J, Kerr DNA, et al.: Hyperparathyroidism in chronic renal failure and dialysis osteodystrophy. *Q J Med* 34:359–376, 1970.
12. Eastwood JB, Bordier PHJ, Wardener HE: Some biochemical histologic, radiologic and clinical features of renal osteodystrophy. *Kidney Int* 4:128–140, 1973.
13. Johnson C, Graham B, Kingsbury CF: Roentgenographic manifestations of chronic renal disease treated by periodic hemodialysis. *Am J Roentgenol Radium Ther Nucl Med* 101:915, 1967.
14. Parfitt AM: Soft tissue calcification in uremia. *Arch Intern Med* 124:544, 1969.
15. Tatler GLV, Baillard RA, Varghese Z, et al: Evolution of bone disease over 10 years in 135 patients with terminal renal failure. *Br Med J* 4:315, 1973.

16. Mathews M, Fu-hsiung S, Lindner A, et al: Septic arthritis in hemodialysis patients. *Nephron* 25:87–91, 1980.

17. Montgomerie JA, Kalmanson GM, Guze LB: Renal failure and infection. *Medicine* 47:1–32, 1968.

18. Cross AS, Steigbigel RT: Infective endocarditis and access site infections in patients on hemodialysis. *Medicine* 55:453–466, 1976.

19. Leonard A, Comty CM, Shapiro FL, et al: Osteomyelitis in hemodialysis patients. *Ann Intern Med* 78:651–658, 1973.

20. Lee YH, Kersten MD: Osteomyelitis and septic arthritis. A complication of subclavian venous catheterization. *N Engl J Med* 285:1179–1180, 1971.

21. Dobbelstein H: Immune system in uremia. *Nephron* 17:409–414, 1976.

22. Caner JEZ, Drecker JL: Recurrent (?gouty) arthritis in chronic renal failure treated with periodic hemodialysis. *Am J Med* 36:571, 1964.

23. Warren DJ, Otieno LS: Carpal tunnel syndrome in patients on intermittent hemodialysis. *Postgrad Med J* 51:450–452, 1975.

24. Vijay JK, Cestero RVM, Baum J: Carpal tunnel syndrome in patients undergoing maintenance hemodialysis. *JAMA* 242:(26)2868–2869, 1979.

25. deBroe, MD, Bosteels V, Wieme RJ: Increased intestinal alkaline phosphatase in serum of patients on maintenance hemodialysis. *Lancet* 1:753, 1974.

26. Avioli L, Teitelbaum SC: Renal osteodystrophy, in Early LE, Gottschalk CW (eds.): *Strauss and Welt's Disease of the Kidney*, vol. 1. Boston, Little, Brown and Co, 1979, pp 307–370.

27. Ritz E, Franz HE, Jahns E: The course of secondary hyperthryoidism during chronic hemodialysis. *Trans Am Soc Artif Intern Organs* 14:385, 1962.

28. Nolph ND, Husted FC, Sharp, GC, et al: Antibodies to nuclear antigens in patients undergoing long-term hemodialysis. *Am J Med* 60:673–676, 1976.

29. Dasgupta MK, Higgins MR, Dossetor JB: Antibodies to DNA in patients undergoing long-term hemodialysis. *Clin Neph* 14(6):288–293, 1980.

30. Craddock PR, Fehr, J, Brigham KL, et al: Complement and leukocyte-mediated pulmonary dysfunction in hemodialysis. *N Engl J Med* 296(14):769–774, 1977.

31. Follis RH, Jackson DA: Renal osteodystrophy and osteitis fibrosa in adults. *Bull Johns Hopkins Hosp* 72:232–241, 1943.

32. Cohen MEL, Cohen GF, Ahad V, et al: Renal osteodystrophy in patients on hemodialysis: A radiological study. *Clin Radio* 21:124, 1970.

33. Ellis HA, Peart KM: Renal osteodystrophy with particular reference to the effect of chronic intermittent hemodialysis. *Nephron* 18:402, 1971.

34. Bishop MC, Woods GC, Oliver DO, et al: Effects of hemodialysis on bone in chronic renal failure. *Br Med J* 3:664–667, 1972.

35. Parfitt AM, Massry, S, Winfield AC: Osteopenia and fractures occurring during maintenance hemodialysis. *Clin Orthoped Related Res.* 87:287–302, 1972.

36. Massry SG, Coburn J, Popvtzer MM, et al: Secondary hyperparathyroidism in chronic renal failure: The clinical spectrum in uremia during hemodialysis and after transplantation. *Arch Intern Med* 124:431, 1969.

37. Schwartz EE, Lantieri R, Teplick JG: Erosion of the inferior aspect of the clavicle in secondary hyperparathyroidism. *Am J Roentgenol* 129:292–295, 1977.

38. Grennfield GB: Roentgien appearance of bone and soft tissue changes in chronic renal disease. *Am J Roentgenol.* 116:749–757, 1972.

39. Steinbach HL, Gordon GS, Eisenberg E, et al: Primary hyperparathyroidism: A correlation of roentgen, clinical and pathologic features. *Am J Roentgenol* 86:329–343, 1961.

40. Pugh DG: Subperiosteal resorption of bone. A roentgenologic manifestation of primary hyperparathyroidism and renal osteodystrophy. *Am J Roentgenol* 66:577–586, 1951.
41. Resnick D, Niwayama G: Subchondral resorption of bone in renal osteodystrophy. *Radiology* 118:315–321, 1976.
42. Meema HE, Oreopoulos G, Rabinovich S, et al: Periosteal new bone formation (periosteal neostosis) in renal osteodystrophy. *Radiology* 110:513, 1974.
43. Johnson WJ, Goldsmith RS, Beabout JW, et al: Prevention and reversal of progressive hyperparathyroidism in patients treated by hemodialysis. *Am J Med* 56:827, 1974.

21

NIH, Kidney Research, and the Patient with Renal Disease

NANCY B. CUMMINGS AND GLADYS H. HIRSCHMAN

The first venture of the Federal government into the support of cata-strophic illness for almost all Americans afflicted with a disease was made on October 30, 1972, when PL 92-603, Section 299(I), known tersely as the End Stage Renal Disease (ESRD) Amendment, was enacted. In 33 lines of succinctly worded public law, it was stated that "every individual who . . . is medically determined to have chronic renal disease and who requires hemodialysis or renal transplantation for such disease, shall be deemed to be disabled for the purposes of coverage under parts A and B of Medicare subject to the deductible, premium, and copayment provisions of title XVIII."[1]

The unpredicted rapid escalation of the costs of this program to over a billion dollars by 1980, as well as the significant human suffering, contrast sharply with the limited level investment in research into means to prevent disorders resulting in end-stage renal disease. These costs are many orders of magnitude greater than the unusually modest investment in renal research. Further, the funding of research into the complications and treatment of end-stage renal disease is of modest proportions also. The ability to arrest or to prevent those diseases resulting in ESRD eventually will be developed by an increase in the understanding of basic mech-anisms underlying these diseases achieved through scientific research. This ability will provide the means to diminish the human and economic costs.

In the late 1960s the concerns of patients' families and of physicians treating patients with chronic renal failure primarily focused upon means

NANCY B. CUMMINGS AND GLADYS H. HIRSCHMAN • National Institute of Arthritis, Diabetes, and Digestive and Kidney Diseases, National Institutes of Health, Bethesda, Maryland.

to provide funds for the available costly treatment modalities: dialysis or transplantation. Recently patients and their relatives have begun to consider that research to avert the final outcome must be emphasized also, even if it is for a future generation of patients. Shortly after the 1980 election, Francis G. Armstrong of Midland Park, New Jersey, a home dialysis patient who had rejected a kidney transplant, wrote to President Elect Reagan: "I beg you to funnel ample funds into research to find a cure for future patients. Whether the answer lies in surgery or medicine, I know not which but there is an answer. This answer will relieve the Federal Government from substantial funding and President Elect Reagan, you will have helped answer many people's prayers." Mr. Armstrong's humanitarian concern for future patients is one that nephrologists would echo. The high costs of caring for these patients is indicated in the Second Annual ESRD Report submitted to the Congress in FY 1980.[2] In 1979 there were 45,565 patients on hemodialysis, up 25% from 1978. There were 4,271 transplants performed in 1979, up 8.2% from 1978; and 4,697 renal transplants performed in 1980.

METHODS

Data about the ESRD population were derived from six sources:

1. For the period through 1976 the ESRD data were based upon the National Dialysis Registry operated by the Research Triangle Institute, Research Triangle Park, North Carolina, under an NIH contract.[3]
2. Beginning in 1977 the data source was the ESRD Medical Information System (MIS), Medicare Program, Social Security Administration.[4]
3. The Second Annual Report to Congress (FY 1980) submitted by the Office of Special Program, Health Care Financing Administration (HCFA) [as mandated by Section 1881 (g) of the Social Security Act] provided the data for 1978–79.[2]
4. The 1980 data were derived from the quarterly statistical report of the ESRD Section, Office of Special Programs, prepared in February 1981[5] with the dialysis population reported as of June 1980 and was supplemented by a special communication from the same office and included information entered up to March 1981.
5. The Naval Medical Data Services Center provided information available about ESRD patients treated in Navy facilities. (Personal communication from Dr. Louis P. Hellman.)
6. The Biometrics Division supplied the data on ESRD patients treated at Air Force facilities. (Personal communication from Colonel Frank J. Perry.)

7. The Renal and Metabolic Diseases Medical Service gave the data relevant to ESRD patients treated by the Veterans Administration. (Personal communication from Dr. Neil S. Otchin.) Data about ESRD patients treated by the Army were not available at this writing.

The analysis of kidney and urinary tract research supported by the National Institutes of Health (NIH) was made utilizing data obtained through the Computer Retrieval of Information on Scientific Projects System (CRISP) operated by the Statistics and Analysis Branch, Division of Research Grants, NIH. All research supported by NIH should be entered in the CRISP system. However, occasional deficiencies are noted, such as failure to find a current grant in the printout or presence of a project no longer funded in the listing. Eighteen broad categories, with related headings, which are called CRISP "indexing terms" or "main indicators," were used to query the system.

These categories were: (1) kidney function, renal medulla, renal tubules, renal cortex, glomerulus, juxtaglomerular apparatus, basement membrane, kidney cells, micropuncture, renal tubular transport, body fluid and electrolyte balance, renal circulation (renal arteries, veins, circulatory disorders); (2) congenital abnormalities; (3) kidney disorders (including hydronephrosis, hyperplasia, necrosis, etc.); (4) metabolic disorders (inborn); (5) polycystic kidney and medullary cystic disease; (6) kidney-related connective tissue disorders; (7) pregnancy toxemias; (8) nephrotic syndrome; (9) glomerulonephritis, glomerulopathies; (10) nephrotoxins; (11) renal hypertension; (12) chronic renal failure (including uremic syndrome, nephrosclerosis, diabetic nephropathy, vitamin D and mineral metabolism, secondary hyperparathyroidism, endocrine derangements, carbohydrate, lipid, protein metabolism, etc.); (13) artificial kidney, hemodialysis, peritoneal dialysis; (14) kidney transplant; (15) lower urinary tract physiology and disorders (ureter, urethra, bladder, sphincters, prostate, etc.); (16) surgery and prosthesis; (17) urolithiasis; (18) lower urinary tract infection and pyelonephritis.

ESRD PATIENTS

The total Medicare outlay in 1979 was about $29 billion for 26.5 million persons enrolled in the program. According to Susan Landicine, Medicare Health Budget Officer, in a personal communication, the ESRD program expenditure took $1.2 billion or 4.13% (Figure 1) of the total Medicare expenditure for 49,844 persons or 0.19% of persons treated through Medicare funds.[9] These reflect per capita expenditures by the

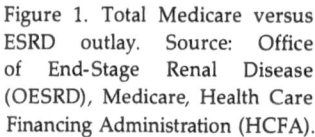
Figure 1. Total Medicare versus ESRD outlay. Source: Office of End-Stage Renal Disease (OESRD), Medicare, Health Care Financing Administration (HCFA).

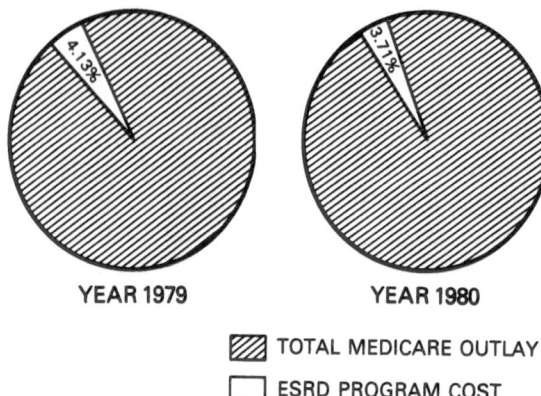

YEAR 1979   **YEAR 1980**

▨ TOTAL MEDICARE OUTLAY

☐ ESRD PROGRAM COST

entire Medicare Program of $1,094 per person, while the ESRD program's per capita figure is $24,075.

In 1980 Medicare outlays rose to $35 billion for 27 million persons, while the ESRD portion rose to $1.3 billion for 53,629 persons, a drop to 3.71% of total Medicare costs. This $1.3 billion (Table I) expended in 1980 represents a figure that has increased annually from $286 million in 1974 through $792 million in 1978 and $984 million in 1979. The projections of costs through 1985 shown in Figure 2 indicate that benefits paid out annually by 1985 will be about $2.68 billion for about 84,000 patients as noted in Figure 3. The Health Care Financing Administration has projected further that the ESRD population will grow to 90,000 by 1995, as Rettig[6] has stated, though "actual numbers have steadily exceeded previous estimates and no one is certain where the equilibrium level is."

Data about the characteristics of the patient population are skimpy. The ESRD MIS never functioned in a fashion to provide clear-cut medical data about etiology of the underlying disease processes. Utilizing other sources such as the California Regional Medical Program's system,[7] the European Dialysis and Transplant Association's Registry,[8] and the Canadian Registry (described in a personal communication from Dr. R. D. Guttman and now in danger of being phased out), one can develop a broad impression of causes of ESRD, but precision is lacking. Cystic diseases are responsible for 9–11% of patients on the ESRD rolls; glomerulonephritis for one third to two thirds of patients; hypertension (as a primary cause) about 20%; diabetic nephropathy about 11%; toxic nephropathies, especially analgesic abuse nephropathy, from 3% to 30%; congenital abnormalities, about 10%; and infections, 5% to 10%. Better data would be useful in planning approaches to research. Rettig, in his study of the ESRD program, analyzes the MIS experience and noted that "at no time in the design, development, or operation of the system was sustained, informed policy direction given to the system" and that the

Table I. Annual Cost of Dialysis and Transplant Services United States 1978–1980

	1978			1979			1980		
	Patients on dialysis (nos.)	Transplants performed[a]	Cost in million $	Patients on dialysis (nos.)	Transplants performed[a]	Cost in million $	Patients on dialysis (nos.)	Transplants performed[a]	Cost in million $
TOTAL									
Medicare patients	36,463	3,949	$951	45,565	4,279	$1,182	49,029	4,697	$1,308
Cost to Medicare program			$792			$985			$1,090
Costs to Medicare beneficiary for treatment			$158			$196			$218
Veteran patients	4,222 Number of dialyses	238	$99	4,042 Number of dialyses	246	$108	3,891 Number of dialyses	311	$113
Military patients									
Air Force				166	22		193	14	
Navy	6,071			5,144			4,024		
Army									

[a] Transplants performed: Figure represents total reported to the NIAID and the Medical Information System, Medicare. Source: Office of End-Stage Renal Diseases (OESRD), Medicare, Health Care Financing Administration (HCFA); Veterans Administration, Renal and Metabolic Diseases Medical Service, and Naval Medical Data Services Center.

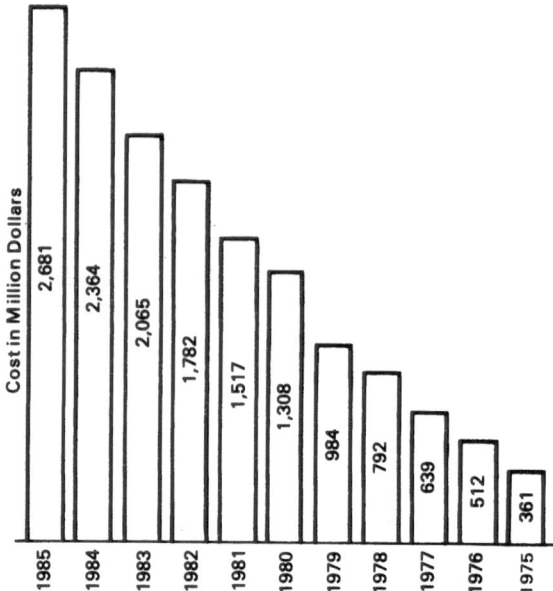

Figure 2. Annual projected costs of medical services, Medicare End-Stage Renal Disease Program, United States, 1975–1985. (Projections are based only on those inpatient and outpatient services covered by Medicare as of March, 1981.) Source: OESRD, Medicare, and HCFA.

"ESRD MIS was never significant to higher level officials."[6] NIH was hopeful that good information might be obtained once the system became functional because it would provide a valuable epidemiologic resource.

The ESRD MIS does provide information about patients that includes type of treatment, number of hospitalizations, and mortality. Figure 4 shows the distribution of center and home dialysis treatment for the years 1978, 1979, and 1980. There has been an extremely modest increase in the percent of patients on home dialysis since the enactment of PL 95-292,[9] which included incentives for home dialysis and removed some of the disincentives. The number of transplants performed has remained almost constant for the three years 1977–79; in 1980 there was a modest increase in numbers. The percentage of cadaver transplants has remained stable at about 70.

RESEARCH

It is helpful to view the distribution of research funding in kidney and urinary tract disease against a background of that of national health research and development (R&D). If one relates health research and

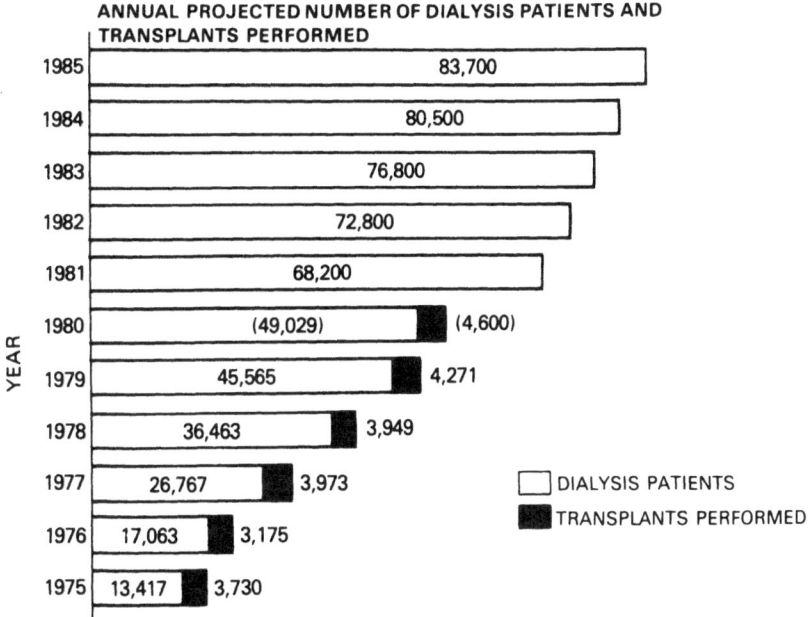

Figure 3. Medicare dialysis and transplant patients, United States, 1975–1985. (Projections are based only on those inpatient and outpatient sources covered by Medicare as of March, 1981.) Source: OESRD, Medicare, HCFA.

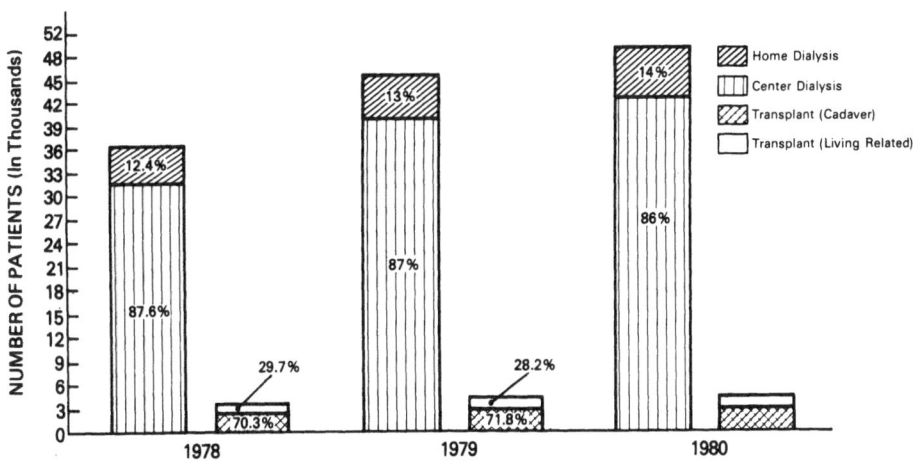

Figure 4. Dialysis and transplant patient population, 1978–1980. Source: OESRD, Medicare, HCFA.

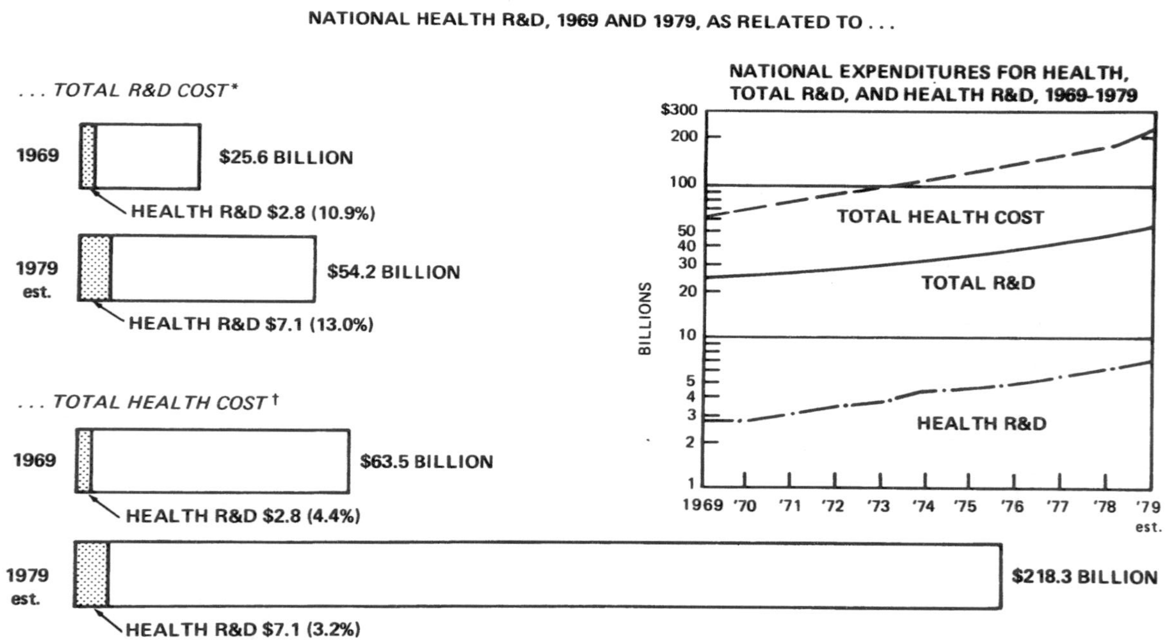

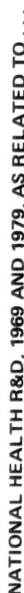

Figure 5. National health R&D, 1979 and 1979. *Source: NSF and NIH. †Source: HCFA, with adjustments of R&D (and therefore of totals) to conform to NIH data.

development costs to total R&D costs (Figure 5), one notes from 1969 to 1979 more than a doubling of total R&D with the percentage devoted to health increasing from 10.9% to 13.0%. However, as a percentage of total health costs, the amount expended for R&D has declined from 4.4% to 3.2%. The dollars for research have more than doubled against a backdrop of total health costs increasing more than threefold. In Figure 6 one notes the national support for health R&D by source. It is noteworthy that NIH has contributed not only the largest amount of any federal agency, but also the largest percentage of any grouping. Since 1974 the NIH share has remained around the 40% mark, while the absolute health R&D figures have climbed consistently in current dollars and very slightly in constant (1969) dollars. It is of interest to compare the federal funding of ESRD treatment with the expenditures in kidney and urinary tract research, and with research related specifically to chronic renal disease and renal transplantation (Figure 7). If one makes this calculation, one sees that all kidney and urinary tract research, exclusive of cancer, supported by NIH totaled just over $57 million in 1979 and was 4.8% of the expenditures for ESRD in 1979.

There is no precise comparable figure for the costs to treat all kidney and urinary tract disease (KUTD). These costs would encompass treatment of such common disorders as cystitis, which is responsible for about 25% of absenteeism among working women; benign prostatic hypertrophy, which affects about 50% of men by age 50 and 80% percent by age 80, of whom about 10% will require surgical treatment; urolithiasis, which has a hospitalization incidence among men in mid-years ranging from 120 to 130 per 100,000 hospitalizations. The expenditures for chronic renal failure and for renal transplantation research, which had a price tag of just over $13 million for 1979, were barely over 1% of the ESRD expenditures for that year.

The distribution of the $57 million of research funding into kidney and urinary tract studies (excluding cancer) at NIH is portrayed in the pie chart (Figure 8) and Table II. This shows that the grouping of kidney structure and function, which includes most of the research not related to a specific disease and primarily laboratory research, utilizes about 38% of the funds. This represents an increase in both percentage of research efforts and dollars since a similar analysis undertaken in 1976.[10] Renal disorders, which would include most of the causes of ESRD, uses about 29% of kidney–urinary tract disease research dollars, a figure representing an increase in dollars although a decrease in percent over those of 1976. The dollar figures in renal failure and in urinary tract infections research have remained almost constant from 1976 to 1979, with a drop in percentage. The investment in research, both in urolithiasis and urinary

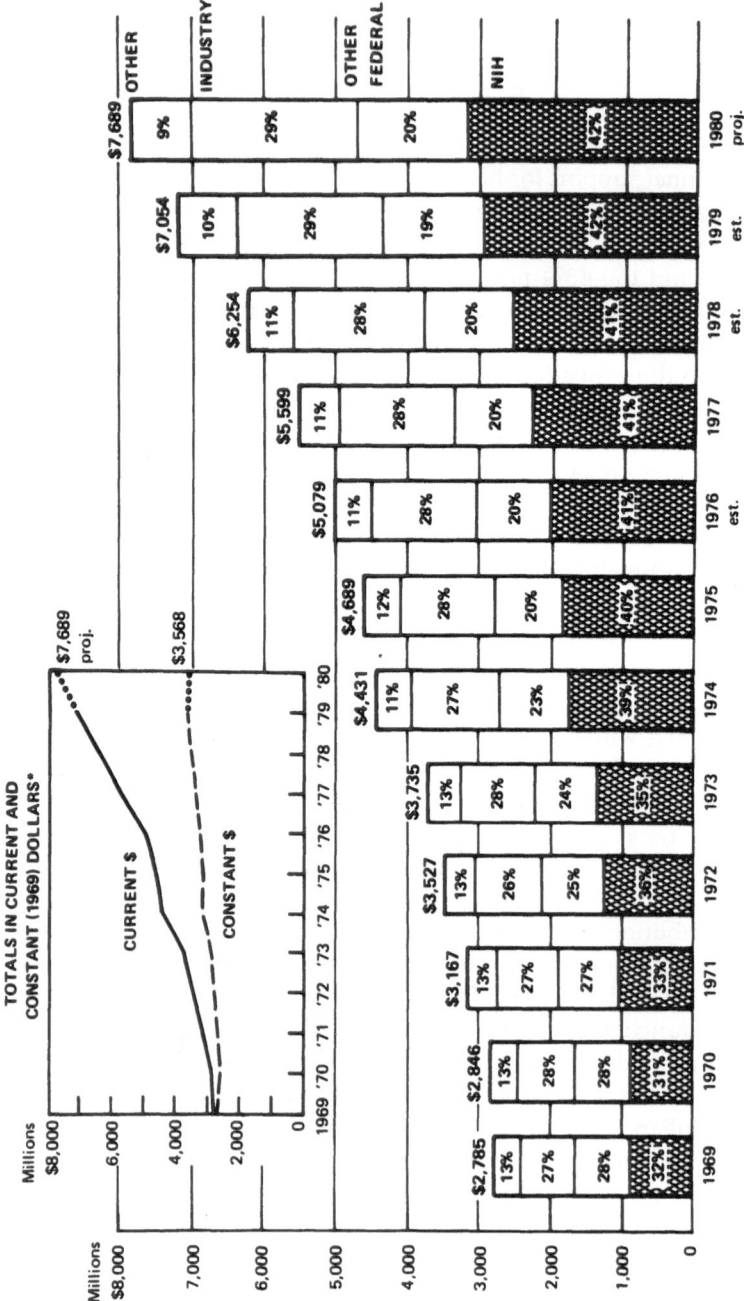

Figure 6. National support for health R&D by source, 1969–1980. (Dollars are in millions.)

*Constant dollars based on biomedical R&D price index, 1969–1979. For 1980, based on percentage increase in estimated GNP implicit price deflator. Projected biomedical R&D price index, 215.5.

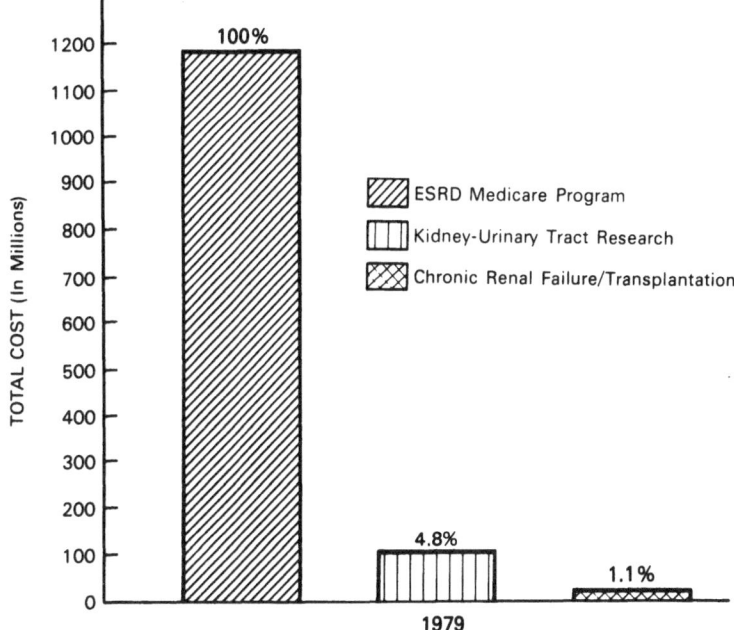

Figure 7. Comparison of funding of ESRD program and federal support of chronic renal failure/transplantation and kidney–urinary tract research (FY 1979). Source: OESRD, Medicare, HCFA, and Computer Retrieval of Information on Scientific Projects (CRISP), Division of Research Grants (DRG), National Institutes of Health (NIH).

tract research, has doubled and the percentages have increased from 3.3% to 5% and 4.3% to 8%, respectively.

The relative distribution of research funding in the different categories among the different NIH institutes is indicated in Figure 9. Most KUTD research, exclusive of cancer, is in the National Institute of Arthritis, Diabetes, Digestive and Kidney Diseases (NIADDKD) and the National Heart, Lung and Blood Institute (NHLBI). The Division of Research Resources (DRR) contribution represents clinical research conducted in the General Clinical Research Centers (GCRC).

The contrast of estimated cost of a few of the diseases resulting in CRF as a rough percentage of the Medicare costs and the research grant support is striking. Although accurate information about the incidence of the diseases resulting in chronic renal failure is not available for the United States, assumptions can be made for purposes of comparing research dollars and ESRD costs (Figure 10). The almost imperceptible portion at the bottom of the bars and the percentage below each bar are that

Table II. Kidney and Urinary Tract Disease Research Funded by NIH—FY '79[a]

Category	Dollar amount	Percent of total ($)	No. of projects	Percent of total (no.)
Kidney structure and function	26,551,169	38.21	378	30.00
Renal disorders	22,475,765	29.34	444	35.23
Chronic renal failure and transplantation	12,323,639	17.73	240	19.04
Urinary tract	5,570,155	8.01	82	6.50
Urinary tract infection	1,188,215	1.71	22	1.74
Urolithiasis	4,638,301	4.96	94	7.46

[a] Source: Computer Retrieval of Information on Scientific Projects (CRISP), Statistics and Analysis Branch, Division of Research Grants (DRG), NIH.

percentage for research as measured against the portion of ESRD costs assignable to each disease entity.

The directions of research are determined primarily by investigators, motivated by opportunities for discovery, available methodologies, expertise, and interest, and often tempered by need in a clinical area. The NIH has many different mechanisms for encouraging research into new areas, such as conferences, workshops, program announcements (PAs), Requests

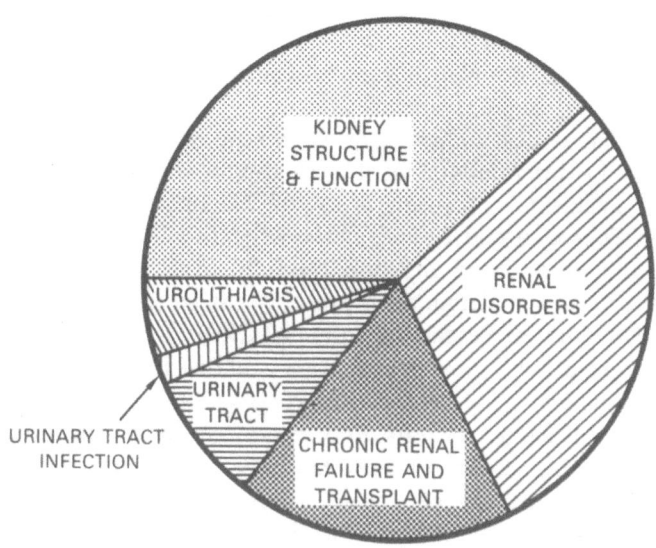

Figure 8. Kidney and urinary tract diseases research funded by NIH, FY 1979. Source: CRISP, DRG, NIH.

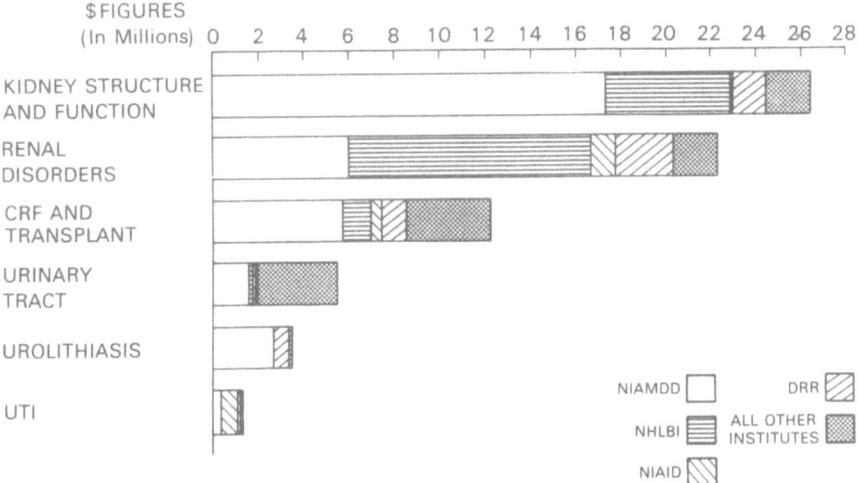

Figure 9. Kidney and urinary tract diseases research funded by NIH, FY 1979 (by institute). Source: CRISP, DRG, NIH.

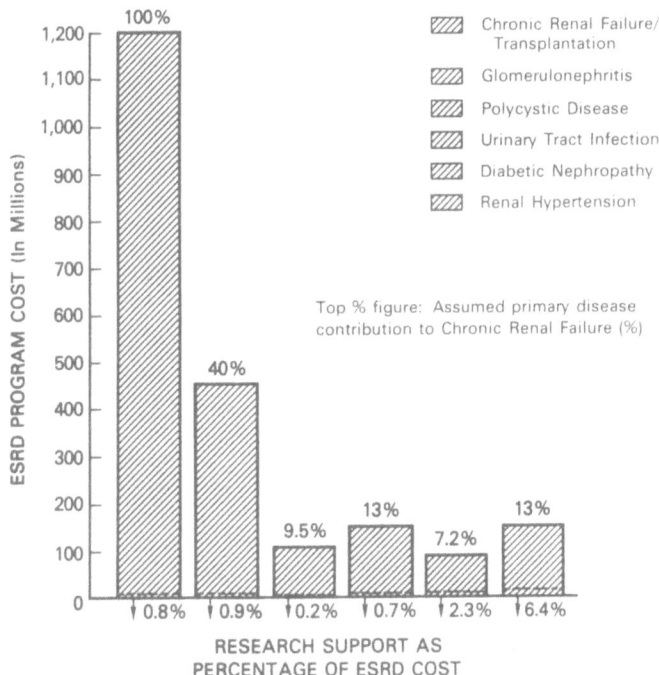

Figure 10. Total ESRD cost, percent contribution of primary disease to chronic renal failure, and research support as percentage of ESRD cost.

for Applications (RFA), and Requests for Proposals (RFP). All of these are dependent upon potential avenues of study, the state of the art, training, and methodology. They can be tempered by concerns expressed by interest groups, pattern of disease, and momentum of a given area.

The economic costs of treatment of chronic renal failure are enormous. The NIH mandate to conduct research to improve the nation's health must be kept in the forefront of our thinking in the encouragement of investigations that will aid in elucidations of basic mechanisms responsible for CRF. The ultimate goal must be to minimize the human costs of ESRD by improvements in the treatment of complications of CRF and by prevention or arrest of the responsible diseases.

REFERENCES

1. Social Security Act Amendments of 1972, Public Law 92-603, 92nd Congress, H.R. 1, Oct 28, 1972, pp 135–136.
2. End-Stage Renal Disease, Second Annual Report to the Congress, FY 1980, Department of Health and Human Services, Health Care Financing Administration, Office of Special Programs.
3. Bryan FA Jr; The National Dialysis Registry: Development of a medical registry of patients on chronic dialysis. *Final Report*, Center for Health Studies, Research Triangle Institute, Research Triangle Park, NC, Aug 1976.
4. ESRD Medical Information System, Office of End Stage Renal Disease, Health Care Financing Administration, Baltimore, Md.
5. *Quarterly Statistical Summary*. End-Stage Renal Disease Program, Division of Information Systems and Beneficiary Entitlement, Health Care Financing Administration, Sep 30, 1980.
6. Rettig RS: Implementing the end-stage renal disease program of Medicare. *R-2505HFCA/HEW*, RAND Corp, Sept 1980.
7. Mann, MM, Strauss DP: A medical and demographic description of 2395 chronic hemodialysis patients in California. California Kidney Disease Information System, June 1975.
8. Robinson BHB (ed): *Proceedings of the European Dialysis and Transplant Association*, vol 15. Pitman Medical, 1978, pp 3–114.
9. Social Security Act Amendments of 1978, Public Lay 95-292, 15th Congress, H.R. 8423, June 13, 1978.
10. Research needs in nephrology and urology, Appendix II, in *Data Book: Research in Kidney and Urinary Tract Disease*. US Dept of Health Education, and Welfare, National Institutes of Health, DHEW Publications No. (NIH) 78-1481, 1976, pp 92–131.

22

Patients on Hemodialysis
for Over Ten Years

ALVIN I. GOODMAN, STEPHEN A. WESELEY,
AND KARIM B. SOLANGI

The first patient to commence chronic hemodialysis at the Westchester County Medical Center began home hemodialysis training in November 1967. The Westchester County Medical Center, at that time known as Grasslands Hospital, was one of 12 demonstration projects supported by the Chronic Kidney Disease Program of the United States Public Health Service. For the remainder of 1967, and in 1968, 1969, and 1970, the program was principally a home training program and no patients were chosen other than those who were going on to home hemodialysis training. Sometime during the first half of 1971 a modest in-center hemodialysis program was also begun. From those early years of our chronic hemodialysis program there remain alive today 17 patients, most of them from the early home program and several from the early in-center program.

It is of interest to review the selection criteria from those early years. They included that patients to be selected must be beyond puberty and no more than 60 years of age. Creatinine clearance must be below 6 ml/min, and there should be no irreversible changes of uremia and no evidence of other diseases that carried a poor prognosis. There should, as well, be no evidence of psychosis and there must be an adult in the home to undergo training with the patient. Since 1973, we have not utilized a rigid set of criteria, such as this one.

ALVIN I. GOODMAN • Division of Nephrology, Department of Medicine, New York Medical College; and Nephrology-Renal Unit, Westchester County Medical Center, Valhalla, New York. STEPHEN A. WESELEY AND KARIM B. SOLANGI • Division of Nephrology, Department of Medicine, New York Medical College, Valhalla, New York.

Of the 17 patients who have survived on chronic hemodialysis for over ten years, 15 are still alive, two having died at about the ten-year period. Of the 15 patients who have survived over ten years, there is still one from our original group. Two patients started in 1967; therefore, our longest patient still on hemodialysis is now 14 years and four months on the program. He is a home patient who began his training program at the age of 32. The average age of the patient commencing home training was 37 years. There were ten males and seven females. Twelve patients were white, four were black and one was oriental. It is of some interest that 16 transplants were attempted by eight patients, including four by one patient. These transplants lasted for several days to several weeks. In effect, they imparted little in the way of the longevity under discussion and contributed a certain amount of morbidity. Interestingly enough, because the transplants were of such ephemeral duration, one gains the impression that there is a virtual inverse relationship between duration of transplant and longevity, certainly in the early years of end-stage renal disease care. This, of course, may well be due to the fact that in the years under discussion, heavy use of immune suppression medication and steroids was the rule, even in the face of certain rejection. The morbidity and mortality that ensued from what we now regard as ill-advised medical tactics in the face of rejection had an awesome significant toll in terms of ultimate prognosis within that group of patients. The paradox that followed is quite clear in this retrospective view of those early years in that this group of 17 patients, 8 of whom underwent 16 transplants, were spared the more injurious effects of heroic efforts at combating rejection since virtually every one of the transplants lasted but a few days. It is also probable that few of us, laboring in those vineyards in those days, could come up with a comparable list of survivors who underwent cadaver transplantation in the period 1967 through 1971 and who had durable and long-lasting renal function and are still alive and well today. The awesome effects of high-dose steroids and immunosuppression are now more clearly understood, and respected and feared. The two deaths that did occur among the 17 patients were of now easily recognizable causes, one at 157 months, or just over 13 years, from severe infection, and one just at ten years from cardiovascular causes. These data are illustrated in Table I.

In Table II some of the predialysis characteristics of these 17 patients are summarized. Three of the patients, two black and one oriental, had malignant hypertension prior to dialysis. Ten of the other patients had a milder form of hypertension when starting on hemodialysis. Nine patients fulfilled electrocardiographic criteria for the diagnosis of left ventricular hypertrophy and eight patients had an enlarged heart as seen on a chest x-ray. It is indeed important to note that hypertension, left ventricular

Table I. Patients on Chronic Hemodialysis Over Ten Years

	Year started	Age	Sex	Race	Death	Tx[a]
1.	1967	32	M	O		2
2.	1968	48	M	C		
3.	1968	29	M	C	157 mo	4
4.	1969	32	M	C		
5.	1969	19	F	C		2
6.	1969	49	F	C		
7.	1969	36	M	C		
8.	1970	25	F	C		2
9.	1970	57	M	C		
10.	1971	31	F	C		2
11.	1971	40	F	C		
12.	1971	33	M	C		1
13.	1971	44	M	B		
14.	1971	40	F	B	120 mo	1
15.	1971	19	M	C		
16.	1971	52	F	B		
17.	1971	44	M	B		2
		37 avg.	M 10 F 7	B 4 C 12 O 1	2	16/8 patients

[a] Number of transplants.

hypertrophy, and an enlarged heart (one or more of these characteristics seen in half or more of the patients) do not place severe restrictions on ultimate prognosis and longevity. The chronic hemodialysis population that lives for long periods of time can be shown to be a paradigm of the now-accepted fact that vigorous treatment of hypertension alters significantly the poor prognosis otherwise conferred by that element of disease. As will be seen in further results, good blood pressure control was an essential characteristic in virtually all of these patients. Nerve conduction, hematocrits, and bone disease did not seem to affect ultimate prognosis in any characteristic fashion. Patients who started with low hematocrits, and even remained with low hematocrits, did not necessarily have a different course from patients with high hematocrits. Most nerve conduction studies were normal predialysis and the three that were abnormal were only mildly so. Even severe bone disease, while imposing a fair degree of morbidity and requiring medical intervention, did not necessarily preclude a good prognosis.

One significant characteristic was that only one patient in this group had angina as a manifestation of coronary artery disease. He was among

Table II. Predialysis Characteristics (before Starting on Dialysis Program)[a]

	BP[a]	EKG	Chest x-ray	NC[b]	Hematocrit (percent)	Bone disease	CAD[c]
1.	M	LVH	EH	N	17	—	—
2.	B	LVH	EH	↓	21	+	ANG
3.	B	LVH	N	N	17	—	—
4.	N	N	N	N	18	++++	—
5.	B	LVH	N	N	19	—	—
6.	B	LVH	EH	N	24	+	—
7.	B	N	EH	N	20	—	—
8.	N	N	N	↓	21	—	—
9.	B	LVH	EH	↓	27	—	—
10.	B	N	N	N	31	—	—
11.	B	N	N	N	26	—	—
12.	B	N	N	N	33	—	—
13.	B	LVH	EH	N	23	—	—
14.	M	LVH	EH	N	30	—	—
15.	N	N	N	N	20	—	—
16.	N	N	N	N	29	+	—
17.	M+B	LVH	EH	N	18	—	—

[a] BP: blood pressure: (M: malignant; B: benign).
[a] NC: nerve conduction (N: normal; ↓: decrease)
[c] CAD: coronary artery disease; ANG: angina.

our earliest patients and was one of our oldest. In fact, this patient was peritoneally dialyzed for several months before being placed on hemodialysis in order to see if, after removal of significant quantities of fluid and weight, the angina would markedly improve. The angina did improve after two months of peritoneal dialysis and, in fact, disappeared prior to the commencement of hemodialysis. It is interesting to note that even in 1967, when our program started, it was presumed that the single most important handicap or prognostic element for longevity was coronary artery disease.

In order to try to define what elements might be involved in long-term survival in patients on chronic hemodialysis, four particular characteristics were reviewed. Since the same physicians have taken care of these 17 patients over the 14 years, an attempt to evaluate these characteristics in a semiquantitative fashion was performed. In Figure 1 the criteria for grading the patients' compliance with dietary instructions and with dialysis instructions are stated. Dietary instructions obviously refer to those limitations placed on the ingestion of salt and potassium at the first level and quantity of protein at the next. Dialysis instructions included such

Diet instructions   5 Does not follow any instructions
                                      4 Infrequently follows instructions
                                      3 Follows instructions $<=1/2$ time
                                      2 Follows instructions most of the time
                                      1 Follows instructions all of the time

Dialysis instructions   5 Ignores all instructions
                                      4 Ignores most instructions
                                      3 Ignores $=>50\%$ instructions
                                      2 Follows instructions most of the time
                                      1 Follows instructions all the time

Figure 1. Compliance scales. Diet and dialysis instructions.

elements as cooperation with the prescription for the number of hours of dialysis, the transmembrane pressure utilized in order to optimize ultrafiltration, and other sundry instructions that were thought to produce good dialysis. Figure 2 contains those criteria used for evaluating blood pressure control and chemical control. The means of three predialysis blood pressures in the same year were reviewed over the life span of the patient on hemodialysis and, most particularly, during the last five years of hemodialysis with 140/90 being considered normal.

Chemical control was judged by our attempt to keep predialysis serum creatinine on an average at below 14 mg%.

Table III, on instant scanning, indicates well that following dialysis therapy instructions, blood pressure control, and chemistries, in that order, were fairly high in the patient compliance scales. Compliance with dietary instructions appeared to be far less important a prognostic measure. While compliance was usually not terrible, it was average for most of the patients. Indeed, our patients were undoubtedly no different than the general population in terms of adhering to a particular diet in a chronic fashion. It is to be noted that somewhat fewer than half of the patients are on center dialysis and, in fact, the last three patient survivors who were accepted onto the program in 1971 have always been center patients. One cannot evaluate the meaning of home versus center since the first three to four years of our program were essentially a home training program.

Of great importance to look at (and a case that should make all of us think before uttering any bold statements concerning the information being presented here) is patient no. 17, who came to the program at age 44. He is a black male. He has scored at the lowest level of compliance or the highest level on the scales in terms of cooperation with all instructions and with blood pressure control. He has had two transplants attempted,

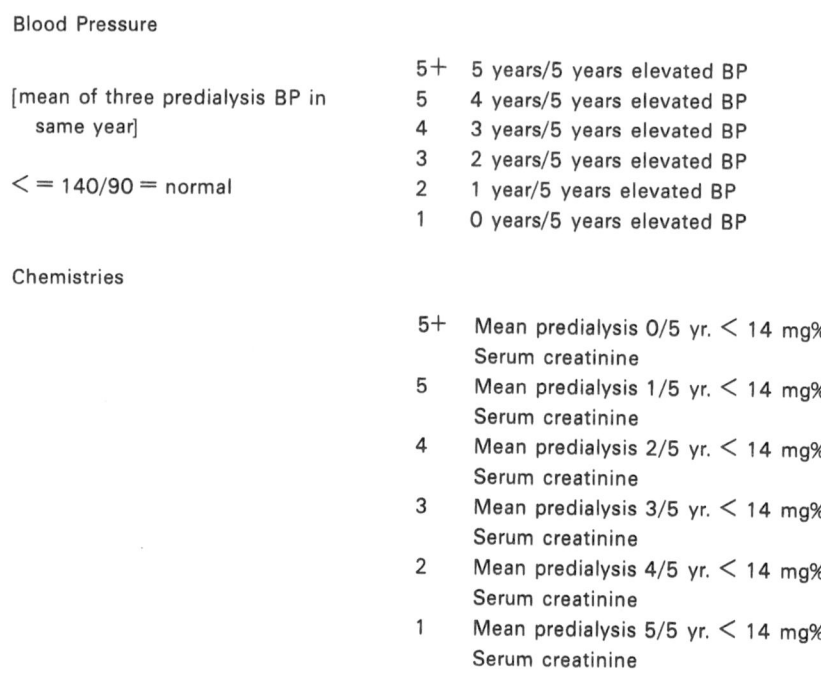

Blood Pressure

	5+	5 years/5 years elevated BP
[mean of three predialysis BP in	5	4 years/5 years elevated BP
same year]	4	3 years/5 years elevated BP
	3	2 years/5 years elevated BP
< = 140/90 = normal	2	1 year/5 years elevated BP
	1	0 years/5 years elevated BP

Chemistries

	5+	Mean predialysis 0/5 yr. < 14 mg% Serum creatinine
	5	Mean predialysis 1/5 yr. < 14 mg% Serum creatinine
	4	Mean predialysis 2/5 yr. < 14 mg% Serum creatinine
	3	Mean predialysis 3/5 yr. < 14 mg% Serum creatinine
	2	Mean predialysis 4/5 yr. < 14 mg% Serum creatinine
	1	Mean predialysis 5/5 yr. < 14 mg% Serum creatinine

Figure 2. Compliance scales. Blood pressure control and chemistries.

which failed. He has dialyzed for no more than about ten hours a week for many years, coming only twice a week at maximum for treatments. His blood pressures are seemingly never close to the normal range and his chemistries vary all over the scale. The patient is quite functional and survives very well and has indeed even been removed from the Medicaid roles because it was discovered that he was surreptitiously earning too much money in gainful employment. We would offer this case up for diligent study to any group or board that wishes to create strict criteria for the selection of patients for chronic end-stage renal disease treatment based on retrospective reviews such as we are conducting.

During this same period of 1968–71, 32 other patients for whom there are good follow-up data, and who were started on dialysis at home or at the center, were reviewed and analyzed in an attempt to compare them with the 17 survivors (Figure 3). There were six females and 26 males. We feel quite sure that these 26 males indeed reflect the greater number of males in general being selected for chronic hemodialysis programs during that period of time. The fact that there were seven females surviving in the group of 17 survivors for over ten years may indeed indicate a mild

Table III. Patient Compliance

	Diet	Dialysis Rx	BP	Chemistry	Home/Center
1.	3	1	2	3	H
2.	1	1	1	1	H
3.[a]	5	3	1	1	H
4.	2	1	2	1	H
5.	3	1	1	1	H
6.	3	1	1	1	H/C
7.	3	2	2	2	H/C
8.	3	2	1	1	H
9.	3	2	2	2	H
10.	1	1	1	1	H
11.	2	1	1	1	H
12.	3	1	3	2	H
13.	3	1	2	3	H/C
14.[a]	3	2	1	1	H/C
15.	3	2	1	1	C
16.	2	1	2	2	C
17.	4	5	5+	5+	C

[a] Deaths.

prognostic influence of sex. The average age at the onset of dialysis for the group of 32 patients who expired may be considered significant. Any group that starts such chronic therapy in the fifth decade of life is undoubtedly starting at a disadvantage as compared with a group that starts in the fourth decade of life, as did our survivors. Certainly the influence of degenerative diseases, particularly cardiovascular diseases,

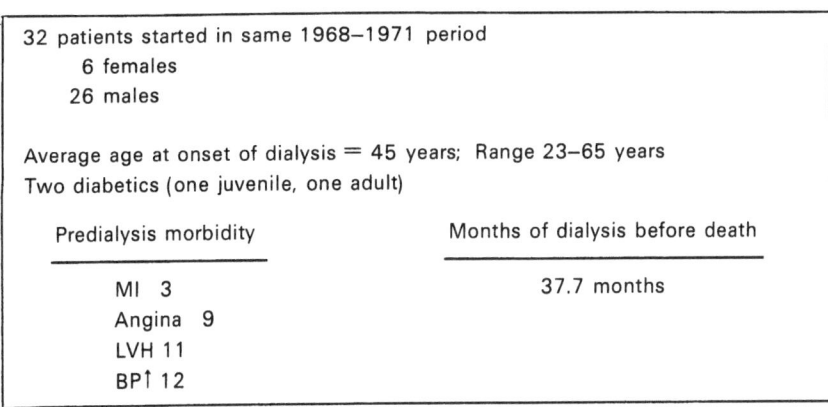

Figure 3. Predialysis characteristics of 32 expired patients.

is known to augment significantly by the fifth decade of life. A review of the predialysis characteristics of these patients shows that three already had a myocardial infarct and nine had angina that persisted or got worse. The patients survived for an average of 37.7 months on dialysis before dying. While this hardly compares to chronic hemodialysis for over ten years, it certainly does not compare poorly with treatments for a variety of other diseases, particularly cancers that require expensive and constant therapy with even a far more dismal prognosis and lesser longevity. After starting dialysis, of the 32 patients, 11 had angina and 13 myocardial infarctions; the causes of death, as may have been predicted and has been well documented in many studies, were cerebro-cardiovascular, infection, and transplant complications (Table IV).

What conclusions can one draw concerning the characteristics of these 17 patients on chronic hemodialysis for more than ten years and in what way can we apply them to the important question that, from a review of this nature, inevitably comes to mind? The obvious question is, of course, how does reviewing the history of these patients aid us in selecting new ones so that they too may live as long? One may begin to give some tentative answers. It would appear that patients with no clinical evidences of coronary artery disease and who have accomplished good blood pressure control during the course of years and adhere well to the dialysis regimen prescribed so as to produce reasonably good chemical results have an excellent chance of surviving ten years or more on chronic hemodialysis. I cannot believe that this summary statement was not well known to us more than ten years ago. In fact, the selection criteria that were originally used by the first dialysis facilities in the United States very closely approximate these results. The compliance scales and the elements involved therein were always those issues considered supremely important by the early nephrologists. We have all lived long enough to have acquired information that would validate our intuitive good clinical sense.

Therefore, the question of selection of therapy of individuals who lie somewhat outside the norms that could easily be established if the end point were to be long-term survival on dialysis still remains a moral and social issue. I submit that this moral and social issue is no different than those that prevail in other areas of medicine. Certainly, within the fields of oncology and cardiovascular surgery one can find significant and important parallel considerations for other disease entities and their therapies. The specific problem that medicine and physicians have in practicing the art is the significant deviations from the norm that seem to defy the very establishment of a standard. Clearly, patient no. 17 in our listing

Table IV. Morbidity and Mortality
of Thirty-Two Patients on Dialysis

Cardiovascular disease:
Angina 11
Myocardial infarction 13
Causes of death:
MI 11
CVA 7
Infection 6
Transplant complications 3
Miscellaneous 5

exemplifies that element of either ignorance or luck, or a combination of both, that defies prognosis.

General conclusions from information such as now being presented could be drawn without regard to particular patients as to the best manner in which to utilize resources in the care of these patients. However, due to the aforementioned lack of precision in our prognostic capabilities this utilization of such information must be carefully circumscribed so that immediate conclusions leading to premature prescriptions and proscriptions would not be warranted. Until more science in this area is available to elucidate the problem, conclusions from such discussions that might lead to public policy should not be the province of physicians alone, nor should physicians and other health care persons rush to embrace criteria and proscriptions established by others in society because they may seem to afford a respite from the struggle that imperfect solutions cause and from the strenuous effort necessary to improve the solutions.

23

Personality and Psychological Factors Influencing Survivorship on Hemodialysis

NORMAN B. LEVY

The notion that psychological factors somehow predispose a person to illness or another to health is well accepted in folklore, poetry, novels, and, more recently, by medical research.

As to the less objective, let me quote the following from a famous novel[1]:

> Cases of typhoid take the following course: When the fever is at its height, life calls to the patient: calls out to him as he wanders in his distant dream, and summons him in no uncertain voice. The harsh, imperious call reaches the spirit on that remote path that leads into the shadows, the coolness and peace. He hears the call of life, the clear, fresh, mocking summons to return to that distant scene which he had already left so far behind him, and already forgotten. And there may well up in him something like a feeling of shame for a neglected duty; a sense of renewed energy, courage, and hope; he may recognize a bond existing still between him and that stirring, colorful, callous existence which he though he had left so far behind him. Then, however far he may have wandered on his distant path, he will turn back—and live. But if he shudders when he hears life's voice, if the memory of that vanished scene and the sound of that lusty summons make him shake his head, make him put out his hand to ward off as he flies forward in the way of escape that has opened to him—then it is clear that the patient will die.

The author essentially states that in the course of the delirium of typhoid fever, a patient who gives up the fight for life will die. However, a patient who continues to struggle may live. This was written by Thomas Mann in the book *Buddenbrooks*, published in 1901 when Mann was only 26 years old and before the days of dynamic psychiatry and chloramphenicol. This book did not produce any objections. In fact, its acceptance and

NORMAN B. LEVY • Departments of Psychiatry, Medicine and Surgery, New York Medical Center; and Division of Liaison Psychiatry, Westchester County Medical Center, Valhalla, New York.

acclaim contributed to Mann's winning of the Nobel prize in literature. Like other great novelists and playwrights, Mann was a keen observer of people and described life the way he saw it and which other people knew.

The observation has been that confidence, joy, and gratification augment good health. But despair, helplessness, and hopelessness predispose to illness. This concept, which tends to find acceptance among laypeople, has not received objective medical attention until recently. Even its application in the past in the medical specialties has been one of "common sense" rather than by objective evidence. For example, most surgeons will not perform elective surgery upon individuals who forecast their own demise and tend to perform surgery with greater confidence in people who are optimistic about their future.

Schmale, initially and later joined by Engel,[2] formulated the concept of the "giving-up given-up complex." This refers to a biological state in which certain depressive emotional states (affects), hopelessness and helplessness, are formulated as making changes in the biological economy of the body, rendering it more prone to physical illness. This concept has not abandoned the germ theory of infectious disease but rather attempts to describe a factor affecting resistance to disease. It essentially states that psychological discomfort is such a factor that produces a decreased resistance to disease. Of course, decreased resistance is not sufficient in itself to cause physical illness, which requires the presence of a pathogen and/or predisposition to that illness. Schmale and Engel formulated that in about two thirds of cases the giving-up given-up complex could be demonstrated as *preceding* the onset of physical illness.

A number of retrospective and prospective studies have verified this concept. Some examples are those of widows and widowers matched with individuals for sex and age. In his study Parkes found a much higher instance of death one year and two years after widowing as compared with the control population.[3] Rahe used naval personnel and engaged in a predictive study as to which individuals would become sick aboard ship on a cruise.[4] He based his predictions entirely upon a study of immediately preceding life events of these people obtained by interviewing them just prior to their going to sea. He was able to predict illness, here usually upper respiratory infections, well within statistical significance.

The notion that emotional factors can affect and alter health is only a small step away from the concept of emotions affecting the course of illness. The latter concept has even wider acceptance, again usually based upon gross observations and "common sense" before systematic psychological studies were available. Physicians who are identified as being psychologically resistive concerning other aspects of medicine, as a rule, accept this view because they have observed it clinically among their patients. It would be the rare nephrologist who did not agree with the title of this chapter, namely, that psychological factors affect a patient's survival on hemodialysis. Aside from the obvious, that psychological factors affect suicide and cooperativeness with a medical regimen, in addition the will to live or the lack of it affects longevity in these patients as it does in others.

PHASES OF ADAPTATION TO HEMODIALYSIS

A study of the phases of adaptation to hemodialysis can shed some light on the issue of long-term survivorship on hemodialysis. In a four-year intensive study of 25 patients undergoing hemodialysis, three phases in adaptation were described after initiating a program of maintenance hemodialysis.[5] These were termed the "honeymoon," the period of disenchantment and discouragement, and the period of long-term adaptation. The observations were made that all 16 of the 25 patients who had experienced a clear-cut "honeymoon" had a distinct and dramatic change in their affective state. The feelings of contentment, confidence, and hope that characterized the honeymoon period decreased markedly or disappeared and were replaced by feelings of sadness and helplessness, which lasted 3 to 12 months. This was termed the period of disenchantment and discouragement. Of the 16 patients, 12 showed a definite chronological relationship between the onset of this period and specific preceding stressful events, the planning or actual resumption of active and productive roles at work, in school, or in the household. Of particular importance was the close time association between these depressive feelings associated with life change and medical complications related to dialysis. The most common of these was clotting of the shunt, which, in those days, was the exclusive avenue of access to the patient's blood stream. Other complications were infections of, or bleeding from, the cannular site and marked venous or arterial spasms of the shunt vessels during dialysis. During this period five patients died.

These data are cited to illustrate the significance of stress on the one hand and medical complications on the other. Further, one is impressed by the fact that the stress during the period of disenchantment and discouragement may largely be iatrogenic, due to unrealistic expectations.

To understand the source of distress, we must recognize that those of us who work in the professions, and more specifically in nephrology, tend to be high attainers in life. As a group we tend to project the expectations that we have for ourselves onto others around us. In addition, the medical model of treatment is inseparably linked with the notion that successful treatment means rehabilitation and that rehabilitation means returning to full work activities that the patient had prior to illness. For these reasons the tendency among medical and other nephrologic professional personnel is to attempt to favor the highest degree of work activity. Often these decisions are made with inadequate psychosocial data. The following case illustrates this.

> J.S. was a 19-year-old black laborer from the South Bronx. In interviewing him it was discovered that he was illiterate, even though he had completed a grammar school education in New York City and had a diploma attesting to it. In addition to treating his renal failure, making him literate became another goal of the hemodialysis unit. Almost everybody joined in this expectation, including the patient, who should have known better but who suspended that knowledge in favor of gratifying his care takers, his family, and himself. Unfortunately, the patient somehow could never manage to make the appointment with his Division of Vocational Rehabilitation counsellor, a necessary person on the road to getting special tutoring. The obstacles somehow were insurmountable. On one occasion he forgot the appointment, on another he started out but didn't have the carfare, and on still another he got lost; finally, he developed a major clotting of his shunt as he was preparing to leave his house, thus requiring a major revision of his shunt. It became apparent to all of us, including the patient himself, that his goal of becoming literate was not a feasible one. The reality was that the factors that inhibited his becoming literate years before were operative now. The patient came from a very deprived background, both economically and, even more important, socially, and for a number of reasons connected with those factors never had sufficient tranquillity to be educable. Had the patient been approached more realistically by staff, the goal of his literacy would never had been set. At best, a goal might be the exploration of its feasibility. The patient, however, joined with the rest of the staff in establishing a totally unrealistic goal, and also joined with the staff in great disappointment, dejection, and depression. He felt he had let the staff down, and the staff in general felt let down also.

This case illustrates how a stressful factor can affect adaptation, psychological as well as medical, and contribute to both physical illness and compromised longevity.

STUDIES OF LONGEVITY OF HEMODIALYSIS PATIENTS

It is not surprising for both lay and medical people to search for psychological factors that play a role in the longevity of patients maintained by hemodialysis. Their usefulness is obvious, both to prognosticate with some accuracy as well as to engage in maneuvers that favor longer life. This is a very difficult notion to examine, even if a very valid one, since a large number of factors affect the course of illness, most of which seem not to be under direct psychological control. Also, psychological factors are not easily measured. They tend to be much more subjective, more difficult to quantitate, and more susceptible to different interpretations. One could test the hypothesis that psychological factors affect longevity of hemo-dialysis patients by testing a group of patients who are long-term survivors and comparing them with a group who did not survive long, examining characteristics of each group and subjecting the differentiation to tests of statistical significance. One such study was reported on factors affecting the survival of 14 and the demise of seven patients studied prospectively over a two-year period.[6] The survivor group contrasted with those who died to a statistically significant degree in relation to a number of measures. The only psychosocial factors were three: having at least one living parent, being a member of the Roman Catholic church, and having a marked indifference to fellow patients.

METHOD

I attempted to isolate factors affecting survivorship by engaging in the following study. Ten nephrologists, ten nurses, and ten patients who had survived ten years or longer on hemodialysis were interviewed. All 30 persons were asked their views about personality factors that affect longevity on hemodialysis. The patients themselves were also examined concerning personality factors common and characteristic to them as a group.

RESULTS

The data, collected over a one-year period, revealed the following. Both the physicians and nurses thought that long-term survivorship seemed to be greater among patients who were relatively aloof from their fellow patients, were good attainers in life, and were people who were generally relatively self rather than outwardly involved.

The patients tended to see longevity as an outcome to their strong desire to survive and/or their ability to adapt to a new life style. Six of the ten said that their ability to adhere to a medical regimen played a role in their survival. They were pleased at their ability to tolerate the frustrations involved in being "good patients".

The following were characteristics that were relatively commonly seen in the personality of these patients: They were people who were not "losers" in life, that is, they tended to have a low propensity for self-destructive behavior and at times could be described as selfish rather than self-sacrificing. Three patients were exceptions to this latter generalization. They were involved in health care professions associated with renal disease. In fact, their work activities could better be described as being somewhat self-sacrificing rather than selfish. All ten surviving patients were further characterized by being relatively independent. Eight could be described as people who did not necessarily accept what was told to them by professional staff but often challenged and questioned them. This contrasted rather greatly with many of their fellow patients, who tended as a group to be relatively compliant. With the exception of the three involved in health care professions, they were people who tended not to be sympathetic toward other patients and to strongly separate themselves from them, seeing themselves as different or unique from most of the other patients. When engaged in patient-related activities, it was usually from the standpoint of understanding but not mimicking the feelings of their fellow patients. For example, presented with the death of another patient, long-term survivors tended to underscore their dissimilarity from the deceased and were often critical of that person's approach to life. Further, all were people who either do not experience, or rarely experience, the emotional states of hopelessness and helplessness, but rather accommodate to life situations in an aggressive and angry way. Presented with a medical problem, their tendency toward despair was minimal. Their emotional outlook more likely would be directed either toward a constructive endeavor or to faulting an external source such as an error made by a member of the professional staff or family care taker. I have previously described this group as being "givers of ulcers rather than getters of ulcers."[7]

As a final note on this theme, I would like to have you regard the matter similarly to the earliest phases of work surrounding personality factors affecting onset of coronary artery disease. The isolation of these factors in coronary artery disease that belong under the heading of Type A behavior has been shown by rather elegant retrospective and prospective studies to play a statistically significant role in the onset of this illness.[8] As a further outcome of this work, there is an attempt to alter coronary personality behavior—that is, Type A behavior—as a method of prevention of coronary artery disease. Currently we are still in a rather early phase of understanding the psychological factors affecting longevity in hemodialysis. Perhaps in the near future not only might we definitively learn which factors play a role in longevity in these patients, but also be able to suggest techniques, which, from the psychological standpoint, will help the longevity of these patients. Until then, we need to encourage psychological work in this area.[9]

REFERENCES

1. Mann T: *Buddenbrooks*. New York, Vintage Books, 1952, p 591.
2. Engel GL: A life setting conducive to physical illness: The giving-up given-up complex. *Ann Intern Med* 69:293–300, 1968.
3. Parkes CM: The psychosomatic effects of bereavement, in Hill OW (ed): *Modern Trends in Psychosomatic Medicine*, ed 2. New York, Appleton-Century-Crofts, 1970, p 71.
4. Rahe RH: Subjects' recent life changes and their near-future illness susceptibility, in Lipowski ZJ (ed): *Advances in Psychosomatic Medicine: Psychosocial Aspects of Physical Illness*, vol 8. Basel and New York, Karger, 1972, p 72.
5. Reichsman F, Levy NB: Problems in adaptation to maintenance hemodialysis: a four-year study of 25 patients. *Arch Intern Med* 130:859–865, 1972.
6. Foster FG, Cohn GL, McKegney FP: Psychologic factors and individual survival on chronic renal hemodialysis—A two-year follow-up—Part I, in Levy NB (ed): *Living or Dying: Adaptation to Hemodialysis*. Springfield, Ill., Charles C Thomas, 1974, p 74–101.
7. Levy NB: Psychological factors affecting long-term survivorships on hemodialysis. *Dial Transplant* 8:880–881, 1979.
8. Friedman M, Rosenman RH: Association of specific overt behavior pattern with blood and cardiovascular findings. *JAMA* 169:1286–1292, 1959.
9. Levy NB (ed): *Psychonephrology I: Psychological Factors in Hemodialysis and Transplantation*. New York and London, Plenum Publishing Corp, 1981.

Section VII

The Transplantation Alternative

Until now we have had little "hard data" concerning transplantation. This section remedies in part this lack of credible information.

Kjellstrand and Simmons review the long-term renal transplant recipient and note "a marked increase in death rate even late after transplantation." The major risks are infection—"forever an important risk of death," cardiovascular disease, liver failure, and, surprisingly, suicide, which accounted for 9% of long-term deaths. There are not literative reports of decade-long transplant survivors for comparison. The results "look quite grim." They observe that over half of the patients surviving a decade are dead, lost, or in serious trouble.

In contrast, Butt and colleagues report progressively improving patient and graft survival over the last eight years, which may foreshadow better long-term survival for the renal transplant recipient. Nevertheless, of the at least 38,000 kidney transplants performed to date, the number of long survivors is quite small. Stenzel and associates, wishing to clarify the events of graft rejection, contend that "long-term survival of renal graft recipients . . . depends on the clarification of molecular mechanisms in T-cell activation." They anticipate that elucidation of vulnerable points in the immunologic response to foreign tissue will permit formulations of new strategies for forestalling allograft rejection.

Prevention, retardation, and management of early, preuremic renal disease is the message of this volume.

M.M.A.

24

Long-Term Survivors After Renal Transplantation

CARL M. KJELLSTRAND AND RICHARD L. SIMMONS

During the past two decades renal transplantation has become an established clinical procedure performed in a large number of hospitals. Over 20,000 transplants were reported to the European Dialysis and Transplant Association as of January 1, 1979,[1] and at least 35,000 transplants were performed in the United States through 1979. The early problems, mainly related to insufficient dialysis preparation, overimmunosuppression, and infections, have been described in hundreds of articles over the past decade. This clinical research has led to a marked improvement in the immediate post-transplant survival. Thus many centers report an improvement from approximately a 10%–20% first-year survival during the early 1960s to a first-year patient survival of around 90% in the late 1970s.[2]

There is much less experience concerning the long-term fate and problems of these patients. In this chapter we review some of the literature and our own experience with patients who survive many years after renal transplantation.

OVERALL SURVIVAL AND CAUSES OF DEATH

Table I summarizes the causes of death early and late after transplantation as reported by the European Dialysis and Transplant Association.[1] It is clear that there is a shift in death. Early after transplantation (zero–three months), of the patients who die almost half die of infection. Between two

CARL M. KJELLSTRAND ● Division of Nephrology, Departments of Medicine and Surgery, University of Minnesota; and Nephrology Division, Regional Kidney Disease Program, Hennepin County Medical Center, Minneapolis, Minnesota.   RICHARD L. SIMMONS ● Department of Surgery, University of Minnesota Hospitals, Minneapolis, Minnesota.

Table I. EDTA 1979 Registry—Deaths per 1000 Patients per Year

Cause of death	Time			
	0–3 months	(Percent total)	2–5 years	(Percent total)
Infection	124	45	8	26
Cardiovascular	59	21	8	26
Gastrointestinal bleed	18	7	0.6	2
Malignancy	0	0	2.3	7
Other	75	27	12.1	39
Total	276	100	31	100

and five years, this decreases to 26%; instead, cardiovascular deaths, deaths in malignancy, and other deaths have increased.

Table II summarizes the long-term experience from four very large transplant centers.[3-6] Of 608 patients surviving between 3 and 14 years, 75, or 12.3%, died after this time. Table III details the deaths in 61 of these 75 patients, where this was described in detail, representing 526 of the 608 patients.[3-5] Infection remains at 26%; cardiovascular deaths have increased to 33%. An important contributor is liver failure, responsible for 11% of the deaths; suicides are the cause of 8% of the deaths. Only four patients, 7%, died of cancer. The other deaths included two patients who died of hyperparathyroidism, and three patients who died of uremia and wasting.

Only Matas and his co-workers[3] had performed cumulated survival statistics in their long-term transplant survivors. When compared with survival curves in the normal population, there was a marked increase in death rate even late after transplantation. Opelz and his co-workers[7] also found that long-term survivors even five–ten years after transplantation have a relentless death rate along an exponential curve, with a T½ of approximately 12 years for recipients of cadaver kidneys, 36 years for recipients of HLA identical kidneys, and 19 years of HLA nonidentical recipients.

Table II. Death in Long-Term Survivors

	Richmond, VA	Denver, CO	Minneapolis, MN	Gothenburg, Sweden	Total
Observation time in years	5–13	5–14	3–12	3–10	—
Patients at risk	82	200	198	128	608
Died	14	24	20	17	75
Percent died	17	12	10	13	12.3

Similarly, the death curves as reported by Kjellstrand et al. summarizing European Dialysis and Transplant Association statistics also show no trend toward leveling, even at ten years. The grim truth is that a recipient of a renal transplant or on chronic hemodialysis is never home safe.

Infectious Deaths

It is clear that infection remains forever an important cause of death in patients. Particularly interesting is the fact that the herpes group virus continues to be responsible for many deaths even very late after transplantation. Thus two patients in the Denver group died of late CMV infection and three patients in the Minneapolis series died, respectively, of cytomegalovirus, chickenpox, and herpes simplex infection.[3,4] This group of infections, which is such a problem during early transplantation, obviously remains so even very late.

Cardiovascular Deaths

There is a slow but steady increase in cardiovascular deaths. It was at one time thought that this would not be the case.[6] Although Thomas and Lee[6] implied that arteriosclerosis was not common, 6 of their 14 patients actually died of cardiovascular problems. Cardiovascular complications were once thought to be the limiting factor of long-term survival of chronic dialysis. Recent articles suggest that this is not the case.[9-12] In dialysis, preexisting hypertension seems to be the most common risk factor. Similar observations have been made in transplantation. Thus Ibels and his co-workers[13] reported that patients who were transplanted because of renal failure secondary to hypertension were particularly prone to vascular complications. If these observations are true, improvements of transplantation or dialysis per se will not be efficient ways of dealing with the problem. Only intensified treatment of the hypertension long before dialysis and transplantation are necessary is likely to influence this factor as an important cause of death both early and late.

The causes of death in dialysis after chronic hemodialysis and transplantation thus show exactly opposite trends. The early deaths following dialysis are overwhelmingly vascular; following transplantation the overwhelming cause of early death is infection. Later infections become the leading cause of death in dialysis, and vascular problems become the most important cause following transplantation. At two–five years after transplantation and dialysis, patients die of the same causes; approxi-

Table III. Cause of Death

	Denver	Minneapolis	Gothenburg	Total
Infection	8	7	1	16 (26%)
Pneumonia	6	0	0	
Herpes group virus	2	3	0	
Other	0	4	1	
Cardiovascular	5	6	9	20 (33%)
Myocardial	2	2	6	
Cerebral	0	4	2	
Other	3	0	1	
Gastrointestinal	2	2	0	4 (7%)
Colon perforation	2	1	0	
Pancreatitis	0	1	0	
Liver failure	4	3	0	7 (11%)
Suicide	3	1	1	5 (8%)
Malignancy	1	1	2	4 (7%)
Other	1	0	4	5 (8%)
Total	24	20	17	61 (100%)
Patients with renal failure	8	4	11	23 (38%)

mately one third of the deaths are due to vascular complications and one third to infections in both groups.

It is difficult to relate all of the vascular deaths occurring late after transplantation to preexisting hypertension, and no scientific analysis of this problem has been done. One would expect that these patients would have already died during preparatory dialysis, or early after transplantation as described by Ibels et al.[13] It is possible that the immunosuppression or some other factor of transplantation induces vascular disease.[14]

If this is correct, the new trend of usage of very-low-dose steroids could improve on this problem. It seems clear that much overusage of prednisone has taken place, and that a much lower dose of this drug can be used from the onset of transplantation without adversely affecting early renal survival and will usually improve patient survival.[15-17] It remains, of course, entirely speculative whether this will improve long-term problems. The most drastic reduction, cessation of prednisone completely, is not possible as it almost inevitably gives rise to rejection and kidney loss.[18]

Liver Failure

The third most common cause of death late after transplantation is liver failure, responsible for 7/61 (11%) of deaths occurring in long-term survivors (Table III). The causes of this liver failure in transplantation remain unknown. Efforts to correlate with viruses hepatitis-A, B, non-A non-B, Epstein-Barr, adenovirus, cytomegalovirus, or with drug toxicity from azathioprine or methyldopa have been unrewarding.[19-22] In spite of several analyses, the cause remains unknown and in all likelihood it will prove to be multifactorial, perhaps a combination of damage secondary to virus disorders, azathioprine toxicity, and alcoholism as described by Shideman et al.[23] One approach to this problem would be to discontinue azathioprine on a trial basis, years after transplantation.

Suicide

The fourth most common cause of death following transplantation is suicide. Five (8%) of the 61 long-term deaths were due to this, and several other patients indirectly committed suicide by refusing retransplantation or return to dialysis after transplant failure. It is known that the suicide rate of patients on dialysis is five to six times that reported for the normal population.[1] Many dialyzed patients probably also commit covert suicide by not participating in their care in dialysis.[1] It seems to be equally clear that living with a transplant is trying, and that some patients cannot stand the pressure of living on borrowed time. Thus five patients of the 526 at risk (Tables II and III) did commit suicide after transplantation for an approximate rate of 0.1% per year. This rate is exactly the one recently described for chronic dialysis patients by the European Dialysis and Transplant Association Registry.[1]

Malignancy

Malignancy has not been a common cause of death after transplantation. Only four patients died of malignancy. As described by us earlier, there does not seem to be any accumulated risk of malignancy even in long-term survivors.[23] All of our malignancies occurred between three and six years following transplantation in our longest survivors.

The four deaths from malignancy described by the large groups are as follows: undifferentiated adenocarcinoma leading to death four years after transplantation in a 52-year-old recipient,[3] multiple squamous cell epitheliomas of head and neck with liver and bone metastasis,[4] epipharyngeal carcinoma in a 58-year-old man occurring five years after transplantation, and cerebral reticulum cell sarcoma in a 51-year-old man, also occurring approximately five years post-transplant.[5]

Thus, although death from malignancy remains important, it has not emerged as an overwhelming problem following transplantation.

Other Deaths

Four deaths occurred because of complications in the gastrointestinal tract. Three patients died of colon perforation and one of pancreatitis. Two patients died of complications of hyperparathyroidism and three of uremia and wasting late after transplantation.[3-5]

The Role of Chronic Rejection

Complications leading to death seem to occur particularly often in patients who experience chronic rejection with a second episode of chronic renal failure. Thus eight of the 24 deaths in the Denver series occurred in patients with renal failure as did four of 20 in the Minneapolis series. Eleven of the 17 patients who died in the Gothenburg series had a creatinine level of 2 mg/dl or higher but only one had been returned to hemodialysis.[3-5]

Our own large experience with approximately 1,500 patients is similar. The death rate in patients returning to dialysis from transplantation is three to four times that of the early death rate in patients who came to dialysis with their first episode of uremia.

Thus, if renal failure ensues after transplantation, one should very quickly taper immunosuppression and not subject a patient to the double threat of being both immunosuppressed and chronically uremic. It does seem logical that one should be able to achieve death rates following transplant rejection that should not be markedly different from that for a patient with a first uremic episode.

FATE OF PATIENTS SURVIVING ONE DECADE

Only our group seemed to have described patients surviving over one decade.[23] In 30 patients who survived more than ten years following renal transplantation, there was no longer any difference in complications or survival of recipients of a cadaver or related kidneys. Four patients died between 10 and 15 years following transplantation—one of gram-negative sepsis following transplantation nephrectomy, one of chronic liver failure, and two suddenly of unknown causes. One of these patients had severe atherosclerosis on autopsy; the other did not. Another three patients, two recipients of related kidneys and one of a cadaver kidney, were undergoing severe chronic rejection.

Three years later another three patients had died. One of these had an accident and may have been a sudden death; details are unknown. The other two patients died from complications of chronic rejection. Thus, of the seven patients who died, three were sudden deaths, all in patients with normal renal function. One patient died with relatively normal renal function in liver failure. Three patients died of complications of chronic rejection. All these patients had had their transplanted kidneys functioning for over ten years, although one had been retransplanted one year after the first kidney. Liver failure occurred in connection with chronic rejection in two of these three patients. It is clear that chronic rejection is a very deadly complication for these patients. Of the remaining 23 patients, four have been lost to follow-up, and two had evidence of chronic rejection. Five of the remaining 19 patients have evidence of severe chronic rejection (creatinine 1.9, 2.3, 2.5, 3.2, 4.9 mg/dl). Thus, of the 30 patients who survived a decade after transplantation, only 14 (47%) have normal renal function now and three of these were retransplanted having had their second or third grafts (three–five–seven years). Only 11 patients have their first transplant kidney still functioning—two are cadaver transplants now 14 and 15 years out with creatinines of 1.2 and 1.4, and nine have related-donor transplants performed between 12 and 17 years ago. The creatinine levels in these patients range from 0.7 to 1.1 mg/dl.

None of the patients have died of malignancy. All malignancies occurred between three and six years after transplantation, and none caused death, attesting to the fact that malignancy does not seem to emerge as a main threat in transplantation.

It is also clear that there is no difference in kidney survival or renal function in patients receiving cadaver or related transplants and surviving beyond one decade. Thus two of seven cadaver transplants, and 9 of 23 related-donor recipients ($p =$ n.s.) continue to do well.

It is clear that the statistics look quite grim. Over half of the patients surviving a decade are dead, lost, or in serious trouble. It may not be, however, that these patients represent a typical group of patients, or will necessarily foretell similar problems for other patients transplanted later. They represent patients done between 1963 and 1968, when dialysis and transplantation were done late when many complications of uremia may have been irreversible, and thus are similar to the dialysis patients described by Lindner et al.[24]

The relatively sudden very late onset of renal failure, described as chronic rejection, has also been seen by other groups.[25] Posborg, Petersen and their colleagues[25] have done a careful morphologic analysis of this problem and believe that this may represent de novo glomerulonephritis. They base this on the fact that the disease has no relation to the original one in the patients and because of morphologic analysis.

Two other groups have, in brief reports, described their experience of long-term (8–12 year) survivors after renal transplantation. Halgrimson and the group in Denver[26] reported four deaths occurring in patients between eight and ten years after transplantation and that another three lost their renal grafts during this time. They also reported no difference between related and cadaver recipients. The same experience—no difference late after transplantation between cadaver recipients and related donors—was reported by Thomas et al.[27]

SUMMARY

Renal transplantation is an established clinical procedure. The early problems have been described and recognized and the result of this clinical research has been a marked improvement in early survival from 10% to 90%.

Late transplantation complications are now beginning to emerge. Although infections remain very important, cardiovascular complications seem to be the leading cause of late deaths after transplantation. The influence of preexisting hypertension and prednisone and other factors remains to be elucidated. Liver failure is the third most common cause of death. The relative contribution of previous or existing viruses, alcoholism, and nephrotoxicity by azathioprine is unknown and worthy of clinical investigation. Particularly disturbing is the fact that a death from any cause is often associated with a second episode of chronic renal failure. This problem should be available to treatment by curtailment of immuno-suppression and early return to dialysis.

Suicide has become as common in transplant patients as it is in dialysis and in this small series is the fourth most common cause of death, more common than the deaths from malignancy. No investigations into the causes or prevention of this seem to have been undertaken.

In our small series of 30 patients surviving for more than ten years after their first transplant, 23% have died and only 48% survive with normal renal function between 12 and 17 years after transplantation.

REFERENCES

1. Brunner FP, Brynger H, Chantler C, et al: Combined report on regular dialysis and transplantation in Europe, IX, 1978. *Proc Eur Dialysis Transplant Assoc* 16:2–73, 1979.
2. Kjellstrand CM, Avram MM, Blagg CR, et al: Cadaver transplantation versus hemodialysis. *Trans Am Soc Artif Intern Organs* 26:611–624, 1980.

3. Matas AJ, Simmons RL, Buselmeier TJ, et al: The fate of patients surviving three years after renal transplantation. *Surgery* 80:390–395, 1976.

4. Weil R, Schroter CPJ, West JC, et al: A 14-year experience with kidney transplantation. *World J Surg* 1:145–149, 1977.

5. Blohme I, Ahlmen J, Sandberg L: Prognosis for recipients of successful renal transplants. *Scand J Urol Nephrol* 38(suppl):89–98, 1976.

6. Thomas FT, Lee HM: Factors in the differential rate of arteriosclerosis between long surviving renal transplant recipients and dialysis patients. *Ann Surg* 184:342–351, 1976.

7. Opelz G, Mickey MR, Terasaki PI: Calculations of longterm graft and patient survival in human kidney transplantation. *Transplant Proc* 9:27–30, 1977.

8. Wing AJ, Brunner FP, Brynger H, et al: Combined report on regular dialysis and transplantation in Europe, 1977. *Proc Eur Dialysis Transplant Assoc* 15:4–76, 1978.

9. Burke JF, Francos GC, Morre LL, et al: Accelerated atherosclerosis in chronic dialysis patients—Another look. *Nephron* 21:181–185, 1978.

10. Lundin AP, Adler AJ, Feinroth MV, et al: Maintenance hemodialysis. *JAMA* 244:38–40, 1980.

11. Vincenti F, Amend WJ, Abele J, et al: The role of hypertension in hemodialysis associated atherosclerosis. *Am J Med* 68:363–369, 1980.

12. Rostad SG, Gretes JC, Kirk KA, et al: Ischemic heart disease in patients with uremia undergoing maintenance hemodialysis. *Kidney Int* 16:600–611, 1979.

13. Ibels LS, Stewart JH, Mahony JF, et al: Deaths from occlusive arterial disease in renal allograft recipients. *Br Med J* 3:552–554, 1974.

14. Kjellstrand CM: Side effects of steroids and their treatment. *Transplant Proc* 7:123–129, 1975.

15. McGeown MG, Douglas JF, Brown WA, et al: Advantages of low dose steroid from the day after renal transplantation. *Transplant* 29:287–289, 1980.

16. Chan L, French ME, Beare J, et al: Prospective trial of high dose versus low dose prednisolone in renal transplant patients. *Transplant Proc* 12:323–326, 1980.

17. Salvatierra O, Potter D, Cochrum KC, et al: Improved patient survival in renal transplantation. *Surgery* 79:166–171, 1976.

18. Zoller KM, Cho SI, Cohen JJ, et al: Cessation of immunosuppressive therapy after successful transplantation: A national survey. *Kidney Int* 18:110–114, 1980.

19. Nielsen V, Clausen E, Ranek L: Liver impairment during chronic hemodialysis and after renal transplantation. *Acta Med Scand* 197:229–234, 1975.

20. Anuras S, Piros J, Bonney WW, et al: Liver disease in renal transplant recipients. *Arch Intern Med* 137:42–48, 1977.

21. Ware AJ: Etiology of liver disease in renal transplant patients. *Ann Intern Med* 91:364–371, 1979.

22. Mozes MF, Ascher NL, Balfour HH, et al: Jaundice after renal allotransplantation. *Ann Surg* 188:783–790, 1978.

23. Shideman J, Najarian JS, Simmons RL, et al: Longterm survival and complications more than 10 years following renal transplantation, in Giordano C, Friedman EA (eds) *Uremia: Pathobiology of Patients Treated for 10 Years or More*, Milan, Italy, Wichtig Editore, 1981, pp. 142–151.

24. Lindner A, Charra B, Sherrard DJ, et al: Accelerated atherosclerosis in prolonged maintenance hemodialysis. *N Engl J Med* 290:697–701, 1974.

25. Posborg Petersen V, Steen Olsen T, Kissmeyer-Nielsen F, et al: Late failure of human renal transplants. *Medicine* 54:45–71, 1975.

26. Halgrimson CG, Penn I, Booth A, et al: Eight-to-ten year follow-up in early cases of renal homotransplantation. *Transplant Proc* 5:787–791, 1973.

27. Thomas F, Lee HM, Wolf JS, et al: Long-term (8–12 years) prognosis in related and unrelated renal transplantation. *Transplant Proc* 7:707–711, 1975.

25

Brighter Outlook
for Kidney Transplantation

KHALID M. H. BUTT, ABDUL G. ARSHAD, JOON H. HONG,
LEA EMMETT, ISMAIL PARSA, ROLAND J. ADAMSONS,
AND ELI A. FRIEDMAN

The emphasis throughout this volume has been on maintenance of renal failure patients with dialysis; nonetheless, it is evident that the best survival, and certainly the best quality of survival for these patients, is dependent on the integration of two complementary therapies: transplantation and dialysis. The surgical contribution to the management of the patient with end-stage renal failure begins with the establishment of an access for dialysis. Once a dependable access has been developed, the best results are seen in a self-dialysis setting, either home hemodialysis or peritoneal dialysis (CAPD). Undoubtedly, access is the backbone of dialytic therapy.

There is little doubt that the optimal physical and psychosocial rehabilitation is seen in patients who have been successfully transplanted. With a view to assessing the progress in successful engraftment and to verify the changing spectrum of the mortality and morbidity of transplantation, we embarked on the following study.

METHODS AND MATERIALS

An average of 100 kidney transplants have been performed every year since 1973 by the Transplantation Service of the State University of

KHALID M. H. BUTT ● Department of Surgery and Transplantation Service, Downstate Medical Center, Brooklyn, New York.   ABDUL G. ARSHAD AND ISMAIL PARSA ● Department of Pathology, Downstate Medical Center, Brooklyn, New York.   JOON H. HONG, LEA EMMETT, AND ROLAND ADAMSONS ● Department of Surgery, Downstate Medical Center, Brooklyn, New York.   ELI A. FRIEDMAN ● Division of Nephrology and Department of Medicine, Downstate Medical Center, Brooklyn, New York.

New York, Downstate Medical Center. For the purposes of this study, we made a comparison of patient survival and functional graft survival of the transplants done in the first two years of this period with that of the last two years. Since there were too few diabetic uremics in the earlier years of our experience, we have excluded them from consideration.

The actuarial patient survival of 86 nondiabetic recipients of living related-donor kidneys from 1973–74 was 76% at two years, as compared with that of 30 recipients from 1979–80 of 100%—a significant improvement ($p < 0.025$) (Figure 1). The corresponding functional graft survival from 1973–74 was 55% at two years, as compared with 90% from 1979–80 ($p < 0.01$) (Figure 2). The patient survival of 106 nondiabetic recipients of cadaver donor kidneys from 1973–74 was 71%, while that of 164 recipients from the 1979–1980 period was 87%, again a significant improvement ($p < 0.005$) (Figure 3). The corresponding functional graft survival of cadaver donor kidneys was 28% in 1973–74, and 61% in 1979–80 ($p < 0.005$) (Figure 4).

DISCUSSION

The remarkable improvement in the patient and graft survival statistics may be ascribed to our programmatic maturation. Detailed

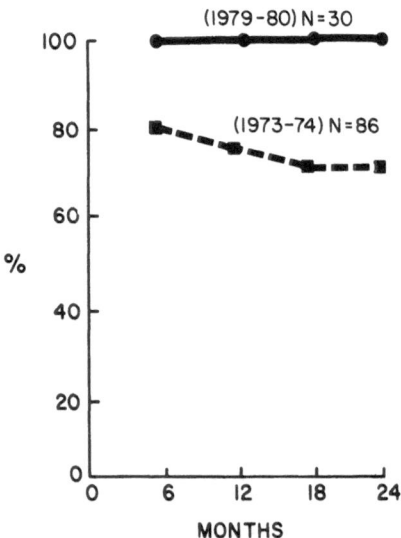

Figure 1. Actuarial patient survival (nondiabetic recipients, living related donors).

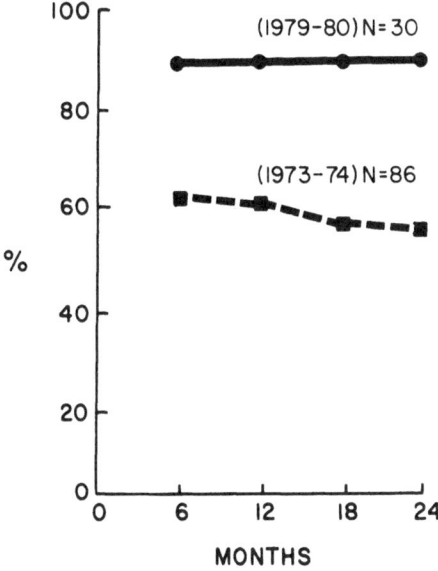

Figure 2. Actuarial graft survival (nondiabetic recipients, living related donors).

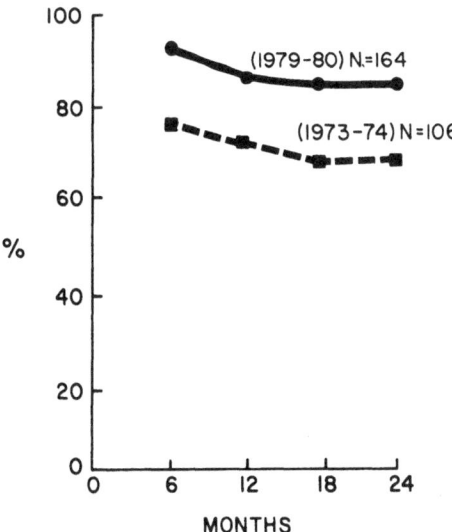

Figure 3. Actuarial patient survival (nondiabetic recipients, cadaver donors).

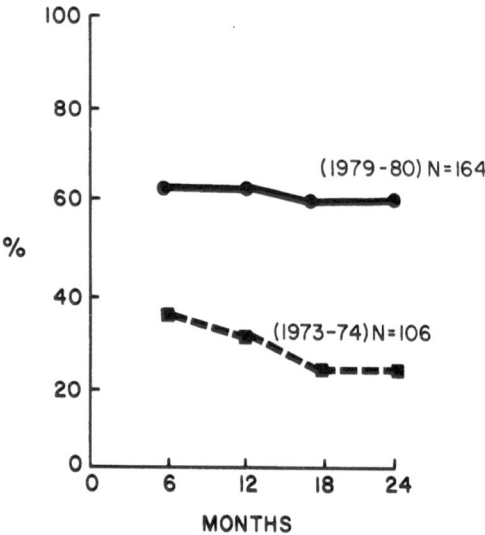

Figure 4. Actuarial graft survival (nondiabetic recipients, cadaver donor).

analysis indicates significant changes in all areas of management of the transplant patient.

Pretransplant Management

Liberal use of blood transfusions during the period preceding transplantation and a methodical periodic check for the development of cytotoxic antibodies are, in all probability, the most crucial factors that have immunomodulated the recipient population in a salutary manner. Systematic prospective screening for antibodies has, in addition, helped us virtually to eliminate hyperacute and accelerated rejections in cadaver donor kidney transplants. The effect of pretransplant blood transfusions in improving the results of cadaver donor kidney transplants has been documented in many retrospective and some prospective studies.[1-4] Donor-specific blood transfusions in one-haplotype matched but strongly MLC-reactive living-related donor-recipient pairs have improved graft survival to nearly 100% in those recipients who do not form cytotoxic antibodies against their blood/prospective kidney donors.[5]

Perioperative Care

Strict adherence to aseptic principles during the operative procedure and perioperative antibiotics have helped eliminate wound infection and ensuing sepsis.[6] Careful ligation of all the lymphatics overlying the iliac vessels in the process of mobilization of the iliac vein has brought the incidence of posttransplantation lymphoceles down to 2–3% from a previous incidence of approximately 16%.

Ureteric necrosis and urinary extravasation therefrom have proven to be avoidable by careful preservation of the blood supply of the ureter. We are now employing our modification of the Lich technique, wherein only a tiny opening is made in the bladder to insert the ureter.[7] Placement of the ureter in an extramucosal tunnel provides us a mechanism for prevention of urinary reflux. We now routinely remove the Foley catheter within 48 hours of surgery without fear of bladder leak. Early removal of the Foley catheter is the single most important factor in the elimination of urologic infections.

Immunosuppression

Conservatism in the use of steroids has been of paramount importance in reducing the infectious complications and mortality of transplantation.[8] Skillful adjunctive use of antithymocyte globulin (ATG) has, in our hands, demonstrably enhanced the survival of kidney grafts.[9] Of the lessons learned from the human transplantation experience of the past decade, none has been so crucial as the acceptance of the irreversibility of rejection in a certain proportion of recipients. Excessive and injudicious use of immunosuppression in such patients is only rewarded by escalation of morbidity and mortality.

CONCLUSIONS

It may be stated without fear of refutation that a kidney transplant recipient today has a much brighter outlook, both in terms of patient survival and function of the graft, compared with that of five to ten years ago. Exciting new techniques and therapies, including cyclosporin A, monoclonal anti-T cell antibodies, and total lymphoid irradiation, hold the promise of a still brighter future.

REFERENCES

1. Opelz G, Terasaki PI: Cadaver kidney transplants in North America: Analysis 1978. *Daily Transplant* 8:167–181, 1979.
2. Van Es AA, Balner H: Effect of pretransplant transfusions on kidney allograft survival. *Transplant Proceed* 11:127–137, 1979.
3. Hunsicker LG, Oei LS, Freeman RM, et al: Effect of blood transfusions on cadaver renal allograft survival. *Transplant Proceed* 11:156–159. 1979.
4. Williams KA, Ting A, Cullen PR, et al: Transfusions: Their influence on human renal graft survival. *Transplant Proceed* 11:175–178, 1979.
5. Salvatierra, O Jr, Amend W, Vincenti F, et al: Pretreatment with donor-specific blood transfusions in related recipients with high MLC. *Transplant Proceed* 13:142–149, 1981.
6. Tilney NL, Strom TB, Vineyard GC, et al: Factors contributing to the declining mortality rate in renal transplantation. *N Engl J Med* 299:1321–1325, 1978.
7. Wasnick RJ, Butt KMH, Laungani G, et al: Evaluation of anterior extravesical ureteroneo-cystostomy in kidney transplantation. *J Urology* 126:306–307, 1981.
8. Salvatierra O Jr, Potter D, Cochrum KC, et al: Improved patient survival in renal transplantation. *Surgery* 79:166–171, 1976.
9. Parsa I, Butt KMH, Sutton AL, et al: HLA-DR, antithymocyte globulin (ATG) and survival of cadaveric renal allografts. *Transplant Proceed* 13:495–498, 1981.

26

Triggering Signals for T-Cell Activation in Renal Transplantation

KURT H. STENZEL, A. L. RUBIN, AND A. NOVOGRODSKY

Long-term survival of renal graft recipients and patients with immuno-logically mediated renal disease depends on the clarification of molecular mechanisms involved in T-cell activation. The lymphocyte membrane serves as a transmitter of external signals that induce cell proliferation and differentiation. The signals that interact with the cell membrane and trigger these events may be either immunologically specific, and induce a monoclonal proliferation, or immunologically nonspecific, and induce a polyclonal proliferation. Most T-cell mitogens, agents that induce poly-clonal proliferation of T-cells, interact with cell surface polysaccharide moieties. These mitogens include certain lectins and the oxidizing agents sodium metaperiodate (IO_4^-) and galactose oxidase (GO). The initial step in the triggering event is mitogen binding to, or alteration of, a cell surface saccharide structure. The nature of this interaction is central to the understanding of the molecular mechanisms responsible for lymphocyte activation, and the subsequent cascade of events that leads either to graft rejection or acceptance.

STRUCTURAL ASPECTS OF MITOGENIC SITES

An oligosaccharide, common to many glycoproteins, can serve as the target for most, if not all, T-cell mitogens.[1] For reasons that are not readily apparent, wheat germ agglutinin (WGA) was originally reported to be nonmitogenic.[2] Recent studies, however, have clearly demonstrated its mitogenic properties.[3] Hepatic binding protein (HBP), a protein that specifically binds asialoglycoproteins,[4] has recently been found to be

KURT H. STENZEL, A. L. RUBIN, AND A. NOVOGRODSKY • Rogosin Kidney Center, The New York Hospital–Cornell Medical Center, New York, New York.

mitogenic for desialyated T-cells.[5] To our knowledge this is the first mammalian lectin that has been found to have mitogenic properties.

The fact that these mitogens can be accommodated in a single megalo-site does not necessarily indicate that there is a unique mitogenic site on the cell surface. Different glycoproteins share similar oligosaccharide structures, and the possibility that different mitogens induce blastogenesis by interacting with different glycoproteins should also be considered. Co-capping studies, however, indicate that several T-cell mitogens with different saccharide specificities interact with membrane sites that are physically linked.[6]

The unique role of saccharide groups as targets for mitogens was substantiated further by studies involving the conjugation of a ligand to the cell surface, followed by assessing the mitogenic activity of the antiligand. Boitin does not serve as a mitogenic site for avidin when conjugated to cell surface protein moieties but only when it is conjugated to saccharide groups.[7] Thus, binding of a lectin to a saccharide group *per se* is not a requirement for mitogenicity, since nonsaccharide moieties can serve as mitogenic sites, provided they are conjugated to a cell surface saccharide. It would appear that the saccharide moiety functions to provide a binding site for lectins at a critical location on the cell surface.

VALENCY OF MITOGENS

Does simple binding to critical surface sites suffice to induce blastogenesis, or is the triggering signal associated with cross-linking of surface sites? Cross-linking can only be directly imposed on cells by agents that have more than one binding site, that is, multivalent agents. In general, most studies have found polyvalency to be a prerequisite for mitogenic activity. Divalent fragments of antilymphocyte or anti-immunoglobulin antibody, for instance, are mitogenic, whereas the univalent fragments are not.[8,9] Ravid et al.[10] have clearly shown that the divalent anti-DNP fragment is mitogenic for DNP conjugated cells, whereas the monovalent fragment is inactive. In some cases lectins fail to stimulate cells, even though they are divalent, and mitogenicity is seen only with polymeric preparations.[11–13]

Nevertheless, reports have appeared indicating that blastogenesis is induced by monovalent antibody[14,15] and lectin.[16] Several possibilities could explain these findings. The mitogen could interact with accessory cells via nonsaccharide binding sites, thus rendering these cells super-mitogens with multivalency. Alternatively, the mitogen could interact with additional, nonsaccharide sites on the same cell to form a cross-linked structure. A hydrophobic binding site for concanavalin A (Con A) has in fact been shown.[17]

COVALENT CROSS-LINKING AND MITOGENESIS

The possibility that covalent cross-linking of membrane sites might be related to mitogenesis should also be considered. We recently found that both Con A and phytohemagglutinin (PHA) increase lymphocyte transglutaminase (TGase) activity.[18] This enzyme is known to induce crosslinking of protein molecules via γ-glutamyl-lysine bridges.[19,20] TGase activity is present in human peripheral lymphocytes and is enhanced up to 15-fold within 10–30 minutes after treatment of the cells with Con A or PHA. The enzyme is not detected when intact cells are assayed; it is detected only in cell lysates. Con A enhances TGase activity only when it is incubated with intact cells; Con A treatment of cell lysates has no effect. α-Methylmannoside specifically inhibits the enhancement of TGase by Con A. Thus the enhanced TGase activity in cells treated with Con A results from the specific interaction of the lectin with its saccharide binding site on the cell surface, rather than by direct interaction with the enzyme itself. The increased activity of TGase in cells treated with Con A, as compared with unstimulated cells, is maintained under assay conditions in which saturating levels of Ca^{2+} are present. TGase may therefore be involved in early cellular events leading to lymphocyte blastogenesis.[21]

CELL–CELL INTERACTIONS IN TRIGGERING T-CELL ACTIVATION

Cellular interactions, in addition to cross-linking of membrane sites, appear to be important in the activation process. Blastogenesis induced by the mitogenic oxidizing agents provides a useful system for the study of cell–cell interactions in lymphocyte activation. The oxidizing mitogens induce blastogenesis by the generation of aldehyde moieties on cell surface glycoproteins.[21–23] Aldehyde-modified T-cells undergo blastogenesis when cultured with unmodified macrophages, and untreated T-cells undergo blastogenesis when cultured with aldehyde-modified macrophages.[24–26] It has also been shown that unmodified lymphocytes undergo blastogenesis when mixed with aldehyde-modified lymphocytes that have been irradiated or treated with mitomycin.[27,28] Macrophages are required for blastogenesis in this latter system. Evaluation of the cellular interactions involved in blastogenesis induced by oxidizing agents is possible since excess oxidizing reagent can easily be removed after brief incubation, and the cells can be cultured in a mitogen-free environment.

Although the mechanism of aldehyde-induced blastogenesis is not known, it has been postulated that cell surface aldehydes might react with amino groups to form Schiff bases.[23] These interactions could lead to the formation of a cross-linked structure. Borohydride reduction of aldehyde-modified cells has been found to inhibit blastogenesis. This inhibition could result from reduction of the aldehyde moiety with consequent interference with a cross-linked structure. Alternatively, inhibition could result from reduction of a Schiff base to a covalently cross-linked structure, a condition that could interfere with the progression of blastogenesis. A cross-linked structure mediated through Schiff base formation could occur either on the aldehyde-modified cell itself, or between adjacent cells. The latter condition would provide a molecular bais for cell–cell interaction. However, another possibility should be considered. Cells treated with mitogeneic oxidizing agents form dense aggregates by a time- and temperature-dependent process that also depends on active metabolism. This finding raises the possibility that cell–cell interactions induced in this system are not a direct result of aldehyde modification or Schiff base formation, but rather result from a secondary process stimulated by surface oxidation. This secondary process could be the generation of a cell-surface site that interacts with receptors on adjacent cells and thereby promotes blastogenesis. Thus cross-linking of sites on individual cells could provide the first signal for lymphocyte activation, and this could lead to the generation of new cell surface structures. These new structures would then constitute the second signal and be dependent on cell–cell interactions. Kinetically, the first signal corresponds to a mitogen-dependent phase of blastogenesis and the second signal to a phase that is mitogen independent.

Similar mechanisms could also be postulated for lymphocyte activation induced by lectins. Analysis of lymphocyte activation involving lectin stimulation is, however, hampered both by the difficulty in removing lectin and by the propensity of the lectin itself to aggregate cells.

SELECTIVE EFFECTS ON BLASTOGENESIS INDUCED BY DIFFERENT MITOGENS

It should be noted that, although polyclonal agents appear to trigger cells to divide by affecting similar metabolic pathways, different agents selectively affect responses induced by different mitogens. We recently found, for instance, that colchicine has differential effects on blastogenesis induced by different stimuli.[29] Proliferation of human lymphocytes induced by IO_4^- is potentiated by a 30-minute exposure to colchicine (10^{-6} M), followed by washing to remove excess reagent, whereas the response to Con A under similar conditions is inhibited. If colchicine is allowed to remain in the culture media, responses to both agents are severely depressed. Treatment with colchicine before or after IO_4^- modification has similar enhancing effects. Lumicolchicine (a photo-inactivated derivative of colchicine that does not disrupt microtubules) does not alter proliferative responses. In addition to the proliferation of IO_4^-- oxidized cells, irradiated IO_4^--modified lymphocytes induce proliferation when mixed with untreated lymphocytes. Enhancement occurs in both these conditions only when IO_4^--modified cells are treated with colchicine. Proliferation in mixed lymphocyte cultures is also potentiated when either stimulating or responding cells are pretreated with colchicine. These findings suggest a selective stimulatory effect of a brief treatment of cells with colchicine on lymphocyte responses induced by cell–cell contact.

Recently we observed a differential effect of removing adherent cells on blastogenic responses induced by different mitogens.[30] Depletion of adherent cells markedly enhances blastogenesis induced by the galactosyl-directed lectins, soybean agglutinin (SBA), peanut agglutinin (PNA), and HBP, but has little effect on lymphocyte blastogenesis induced by phytohemagglutinin (PHA) or Con A. Treatment of unfractionated lymphocytes with indomethacin, an inhibitor of prostaglandin synthesis, mimics the selective effect of removing adherent cells. Following depletion of adherent cells, indomethacin no longer affects mitogen-induced blastogenesis. Treating lymphocytes depleted of adherent cells with prostaglandin E_1 selectively suppresses responses to HBP, PNA and SBA, while responses to PHA and Con A are less affected. Cyclic AMP analogues, such as dibutyryl cAMP and 8-bromo cAMP, and an inhibitor of cAMP phosphodiesterase, methyl isobutyl xanthine, also selectively suppress responses to the galactosyl-directed lectins. Prostaglandin E_1, the cAMP analogues, and methyl isobutyl xanthine are effective only when added within the first 24 hours after mitogen stimulation. The galactosyl-directed lectins do not selectively stimulate prostaglandin production nor do they selectively elevate intracellular cAMP levels. The data thus indicate that cells stimulated by different mitogens differ markedly in their sensitivity to suppression by similar concentrations of prostaglandin and of cAMP.

It is not yet known whether the selective effects of cAMP on blastogenesis induced by the galactosyl-directed lectins result from stimulation of a selective subset of lymphocytes by these lectins, or whether the mitogens impose an enhanced sensitivity to cAMP on the cells. The latter mechanism could be mediated by a modification of cAMP-dependent protein kinase components by the galactosyl-directed lectins.

In addition to the selective effect of different agents on stimulation induced by various mitogens, similar mitogens induce different enzymatic activities in lymphocytes derived from different species. Gamma glutamyl transpeptidase activity is markedly stimulated by a variety of T-cell mitogens in human and rat lymphocytes, whereas these mitogens do not stimulate gamma glutamyl transpeptidase activity in mouse or guinea pig lymphocytes.[31]

Selective effects on blastogenesis induced by different stimuli provide a useful tool to study mechanisms of lymphocyte activation. cAMP, for instance, has many effects on cellular metabolism that may or may not be related to lymphocyte activation. Since we found a differential effect of cAMP on blastogenesis induced by different mitogens, the cAMP-dependent metabolic pathways that are relevant to blastogenesis can be evaluated. Selective effects on lymphocyte activation induced by different agents might also be of clinical importance in developing strategies for modulating specific immune responses. We have recently found, for example, that simple organic compounds, known to induce differentiation in Friend leukemia cells, inhibit lymphocyte mitogenesis and allogeneic responses.[32,34]

CURRENT PROBLEMS IN LYMPHOCYTE ACTIVATION

The nature of the primary membrane events that are associated with the triggering signal for lymphocyte activation remains obscure. A detailed analysis and comparison of blastogenesis induced by widely differing classes of mitogens, such as lectins, oxidizing agents, and the mitogenic agents that react with grafted mitogenic sites (e.g., biotin), could reveal the critical triggering events in lymphocyte activation. That is, the various mitogens might induce many changes not necessarily relevant to blasto-genesis, but alterations induced in common by all these varying stimuli could be identified and might be relevant to the triggering signal. Similarly, the relevance of any particular metabolic alteration that occurs in lymphocytes following stimulation with various agents to the activation of cells, and their progression to blastogenesis, remains to be clarified. The study of selective effects of different agents on blastogenesis induced by different mitogens might facilitate our understanding of these difficult problems.

It is now apparent that blastogenesis depends on interactions among cells and might depend on more than one signal. The social aspects of lymphocyte behavior are now coming under intense scrutiny in several laboratories. These studies take the form of determining interrelationships among triggering signals, kinetics of cell commitment to DNA synthesis, and the nature of the cell–cell interactions themselves. Further understanding of the metabolic pathways leading to lymphocyte activation will allow the development of specific immunosuppressive agents.

REFERENCES

1. Toyoshim S, Fukuka M, Osawa T: Chemical nature of the receptor site for various phytomitogens. *Biochemistry* 11:4000, 1972.
2. Boldt DH, MacDermott RP, Jorolan EP: Interaction of plant lectins with purified human lymphocyte populations: Binding characteristics and kinetics of proliferation. *J Immunol* 114:1532, 1975.
3. Brown JM, Leon MA, Lightbody JJ: Isolation of a human lymphocyte mitogen from wheat germ with N-acetyl-D-glucosamine specificity. *J Immunol* 117:1976, 1976.
4. Hudgin RL, Pricer WE, Ashwell G, Stockert RJ, Morell AG: The isolation and properties of a rabbit liver binding protein specific for asialoglycoproteins. *J Biol Chem* 249:5536, 1974.
5. Novogrodsky A, Ashwell G: Lymphocyte mitogenesis induced by a mammalian liver protein that specifically binds desialylated glycoproteins. *Proc Nat Acad Sci (USA)* 74:676, 1977.
6. Hellstrom U, Dillner ML, Hammarstrom S, Perlman P: The interaction of nonmitogenic and mitogenic lectins with T lymphocytes: Association of cellular receptor sites. *Scand J Immunol* 5:45, 1976.
7. Wynne D, Wilchek M, Novogrodsky A: A chemical approach for the localization of membrane sites involved in lymphocyte activation. *Biochem Biophys Res Commun* 68:730, 1976.
8. Woodruff MFA, Reid B, James K: Effect of antilymphocytic antibody and antibody fragments on human lymphocytes *in vitro*. *Nature* 215:591, 1967.
9. Fanger MW, Hart DA, Wells JV, Nisonoff A: *J Immunol* 100:1484, 1970.
10. Ravid A, Novogrodsky A, Wilchek M: The stimulation of DNP-conjugated lymphocytes by anti-DNP antibody. *Eur J Immunol* 8:289, 1978.
11. Schechter B, Lis H, Lotan R, Novogrodsky A, Sharon N: The requirement for tetravalency of soybean agglutinin for induction of mitogenic stimulation of lymphocytes. *Eur J Immunol* 6:145, 1976.
12. Bessler W, Resch W, Ferber E: Valency-dependent stimulating effects of lima bean lectins on lymphocytes of different species. *Biochem Biophys Res Commun* 69:578, 1976.
13. Prujansky A, Ravid A, Sharon N: Cooperativity of lectin binding to lymphocytes, and its relevance to mitogenic stimulation. *Biochem Biophys Acta* 508:137, 1978.
14. Sell S: Studies on rabbit lymphocytes *in vitro*. VII. The induction of blast transformation with the F(ab') and F ab fragments of sheep antibody to rabbit IgG. *J Immunol* 98:786, 1967.
15. Sela B, Wang JL, Edelman GM: Lymphocyte activation by monovalent fragments of antibodies reactive with cell surface carbohydrates. *J Exp Med* 143:665, 1976.
16. Wang JL, Edelman GM: Binding and functional properties of concanavalin A and its derivatives. I. Monovalent, divalent, and tetravalent derivatives stable at physiological pH. *J Biol Chem* 253:3000, 1978.

17. Edelman GM, Wang JL: Binding and functional properties of concanavalin A and its derivatives. III. Interactions with indoleacetic acid and other hydrophobic ligands. *J Biol Chem* 253:3016, 1978. .

18. Novogrodsky A, Quittner S, Rubin AL, Stenzel KH: Transglutaminase activity in human lymphocytes: Early activation by phytomitogens. *Proc Nat Acad Sci (USA)* 75:1157, 1978.

19. Clark DD, Neidle A, Sarkar NK, Waelsch H: Metabolic activity of protein amide groups. *Arch Biochem Biophys* 71:277, 1957.

20. Lorand L, Weissman LB, Epel DL, Bruner-Lorand J: Role of the intrinsic transglutaminase in the Ca^{2+}-mediated crosslinking of erythrocyte proteins. *Proc Nat Acad Sci (USA)* 73:4479, 1976.

21. Novogrodsky A, Katchalski E: Membrane site modified on induction of the transformation of lymphocytes by periodate. *Proc Nat Acad Sci* (USA) 69:3207, 1972.

22. Zatz MM, Goldstein AL, Blumenfield OO, White H: Regulation of normal and leukaemic lymphocyte transformation and recirculation by sodium periodate oxidation and sodium borohydride reduction. *Nature (New Biology)* 240:252, 1972.

23. Novogrodsky A, Katchalski E: Induction of lymphocyte transformation by sequential treatment with neuraminidase and galactose oxidase. *Proc Nat Acad Sci (USA)* 70:1824, 1973.

24. Biniaminov M, Ramot B, Novogrodsky A: Effect of macrophages on periodate-induced transformation of normal and chronic lymphatic leukemia lymphocytes. *Clin Exp Immunol* 16:235, 1974.

25. Biniaminov M, Ramot B, Bosenthal E, Novogrodsky A: Galactose oxidase-induced blastogenesis of human lymphocytes and the effect of macrophages on the reaction. *Clin Exp Immunol* 19:93, 1975.

26. Greineder DK, Rosenthal AS: The requirement for macrophage-lymphocyte interaction in T lymphocyte proliferation induced by generation of aldehydes on cell membranes. *J Immunol* 115:932, 1975.

27. O'Brien RL, Parker JW, Paolilli P, Steiner J: Periodate-induced lymphocyte transformation. IV. Mitogenic effect of $NaIO_4$, treated lymphocytes upon autologous lymphocytes. *J Immunol* 112:1884, 1974.

28. Beyer CF, Bowers WE: Periodate and concanavalin A induced blast transformation of rat lymphocytes by an indirect mechanisms. *Proc Nat Acad Sci (USA)* 72:3590, 1975.

29. Stenzel KH, Schwartz R, Rubin AL, Novogrodsky A: Potentiation of lymphocyte activation by colchicine. *J Immunol* 121:863, 1978.

30. Novogrodsky A, Stenzel KH, Rubin AL: Stimulation of human peripheral blood lymphocytes by periodate, galactose oxidase, soybean agglutinin, and peanut agglutinin: Differential effects of adherent cells. *J Immunol* 118:852, 1977.

31. Novogrodsky A, Tate SS, Meister A: γ-Glutamyl transpeptidase, a lymphoid cell-surface marker: Relationship to blastogenesis, differentiation, and neoplasia. *Proc Nat Acad Sci (USA)* 73:2414, 1976.

32. Stenzel KH, Schwartz R, Rubin AL, Novogrodsky A: Chemical inducers of differentiation in Friend leukaemia cells inhibit lymphocyte mitogenesis. *Nature* 285:106, 1980.

33. Novogrodsky A, Rubin AL, Stenzel KH: A new class of inhibitors of lympocyte mitogenesis: Agents that induce erythroid differentiation in Friend leukemia cells. *J Immunol* 124:1892, 1980.

Author Index

Subject Index